*To my husband, Rudy,
whose unconditional support for me has
made my professional endeavors possible
and my personal life complete.*

CONTRIBUTORS

Carmella A. Bocchino, MBA, RN
Senior Washington Representative
Group Health Association of America
Alexandria, VA

Carolyn C. Boyle, MBA, RN
Vice President, Patient Care Services
Summit Medical Center
Oakland, CA

Eula Das, PhD, RN
Adjunct Faculty
Indiana University School of Nursing
Treasurer/Governing Board
    Member—Midwest Alliance
    in Nursing
Diplomate—American College of
    Healthcare Executives
Member—AOEN, IONE, Kiwanis
Indianapolis, IN

Patricia T. Driscoll, MS, JD, BSN
Assistant Professor
Health Care Administration
Texas Women's University
Dallas, TX
Private Law
Dallas, TX

Nannette L. Goddard, RN, MS
Senior Partner, Consulting
Goddard Management Resources
Houston, TX
Assistant Professor
Graduate Program in Nursing
    Administration
University of Arkansas for Medical
    Sciences School of Nursing
Little Rock, AR

Karen F. Gross, JD, RN, BS
Owner, Care Management Consulting
Eugene, OR

Joyce E. Johnson, RN, DNSc, FAAN
Senior Vice President, Nursing and
    Patient Care Services
Washington Hospital Center
Washington, DC

**Karlene Kerfoot, PhD, RN,
CNAA, FAAN**
Executive Vice President
Patient Care & Chief Nursing Officer
St. Luke's Episcopal Hospital
Houston, TX

Nancy R. Kruger, DNSc, RN
Director of Nursing
Pennsylvania State University
The Milton S. Hershey Medical
    Center
Hershey, PA

**Mary Elizabeth Mancini, RN,
MSN, CNA**
Senior Vice President
Nursing Administration
Parkland Memorial Hospital
Dallas, TX

**Diane M. McDonald, RN, BSN,
MSN**
Northeast Director
Work Transformation Services
Hay Management Consultants
Boston, MA

Ruth S. Miller, RN, FACHE
Director of Quality and
  Accreditation
St. Luke's Episcopal Hospital
Houston, TX

Linda Myers, RN
Nursing Education and Quality
  Improvement
Methodist Hospital of Indiana,
  Inc.
Indianapolis, IN

Deborah A. Proctor, RN, MSN
Work Transformation Services
Hay Management Consultants
Los Angeles, CA

Catherine Robinson, MBA
Executive Director
The Western Network
Berkley, CA

Susan C. Roe, DPA, RN
Health Care Consultant
Phoenix, AZ

Nancy J. Sharp, MSN, RN
President
Sharp Legislative Resources
Bethesda, MD

**Donna Richards Sheridan, RN, MS,
MBA, PhD**
Associate Professor
University of California,
  San Francisco
Director of Nursing/Chief Nurse
Executive
Saint Francis Memorial Hospital
San Francisco, CA

Roy L. Simpson, RN, C
Executive Director
Corporate Nursing Affairs
HBO & Company
Atlanta, GA

Beth Tamplet Ulrich, EdD, RN
Vice President
Clinical Information Development
UniHealth America
Burbank, CA

William M. Warfel, PhD, RN, CNAA
Adjunct Lecturer
University of Pennsylvania,
  School of Nursing, Adjunct Faculty
LaSalle University, School of Nursing
Associate General Director
Albert Einstein Medical Center
Philadelphia, PA

PREFACE

It is an exciting time to be entering nursing—a time full of complex change, high expectations, and professional challenges. It seems the world is changing faster than we can keep up, and health care is no exception. Health care reform in the United States and internationally is setting the stage for a major restructuring of health care delivery for all people. The magnitude of the changes will be so great that you will find your job, your work organization, and your own family will all be part of making a difference in a new way.

As a new nurse, you are filled with expectations and apprehension about entering the work world. On one hand, you are lucky that you bring with you very little baggage from past practices, so new practices will be a positive challenge. On the other hand, your professional responsibilities and accountabilities will be heightened as the role of the professional nurse is elevated in the new delivery systems. You, like other nurses, will find the complexity of your professional role to be a challenge minute to minute, day to day, and year to year.

This book focuses on the aspects of your professional role that require management skills and competencies. Although your job may focus primarily on clinical responsibilities, there will be substantial expectation for you also to incorporate management, education, and research skills into your practice. Many nurses think that nurses in management positions, manage, and that nurses in clinical practice, practice nursing. This view can no longer be supported.

In the role of a staff nurse, whether in a hospital, ambulatory, home care, or long-term care setting, a nurse must both recognize and perform the managerial aspects of the job. In a constant struggle to be more effective and efficient in delivering services, organizations today expect that all professionals will play a role in managing the services provided. In fact, organizations are committing themselves to increasing employee involvement in decision making, team work, and support of the work environment.

Nursing Management describes the managerial role of the nurse in complex organizations, the management of one's professional career, and the issues related to contemporary professional nursing practice. The content is focused on both the theoretical base of management practices, and the practical approaches to successfully integrating the concepts into practice.

The expert contributors to this book have all lived the advice they give you. They are familiar with the hands-on needs of new nurses and have shared practical suggestions to ensure your success. This book would not have been possible without their generosity in sharing their thoughts and knowledge.

This book is also the result of the time and attention of my associate, Maggie Tollefsbol. She spent countless hours with contributors, editors, and me keeping all the details straight and on track. Last, but not least, the most patient editor, Jennifer Brogan, proved that flexibility is an art, not a science. To all who helped, I thank you.

Katherine W. Vestal

CONTENTS

xi

xii CONTENTS

III. FOCUS ON CONTEMPORARY NURSING ISSUES

NURSING
MANAGEMENT
Concepts and Issues

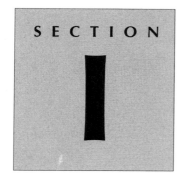

S E C T I O N

I

FOCUS ON MANAGEMENT

The Management Role of the New Nurse

Katherine W. Vestal

LEARNING OBJECTIVES

At the completion of this chapter, the reader will:

1. Understand that management is one facet of the professional nurse role.
2. Delineate several approaches to building self-confidence in the professional nurse role.
3. Describe the changing roles of management in health care.

Vestal, K.W. Nursing Management:
Concepts and Issues, 2 ed.
© 1995 J.B. Lippincott Company

This book is based on the premise that all nurses, regardless of their primary job, must assume responsibility for the management functions that are inherent in every nursing job. It is often said that the role of the professional nurse is becoming increasingly bureaucratic. If bureaucracy includes managing others, managing paperwork, and managing the multiple agendas of the health care enterprise, then there is truth in that statement. The increasing complexity of delivering patient care requires a multifaceted role for the professional nurse that includes managerial responsibilities.

These managerial activities differ depending on the specific job and situation, but they always include effective communication, delegation, human relations, and the management of people, time, and resources. The professional nurse also plays an important role in managing change, resolving conflict, and meeting organizational goals. The role of the nurse is composed of a multidimensional set of activities that focus on care of the patient, support of the organization, and support of the profession and oneself as a professional.

For decades, nursing has rigidly adhered to the categorization of nurses as clinicians, educators, managers, or researchers. These role categories have referred to the *primary* focus of the job. A clinical nurse's job, for example, has been seen as primarily delivering direct patient care. Although the job categories have served to differentiate primary responsibilities, they have created the misconception that these activity boundaries are rigid and that activities are included or excluded by the nature of the job title.

These misconceptions can have an adverse effect on nursing performance. For example, if a staff nurse views herself as involved only in direct patient care, she may consider necessary activities such as solving interdepartmental problems or making the staffing schedule to be the responsibilities of the "manager." Therefore, the ability of the staff nurse to engage in the activities needed to perform her job well is limited because so many of the day-to-day issues are considered outside the boundaries of the staff nurse's job.

BLURRING THE LINES

The time has come to blur the lines that divide nursing roles. The movement in health care to include and to involve staff at appropriate points in decision making requires that jobs be rounded out with a full array of responsibilities from clinical, managerial, educational, and research domains. The rigid roles described above cannot meet the demands of today's complex health care delivery system. Changes must occur in the delivery of health care services to ensure adequate patient care. The nurse who is entering practice can initiate these job changes without the biases of the past and can model this enriched role of the professional nurse for others to emulate.

The new nurse is under intense pressure to perform at a level acceptable to the hiring organization. An effort is made to describe the level of competence needed to work in the organization and to help new nurses acquire these competencies as quickly as possible. If a nurse is not functioning at 100% of expected productivity, the organization must compensate for the lost percentage of work. Orientation and training programs are designed to support the acquisition of competencies and thus the independence of practice needed to provide high-quality and cost-effective services.

Experiencing this pressure, the new nurse concentrates first on learning and performing clinical activities—the primary role she was hired to perform. If the role were purely clinical, this concentration would result in a clear learning pathway. However, other factors immediately begin to emerge. Not only must the nurse conduct a procedure, she must also charge for it, chart it, and direct others to perform the task and possibly to treat the patient. For each simple nursing activity there are innumerable compounding issues to be addressed.

What often results is a frustrated nurse who proclaims that she was hired to be a *nurse*, that is, a clinician, not an accountant, secretary, or housekeeper. Reality sets in as the nurse recognizes that the role of a clinical nurse encompasses much more than clinical care. It is often the accomplishment of the peripheral activities that ensures good patient care and a sound organization.

New nurses do not work in isolation, surrounded only by their patients. Instead, they find a vast array of health personnel, physicians, managers, families, and others who demand their time and attention in coordinated events. New nurses also find that, despite their lack of job experience, they are expected to manage the work flow and activities of other personnel, who may have less formal preparation but usually have more practical experience. Therefore, the responsibility to manage others becomes a challenging human resource agenda that is crucial to the total care of patients.

The new nurse must have a sound management base from which to operate. This aspect of the clinical work role cannot be delegated or relegated as a low priority. Management is a key to success in the professional nursing job. The issue becomes one of managing many aspects of the job—clinical, managerial, educational, and research—with overall consistency. As with most learning, it is easier to start with the simple and move to the complex. The new nurse can identify the basic managerial behaviors necessary for success and practice these until mastery is achieved. She can then move toward the more complex managerial activities that ultimately may result in a change in her primary role from clinical nurse to manager.

Becoming proficient at managerial activities is not easy. However, it becomes reasonable if the managerial activities frequently assumed by staff nurses are defined. This book defines these managerial activities and discusses pragmatic approaches that will familiarize the new nurse with common managerial challenges. These challenges are important aspects of nursing and demonstrate why professional nurses must be able to make initial judgments and provide leadership—activities far beyond a basic task approach to care.

HUMAN EFFECTIVENESS

An individual's behavior stems from her interpretations of what she *thinks* she perceives. Other perceptions influence and help crystallize these individual values and behaviors. In time, these behaviors operate as a person's individual theories and govern her actions as though they were law. Theories in general are guidelines for behavior, and there are many that govern human effectiveness. Management books devote a great amount of attention to the theorists who founded the managerial practices followed today.

Busy managers are understandably impatient with theory, often preferring to apply practical solutions to crises as they arise. However, Kurt Lewin has said that "there is nothing so practical as a good theory," especially when the nurse wants to improve things and needs a useful method of doing so.

The application of theory requires an awareness of a problem, an understanding of the need to change, a commitment to change when practice differs from theory, and an establishment of new habits as the theory is applied. Therefore, application of the managerial theory discussed in this textbook requires an intellectual conditioning experience and an active process of behavioral changes.

Theories of leadership, motivation, and values clarification are important as the new nurse assumes managerial responsibilities. If nurses believe that, as clinicians, they are assuming managerial responsibilities for a job, then the acquisition of a theory base is essential. These theories, then, can be translated into practical methods of enhancing human effectiveness. Health care is undeniably a complex business, and the care delivery system supported by nurses is itself a mesh of complexity.

Just as persons may choose complex or simple life-styles away from the job, so do individuals differ in their preferred vocational roles on the job. At one extreme, some desire complex and continuously challenging positions; at the other extreme, some prefer simple routine jobs. However complex or simple the job, nurses have one desire in common—the freedom to choose the kind of work they prefer and to relate to it in a way that is compatible with their personal values. Hence, the concept of "every employee a manager" can have meaning for persons at all levels of talent, although their preferred job roles may differ substantially in terms of scope and variety.

Although "every employee a manager" is a universally applicable concept, it depends on appropriate job conditions for its fullest implementation. Every nurse has the potential for managing some jobs, although not for managing every job. However, every nurse has the potential for managing certain components of any job or combinations of several jobs. The realization of this potential depends on matching the nurse's talents and aspirations with the appropriate job, which includes the work itself, the style of supervision, procedural constraints, peer relationships, and other climate factors in the workplace.

THE NEW KID

Every nurse is "the new kid on the block" at least once in her career, and probably many times. The feeling of being a neophyte recurs with each new job or new role. Although it is never easy to handle, more experienced nurses find that the feeling dissipates more rapidly. Being a new nurse breeds multiple issues to be considered. First, you are a new kid because, clinically, you are new to the profession. Second, you are a new kid because, as a professional nurse, you will automatically be expected to assume some leadership and managerial roles, thus making you a "manager" before you are even comfortable being a nurse.

It is helpful to consider carefully the dilemma of the new kid structure and ways to deal with it. Generally, your fellow employees will react in one of three ways when you begin working with them. Some will be glad you are there, others will resent you for varying reasons, and others will test you before making any decision about you. Hopefully, most will adopt a wait-and-see attitude by not condemning or praising you until they see how you perform. The latter attitude is healthy and all that you can reasonably expect.

You will be measured initially against your predecessor in the position. If that person's performance was miserable, you will seem far better by comparison. If you follow a highly capable performer, your adjustment will be more difficult. In any event, you must be yourself and decide how you can best integrate yourself into the work setting.

It is a time to move slowly with changes, to communicate effectively downward and upward, and to listen intently to what others tell you. Make it a point to have a personal conversation with each of the persons working in your area sometime within the first 60 days on the job. Do not do it the first week or so, but once you have begun to know your colleagues, find a way to know them better. You must be genuinely interested in people, care about them as individuals, and help them achieve their goals. Eventually, your interpersonal abilities may prove to be more important than your technical abilities.

In time, you will expand your influence from the formal group to the informal group as you become an accepted member of the team. Soon you will lose your status as the new kid, and others will step into that role. At that point, you are well on your way to assuming more managerial responsibilities because your increasing seniority will dictate such activities. Still a new nurse? Yes, but growing, both clinically and managerially.

THE ADJUSTMENT PERIOD IS OVER

Fortunately, most new jobs have an adjustment period. That is the time you have to adapt to the new setting and begin to reach full productivity. This adjustment period is undefined in length. In some organizations it may be several days, whereas in others it may be several months. It is during this time that the phrase "I don't know, I'm new here" holds a valid place in your communication.

Predictably, the adjustment period will come to an end and the real partnership between you and the organization will begin. You will discover good aspects, bad aspects, and puzzling aspects of the work setting. It is comforting to realize that there is no employee utopia and that every work setting has its pluses and minuses, so that you can begin fitting in as effectively as possible.

Once the adjustment period is over, the difficult decisions that might have been deferred will surface for action. As a new nurse, you are concentrating on becoming clinically competent, learning the expectations of physicians, supervisors, and colleagues, and finding your way in the complex organization. But as a professional nurse, you are in the spotlight and required to provide some managerial supervision to other employees, including newer registered nurses, licensed practical nurses, and patient care associates. In addition, you must coordinate the activities of many persons and processes from other departments. You will begin to understand fully why health care is considered one of the most difficult settings to manage—it is a people business. People dealing with people in an atmosphere of great stress and confusion can only lead to one thing—a difficult role to fill.

As a new nurse, you will find your managerial responsibilities frequently relate to *people*. You will discover personalities you would like to change, persons who do not give positively to the organization and do not get along with the group, and persons who consistently give their very best. Although specific approaches to these situations are discussed later in this text, the initial need is to develop priorities for your own role.

The process of developing priorities begins with determining what *is* most important. As a new graduate you probably feel that it is *all* important. This places you in the position of deciding what should be done at what time. Subtle shifts repeatedly occur when defining the workload and its importance, and you will find yourself constantly juggling your priorities and those of your colleagues. The pressure of prioritizing activities is a major source of frustration for new nurses, because inevitably some things must go undone, leading to feelings of guilt and inadequacy.

During the initial phase of a new job, sit down with your manager and have a private discussion about priorities. Relate your needs, learn the needs of the unit, and understand the needs of the organization. Then, in concert with the manager, set realistic goals for the next few weeks. Frequent reappraisal is important, and the resetting of priorities will follow as you increase in competence and confidence.

BUILDING CONFIDENCE

Building confidence is a gradual process that is usually the result of successes. As you experience success, you build mastery, and mastery leads to confidence. The learning curve of a new nurse is steep, with almost every encounter with patients, families, and employees becoming a new learning experience. It is important to take the time each day to review your successes. What did you do well, how did that feel, and how can you do even better tomorrow?

At the same time, as a professional nurse, you will need to develop the confidence of your fellow employees, both in their abilities and in your performance. They must be confident that you are competent in your job and that you are fair. Following the same process, as you review your successes, consider the successes of your fellow employees. By assigning new employees tasks that they can master, you will build in them the habit of being successful, starting small with small successes.

Occasionally nurses will perform a task incorrectly or incompletely. Handling such situations is a delicate issue that has great impact on the confidence of employees. "Praise them in public, criticize them in private" is a good credo to follow and is a basic managerial concept. Even when you talk to a nurse in private about an error, your function is to train that person to recognize the nature of the problem so that the error will not be repeated. This is not a personal judgment intended to make the nurse feel inadequate, but rather to isolate the incident and to correct it.

The fact is, nurses are not perfect. Expecting perfection may, in fact, defeat your purposes, because persons can become so self-conscious about making a mistake that they slow their performance to a crawl to make absolutely sure they do not make a mistake. As a result, the volume of work cannot be completed. As a new nurse, being correct as often as possible is important but, by the same token, mistakes will happen. Handle the error with as much attention as needed, and then move on. Nobody is perfect, but the odds for success should be made as high as possible.

Another area that affects the building of confidence is the issue of power. In today's workplace, there are many qualified and experienced individuals. They tend to question instructions and decisions and to associate power with leaders who are persuasive rather than dictatorial. When you are in a leadership role, your attitude will be important in building confidence. The persons working with you will sense your mood and determine your trigger points. Consequently, one of the most important and powerful attributes you can develop is consistent behavior so that other personnel are not continually surprised by your fluctuating attitudes and actions.

You will find that your concern and efforts toward building your fellow employees' confidence will do a great deal in fortifying your self-confidence. You can also build self-confidence by making correct decisions. Each time you make a good, sound decision, confidence in your ability to make judgments is reinforced.

Decision making in nursing is a crucial component of self-confidence because most decisions you make will be a matter of public record. Your decisions will be discussed with colleagues, reviewed at report, and recorded in the patient record. New nurses agonize over every decision because they are not sure they have all the information necessary to make that decision and because they are afraid of making a mistake and possibly injuring a patient.

It is unlikely that you will ever have 100% of the information that might apply to a given situation. If you have made a reasonable and prudent search for data, use the 95% of the information that you have to make a judgment and move on. As you gain more experience, you will find that you are making correct decisions 99% of the time, because the answer is obvious in most situations or you are being asked to reinforce someone else's judgment. Many problems will be brought to you because a colleague wants your agreement and approval before proceeding. This simple act by others will continually reinforce your confidence in your abilities.

Building confidence in yourself and for yourself by working with others is an important process for a new nurse. You will not be able to depend on someone else to do it for you. Think in terms of what you do well, the activities you performed correctly, and the amount of new information that you are learning daily. Continuous review and evaluation will reinforce the competencies you are gaining and will become the framework for self-confidence that will support you for years to come.

PREPARING AND IMPROVING YOURSELF

As a new nurse, one of your major interests is to do well and be successful. It is difficult to determine exactly how to accomplish these tasks because of the complexity of your role as a professional nurse. But when you look around, it is easy to identify many nurses who are successful and from whom you can learn.

One aspect of success is to feel comfortable with your self-image. Having a good opinion of yourself is a positive step in beginning a professional career. If you think success, if you look successful, if you are confident of being successful, you greatly increase your chances of achieving success. Success is primarily a matter of a positive attitude reinforced by a series of building blocks of achievement.

This success model must be tempered by reality. Realizing that you do not know everything, avoiding the impression of arrogance, and handling mistakes well are important parts of your image. Identifying your learning and practice needs is equally as important. Be willing to admit these needs, and do all you can to meet them. For example, the things you do not do well are frequently the things you do not like to do. That can hardly be a coincidence. Recognize your shortcomings and objectively determine a course of action to become proficient. View yourself as honestly as you can and help yourself to move ahead. Planning your future and your career is crucial to designing a reasonable career path. Although mastery of your current job is the number one priority, the second priority should be working on the path to your future development.

Other aspects of your improvement program may relate to communicating more effectively, managing your time more effectively, and participating successfully in organizational groups and efforts. These activities will, in time, lead to chairing committees, public speaking, and a highly visible profile. Any preparation you make along the way that can ultimately boost your future visibility will pay off later.

MANAGING INNOVATION

All management involves the stimulation and management of innovation. Without innovation, the workplace is stagnant and cannot possibly survive in the turbulent times that health care is experiencing today. Creativity is a form of spontaneity that finds expression in an atmosphere of freedom. Therefore, an effective organization encourages its members to assert themselves as individuals in ways that meet the organization's goals. To ensure that anarchy does not reign, a certain degree of managerial guidance is always required to help individuals function within the organizational framework.

In the past, innovation was often regarded as the exclusive realm of the managerial group. Today's nurse expects and accepts involvement in changes as a part of the job. Staff nurses, nonetheless, probably remain the greatest reservoir of untapped resources in the health care field.

Innovation can thrive if the work climate supports and promotes it. Certain work conditions, such as good job design, group participation, employee involvement, and managers whose roles are to advise, consult, and coordinate, must be met before nurses can actually accept roles as managers of their areas of responsibility. When innovation is introduced, it is this final level of involvement that ensures a commitment to successful change.

Working in groups is a key factor in innovation. Natural work groups are the primary work systems through which creativity can find expression. These systems consist of a group of peers who work together with their common leader. Moreover, because of its established relation to other parts of the organization, a natural work group channels creativity toward the attainment of organizational goals.

Because work groups are important, managers must include team building as a component of the managerial job. In turn, the new nurse needs to learn to be a team player, team member, and, eventually, team manager. As a new professional, new hire, and new team member, defining and enacting your role may take a good deal of thought, work, and sheer guts to carve out a place for yourself.

Innovation is essential to organizational growth and development. Supporting a framework on which practices and systems for innovation can be built is one of the managerial roles of the professional nurse.

QUALITY OF WORK LIFE

During the 1960s, managerial journals emphasized the concept of "job enrichment" as the key to happy workers. In the 1970s, this concept was enlarged to that of "life enrichment" or "quality of work life." This broadened emphasis was the result of the realization that work itself, important as it is, is not the only medium through which meaning is given to life in the workplace. Systems peripheral to the work itself also needed modification. Both the work itself and the peripheral systems are influential in shaping attitudes and improving performance.

Moreover, life-enrichment programs cannot be perceived to be paternalistic or manipulative ploys if they are to have a positive impact on the work force. If managers feel that job-enrichment efforts for staff further diffuse their already overwhelming responsibilities, they are not likely to support the efforts. It is clear, then, that any attempt to improve the qualify of work life for nurses must be supported by the nurses and their managers, and must not be done at the expense of the organization's success. In short, the long-term success of an organization depends on the pursuit of organizational goals that are synergistically related to the needs of its members.

Examination of the quality of work life usually begins with a review of Maslow's hierarchy of needs. When living is precarious, humans devote most of their attention to survival. As security increases, they are free to set their own standards and goals and to examine the rewards of achievement. This simplistic view of Maslow's model must be coupled with the managerial theory that evolved from scientific management, through the human relations era, to emerge into the organizational democracy that institutions strive for today.

Organizational democracy is a model based on the free society that exists outside the hospital doors. This model is a matrix of conditions in the workplace in which all members of the work force have an opportunity to participate in the democratic processes—creating profit, establishing systems for equitable sharing, changing the climate of the organization, and enabling nurses to take charge of their careers.

This democratic organizational model establishes a set of conditions in which responsible, creative, and productive individuals and groups reap higher rewards than the less effective members of the organization. Moreover, these conditions result in a competitive advantage in the business sector, and cost effectiveness in the public sector.

The quality of work life for nurses may be improved by ensuring meaningful work, reducing the management–labor (we–they) dichotomy, and improving the peripheral work systems that seem to encumber nurses in their jobs. Issues of organizational climate can then be addressed.

Every organization has a climate that colors the perceptions and feelings of persons within the work environment. A company's climate is influenced by innumerable factors such as number of employees, nature of the business, age, location, composition of the work force, management policies, rules and regulations, and values and leadership styles of management. Many of the factors influencing an organization's climate are dynamic and interactive, resulting in ever-changing "weather" within the organization. However, some factors remain relatively constant, and this tends to stabilize the characteristic climate for the organization. These pivotal factors are such things as growth rate, delegation tendencies, innovative processes, communication patterns, and stability of the organization. These variables can be analyzed individually for any organization and can provide guidance to new employees in determining what to expect.

New nurses must concern themselves with the quality of work life. Health care organizations are neophytes in the process of converting from outdated organizational styles to more contemporary managerial models. The complexity of this change is compounded by the numerous factions that must be coordinated into a new model. Change will not be easy, but it is essential to the survival of the health care organization. The new nurse will be the change agent in this process.

CHANGING ROLES OF MANAGEMENT

Managerial roles are the key to coordinating effort and technology. This responsibility is not new, but it is becoming increasingly complicated by the accelerating rate of change in health care. Because change requires adaptation at all levels of the organization, new nurses are confronted with the circular problem of encouraging innovation and then of introducing change in a manner that will not threaten the innovator. Being human, new nurses are vulnerable to the threats of change and must be able to monitor and evaluate their effectiveness and to take measures to prevent their obsolescence. Through capable supervisory style, management systems, and other factors affecting organizational climate, the source of influence must shift from official authority to people power, so that initiative and freedom at all levels of the organization will find responsible expression.

The environment in which every employee is a manager provides a realistic opportunity for each employee to be responsible for his or her job. Although many jobs cannot be fully enriched in their present form, most can be improved, fused with others, or more uniquely matched with individual aptitudes and attitudes. Whether the manager's mission is to modify the job or to match it to the right person, it is best achieved by recognizing the talents of those he or she supervises.

Nurses in managerial roles must be able to understand the conditions promoting and inhibiting the expression of talent among team members. This understanding requires a close look at the new responsibilities and activities with which managers should be involved and an equally close look at which of the traditional roles must be modified to accommodate the ever-evolving changes.

It has been said that the most valuable characteristic for those who want to succeed is flexibility. This is certainly true for nurses today. As the health care industry has changed dramatically in the past few years, so have the roles of nurses. These changes have led to role ambiguity as nurses search for models that will meet changing demands. The managerial roles being assumed by clinical nurses are the result of requirements to push decision making lower in the organization and to encourage staff nurses to determine the ways in which the delivery system can best function. The contemporary manager is finding that the pure managerial role is changing. No longer an authoritarian order-giver, today's manager concentrates on providing a climate in which individuals have a sense of working for themselves. Thus, the role of the manager should be to:

- Provide visibility for organizational goals
- Provide resources and define constraints
- Mediate conflict
- Serve as a coach or mentor
- Monitor results
- Stay out of the way so that individuals can manage their work.

This redefinition of the manager's role to provide opportunities for persons to manage their own work gives clear direction to the staff nurse to assume responsibility, whether clinical or managerial.

The new staff nurse must be prepared to see examples of all types of management. Some managers have made the transition to newer styles and others have not. Keep in mind that the requirements for change and organizational growth will always be with us and, in the future, those nurses who are flexible and competent will emerge as leaders. Also keep in mind your ultimate goals and work toward them.

SUMMARY

Managerial concepts needed by the new nurse focus on how to deal with people, how to manage resources, and how to manage one's job. No resource of this type can be all inclusive, but it can offer insights that offset the unknown. This preparation is important in making that first job more meaningful and understandable.

Your attitudes, how you view yourself, and exactly where your successes or failures lie will be determined by *you*. It is important to recognize where you are and what you feel capable of accomplishing so that you do not become controlled by events. Rather, *you* will control how you think and what you think and thereby control your reaction to events.

It is not enough to expect that, if you work hard, you will rise to the top. The process is so complex that predictability is difficult. It is certain, however, that if you follow some basic concepts of managing yourself, you have a better chance of success.

You must make a commitment to grow, both as a total person and as a nurse. Your attitude is the key element, as was beautifully stated by Abraham Lincoln: "Most people are about as happy as they make their minds up to be."

It is possible to be incredibly happy and satisfied in nursing. Over time you will not necessarily become smarter, but you will become more experienced. This experience leads to more effective behaviors and outcomes. Your success as a nurse starts with you and your attitude toward that responsibility. If this book is of some value to you in that process, then the authors will be deeply gratified.

DISCUSSION QUESTIONS

1. Describe several examples of management activities you have performed as a student nurse.
2. Discuss the changing role of the nurse manager and its impact on the changing role of the staff nurse.
3. Develop three different scenarios that demonstrate the staff nurse's role in managing a difficult patient encounter, managing an employee conflict, and developing a staffing schedule for a patient care unit.

REFERENCE

Lewin, K. (1947). Frontiers in group dynamics. *Human Relations*, June, 37.

SUGGESTED READING

Benveniste, G. (1987). *Professionalizing the organization.* San Francisco: Jossey-Bass.
Byham, W. (1988). *ZAPP!* New York: Harmony Books.
Conger, L. (1992). *Learning to lead.* San Francisco: Jossey-Bass.
Covey, S. (1989). *The 7 habits of highly effective people.* New York: Simon & Schuster.
Myers, M. (1981). *Every employee a manager.* New York: McGraw-Hill.

Assessing the Organization

Joyce E. Johnson

LEARNING OBJECTIVES

To choose a health care facility within which you can best "fit," you must be able to understand and assess an organization. This chapter will enable you to:

1. Describe the history of organizational theory and relate it to the health care setting.
2. Understand the basic principles of systems theory and how they relate to health care organizations.
3. Describe organizational behavior in terms applicable to health care facilities.
4. Identify the critical variables used in assessing an organization.
5. Identify key characteristics of learning organizations.
6. Identify key strategies that can be used for improving organization effectiveness.

Vestal, K.W. Nursing Management:
Concepts and Issues, 2 ed.
© 1995 J.B. Lippincott Company

One of your tasks as a newly employed nurse is to understand the behavior of individuals in your organization. The way your coworkers respond to their jobs reflects their expectations and the organization itself. Each organization has a purpose and a unique style of achieving that purpose known as its "culture" or character. That culture is clearly and quickly transmitted to you when you join.

Both formal rules and regulations and informal expectations make up the organizational culture. Patterns of thinking are, in some instances, more powerful than the formal rules and can have a positive or negative impact on your performance and on the organization's productivity.

Because the character of an organization can affect you as a professional nurse, you need to understand the formal and informal structures and these patterns of thinking. Such understanding can assist you in developing your role as a professional nurse in a way that coincides with and complements your organization's expectations of you.

CLASSIC ORGANIZATIONAL THEORY

Classic organizational theorists believe that the size, structure, division of labor, number of supervisory levels, and span of control are key variables in determining the success or efficiency of an organization (Weber, 1947). Figure 2-1 is an example of this organizational structure, which is used by many health care facilities. It is based on the belief that breaking down the operation into *specialized* components is necessary for the assignment and completion of responsibilities. Creating these specialized segments demands coordination that is best handled by *delegation of authority* to supervisory personnel such as the nursing administrator or a head nurse. *Structure* is essentially the height of the organization as compared to its width, whereas *span of control* defines the number of employees managed by the supervisor.

A flatter organization (Figure 2-2) may increase the span of control while decreasing levels of authority. Most health care facilities are moving in the direction of a flatter organizational design.

Classic organizational theory differentiates staff and line relationships. Those with *line* roles, such as the head nurse, have direct responsibility for employees and services. Line authority has traditionally been defined as the right to hire and fire. In contrast, the *clinical specialist* has traditionally held a *staff* position, indirectly responsible for the same services through employee education, consulting, and role modeling. Figures 2-1 and 2-2 depict both line and staff positions.

20

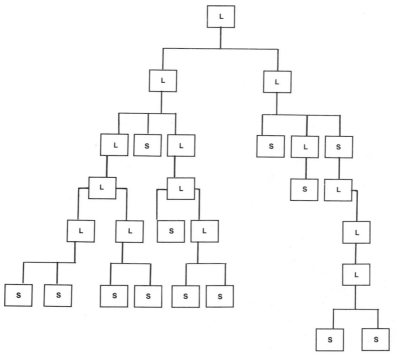

FIG. 2-1. Example of the classic organizational structure used by many health care facilities.

One of the major criticisms of the classic organization theory is that the lack of decision-making opportunities for employees is a result of the structure itself. Often the individual who *makes* the decisions and the individual who implements them occupy different positions on the organizational chart. This criticism has led to study of the psychology of work behavior and research into employee participation as a means of increasing motivation and commitment.

Today, most organizations, including health care facilities, have progressed beyond the classic model to models that reflect the modern approach to organizational structure and design.

MODERN ORGANIZATIONAL THEORY

Modern organizational theorists suggest that an essential element in understanding and predicting organizational behavior is the ability

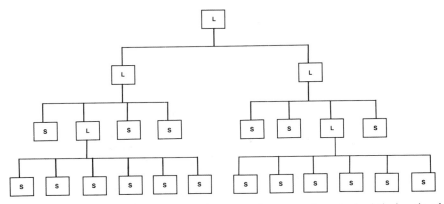

FIG. 2-2. A flatter organization may increase the span of control while levels of authority decrease.

to predict the behavior of the persons within an organization. These theorists contend that motivation, satisfaction, leadership, and the manner in which conflicts are resolved are key to organizational harmony and success. Unlike the classic approach, which focuses on structure and function, this approach maximizes the value of the individual. It recognizes that each employee has a set of unique processes, feelings, and thoughts that may not "fit" with those of the organization and may create tension between employer and employees. The supervisor's role becomes one of initiating activities that help the employee and supervisor to succeed together.

Helping employers and employees to work together has been the focus of a variety of theorists who are convinced that the structure and process of an organization is a single phenomenon (Landy & Trumbo, 1976). For instance, Douglas McGregor (1960) developed two fictional supervisory belief systems, labeled *Theories X and Y,* to describe relationships between supervisors and their employees. Supervisors who believed in Theory X controlled and directed the behavior of employees, whereas those who believed in Theory Y provided an atmosphere that encouraged participation in decision making by controlling not the employee but the surrounding work environment.

Whereas McGregor's work attempted to integrate the goals of the organization with those of the employees, Argyris (1972) pointed out the ways in which organizational structure restricts employee development. For instance, one nurse may be better suited to work in the technical atmosphere of the operating room, whereas another achieves and succeeds as a professional in psychiatric nursing care. A mismatch in either case would inevitably lead to tension between the nurse and the health care facility. These tensions require employer action to be resolved. Issues the supervisor might consider include the rates of absenteeism, turnover, and the role of labor unions. The employer may suggest relocating an employee to another section to give that individual a better chance of succeeding. One of the most important beliefs in modern organizational theory is that the individual must fit the organization and the organization must fit the individual.

Another central belief is that organizations are systems that function through the relations of many parts. According to Senge (1990), "systems thinking is a discipline for seeing wholes." Drawn from fields such as engineering, social sciences, and cybernetics, systems thinking focuses on relations rather than on direct cause and effect, and on change over time rather than on single events.

Such relations within organizations are subtle, complex, and important to understand. In simple terms, systems thinking suggests that individual behavior can have collective consequences within an organization. In health care organizations, this means that everyone within the organization influences the effectiveness of the organization as a system.

Understanding the complex patterns within the system as a means of diagnosing organizational problems and improving productivity often requires a shift in thinking away from the linear cause and effect models so typical in health care organizations in the past.

ORGANIZATIONAL CHARACTERISTICS

Identifying health care facilities where you can find the best organizational "fit" for yourself depends on your ability to define what you value in a work situation. Factors that have been identified in the past as important in many organizations include organizational size, formalization, and centralization of authority. Recently, the focus on organizational productivity has added another characteristic: the ability and willingness of the organization to learn.

Size refers simply to the number of employees and scope of activities sponsored by the organization. Formalization is the degree to which the communications and procedures are written, and the extent to which rules, instructions, and communications are documented. Centralization of authority is the amount of power delegated to departments or subunits. This represents the delegation of responsibility from top management, such as the nurse administrator to the middle manager, or in most cases, first line supervisor or head nurse. Ability to learn is the organization's interest in and commitment to growing and developing.

You should be able to assess organizational characteristics during your interview process or early in your employment. Suggested assessment methods are discussed later in this chapter.

ORGANIZATIONAL CLIMATE

You can quickly develop an impression of an institution's **personality.** Although difficult to conceptualize, this variable is an important barometer for determining your fit in an organization.

You may, for example, perceive a large health care facility as "busy or cold," whereas a smaller community hospital might be seen as quieter, calmer, and more "homelike." You should be able to articulate other perceptions such as efficient, bustling, easygoing, or human. In a learning organization, for example, you may sense a creative, energized spirit in the employees and a feeling of shared commitment.

Although the organizational climate is a variable difficult to quantify, it can have a significant impact on staff turnover, employee satisfaction, and individual and organizational productivity.

ORGANIZATIONAL EFFECTIVENESS

The ability of an organization to achieve its mission or goals, or the degree of its "success," is termed its *organizational effectiveness.* This effectiveness depends on communication patterns, centralization of authority, supervisory styles, employee morale, productivity, and what Senge calls "shared vision."

Organizational effectiveness is built on two central concepts. One is the ability of the organization to define its mission and shared goals. If these are clear, understood, and shared by the staff, the organization's direction and mission will be apparent in everyday activities.

The second concept is the prevalence of team learning in the organization. Team learning, according to Senge, is the phenomenon that occurs when a group functions as a whole along three critical dimensions: the need to think insightfully about complex issues, the need for innovated and coordinated action, and the movement of workers from one team to another to increase learning within the organization.

Historically, health care institutions have adopted mission statements that proclaim a commitment to delivering quality patient care. In recent times, this commitment has been expanded to include the words *total quality management,* reflecting the recognition that quality care is a result of shared vision and collective actions driven by an institution-wide commitment to quality at every level of the organization.

ORGANIZATIONAL CONFLICT

Tension within the organization creates conflict, which can lead to hostility or unintentional efforts by a person or group to prevent others from achieving goals, ultimately decreasing the chances of organizational success. More important than the conflicts themselves is the manner in which they are resolved within an organization. Historically, the standard approaches to conflict resolution have revolved around problem solving and persuasion.

Problem solving encourages individuals to identify a common objective, gather information, and devise and implement a plan to achieve that objective. Participation is encouraged in an atmosphere that focuses on the problem, not on the conflict. Take, for example, the addition of a new patient population to a nursing unit. The nursing personnel may believe they lack the clinical experience needed to provide care to the new patient population, whereas management may believe the nurses are prepared. To resolve the conflict, the nursing staff and management together develop and implement an educational program to provide the appropriate care.

Persuasion is the process by which conflicting individuals or groups are brought together. Although two groups may believe they share the same beliefs, at some level they work toward goals specific to their level of agreement (Landy & Trumbo, 1976). For example, employees and management may agree there is a need for a raise but disagree on the percent of wage increase needed to achieve equity in the marketplace. The amount then may be determined by each group testing its respective rationales associated with salary increases, such as salaries attached to a clinical ladder for advancement versus an across-the-board increase. Problem-solving and persuasion techniques encourage individuals to participate in problem resolution and limit disruption in the organization.

Senge (1990) and Argyris (1985) have suggested that the successful resolution of conflict in an organization is inherently linked to the ability of the members of the organization to learn together as a team and to deal with forces opposing productive dialogue and discussion—the key to effective team learning. Argyris suggested that such opposition takes the form of "defensive routines" that protect workers from embarrassment or threats but limit their ability to learn from the experience. Argyris' studies of management teams suggested that the difference between great and mediocre teams was the degree to which the group dealt with the defensiveness inherent in conflict. Thus, successful management of conflict within organizations depends on decreasing defensiveness through mutual inquiry and reflection. These skills require training and practice to overcome habitual but ineffectual ways of managing conflict.

HOW TO DEFINE AND USE THE SYSTEM

In health care facilities in the United States, nursing is usually the largest division or department. The placement of the nursing department in the hospital's organizational structure should be of utmost importance as you begin to assess the organization in which you are or may be employed. Review the hospital and nursing organizational charts. This can be accomplished during your interview with the personnel department or your prospective supervisor. Structures that are "flat" usually permit decentralized participative decisions and limit bureaucratic "red tape."

Keep in mind that the health care facility's chief nursing administrator should be on peer level organizationally or formally with the hospital's chief medical director and the director of all major service departments and should report to the chief hospital administrator. This permits direct representation of nursing's interest to those responsible for delineating the institution's mission and goals.

THE NURSE EXECUTIVE

As part of this analysis, it is important to understand the nurse executive's role. Nurse executives assume a variety of roles depending on the environment in which they find themselves, their background and level of expertise, and their beliefs about what constitutes good administration. Their roles also depend on the size of the hospital, its philosophy, and other variables. A person new to an organization needs to analyze this role thoroughly to understand what is expected and what is acceptable and unacceptable professional behavior.

Nurse executive management styles range from centralized to decentralized. Centralized management systems appear on paper as "tall" organizational structures with many layers between the staff nurse and the nurse executive. Most of the decision making is centralized in the nurse executive, and there are few forums and councils in which staff nurses and head nurses can participate. What councils and forums there are in a centralized structure will not be decision-making bodies but systems for the nurse executive to deliver information.

Decentralized structures, by contrast, are "flat" and have very few levels between the staff nurse and the nurse executive. The role of the staff nurse is expanded in this structure and includes participation in the governance of the organization. In a decentralized structure, persons in administration are seen as those who can facilitate rather than direct the work of the professional staff nurse. Decentralized structures use a "bottom up" style of organization versus the "top down" style seen in more centralized organizations. The power over clinical decisions in the decentralized organization resides in the highly developed role of the professional nurse rather than in the nurse executive. Decisions about nursing care are delegated to the professional nurse and supported by the nurse executive.

In a centralized style of management, the power resides in the nurse executive. Patient care decisions are made at this level and implemented by the staff nurse whose role is seen as that of a doer and not a thinker. There are many gradations of these two models, and, in practice, it is virtually impossible to find the pure form of either structure.

Nurse executives play a leading role in defining the culture of the nursing organization. They blend their personal styles of management with factors specific to the particular work setting. These include the management style of the chief executive officer and the governing board, the sophistication of the nursing staff, and other aspects of the working environment. The professional nurse should be cognizant of these variables and understand how they might influence the nurse executive's actions.

MIDDLE MANAGEMENT

One management level down from the nurse executive is, depending on the organization, the assistant director, vice president, clinical coordinator, or divisional director. These positions exert supervisory responsibilities over a variety of clinical units within the hospital setting.

The role of the nurse in middle management depends on factors similar to those influencing the management style of the nurse executive. In some settings, the organization is decentralized to the point of allowing this person great freedom to assume the management style with which he or she is most comfortable. In other organizations, roles and behaviors are more standardized according to function, and there is less responsibility and accountability.

In both models, there is great variation in the way individuals perform in their assigned position. Those who are well prepared through education and experience and who feel comfortable with the organizational structure will perform well in this role. Others with differing management styles and perceptions may not be able to function as effectively. The responsibility of the staff nurse is to analyze how this role is being performed in the division and act accordingly.

THE HEAD NURSE

The position traditionally known as the "head nurse" probably has more titles than any other in nursing organizations. The individual may be called unit manager, nurse manager, clinical coordinator, or many other titles. The role of the head nurse ranges from being a simple charge nurse to that of department manager with 24-hour accountability, a budget to manage, and hiring and firing responsibilities. In such situations, the need for assistant directors is minimized and the expertise of the head nurse is maximized. The head nurse may be involved in direct patient care at times or may perform no direct patient care at all.

There are no consistent standards for the credentials required of a head nurse. Some institutions require a master's degree in clinical or administrative nursing, whereas others require only excellent performance as a staff nurse as a prerequisite. Head nurses' philosophies of administration can be quite varied. Some believe in delegating the governance of the unit to the staff nurse, whereas others keep tight centralized control of management functions. Some head nurses have a keen interest in patient care and others emphasize the management role. A key to successful administration of a unit is the communication of expectations by the head nurse to others on the unit. Analyzing these expectations and understanding the "lay of the land" determine the success or failure of the staff nurse. Expectations usually are not communicated directly. The staff nurse often must infer from the actions of the head nurse the beliefs that person holds.

The staff nurse should be alert to the number of employees under the control of one supervisor. Although management theory varies regarding the "correct" span of control, a head nurse responsible for 50 nursing personnel may not be able to provide individual guidance unless assistant supervisory staff is available. Ask how many and what categories of personnel report to the head nurse. Are assistants provided in her absence?

STAFF POSITIONS

In assessing an organization, you should assess the role of staff positions such as clinical specialists, nursing researchers, and educators. In some settings, these staff members work closely with the nursing staff, provide training, and assume supervisory responsibilities. In other settings, these positions assume very specialized functions and have only limited involvement with the nursing staff.

It is therefore important for you to determine the nature and extent of your interaction with other staff in the direct delivery of patient care and in committee and project activities.

THE STAFF NURSE

The staff nurse plays a variety of roles depending on the institution. In some sophisticated systems, the staff nurse is seen as the professional with the greatest amount of decision-making power concerning clinical practices. A shared governance system supports this belief, and staff nurses are involved in the control of clinical practice through a system of peer review and credentialing. Councils or forums are the vehicle through which information and decisions flow from the bottom up. At the opposite extreme, a more technical model views the staff nurse as more of a "worker bee" who carries out the directives of the head nurse and assistant director.

Defining the nursing care delivery system in which you will work is crucial to understanding your organizational role. This can be done with the help of the head nurse and the staff nurses. Within the context of health care delivery, many individuals other than nurses provide patient care. To coordinate all aspects of patient care, the nurse must be able to work effectively with many different types of people. Nursing aides, technicians, licensed practical or vocational nurses, and unit secretaries are some examples of unit-based staff. Within the hospital-wide system, many others work directly with nurses in the care of patients, including pharmacists, laboratory technicians, social workers, and volunteers.

Because the work of all these individuals has an impact on the care of patients, the professional nurse must possess a clear understanding of systems theory to coordinate the work of others. The nurse must know how to train, motivate, and monitor ancillary staff who are directly and indirectly involved with patient care. The nurse must know how to communicate effectively and how to develop collaborative relations with the large number of staff members.

As the cultural diversity of the work force increases, cultural differences can present considerable challenges to effective working relationships among staff members. As coordinators of patient care activities, nurses must develop their cross-cultural competencies and those of ancillary staff members who support the delivery of patient care.

ROLE EXPECTATIONS

Adjusting to the management aspects of the nurse's role requires adjusting to the expectations of that role. For example, a nurse who is put in charge of a unit must develop thinking skills that extend beyond the direct care of individual patients. These skills involve knowing what is expected from the management role and how that role fits into the hospital system.

Nurses who are new to the profession often confuse role expectations with personal needs. For example, an inexperienced nurse might place the need to be liked above the need to require top performance from others. Personal relationships could then become more important than the care of the patient. Such a situation is filled with inefficiencies that ultimately compromise the delivery of direct patient care.

Valuable employees are those who understand the tasks and inherent outcomes of the role that they fill. Success means completing the tasks and, in the process, meeting personal needs related to achievement, affiliation, and recognition. Every nurse must remember that, in health care settings, professional relationships revolve around the delivery of quality patient care and not around personal friendships. To assess professional competence, every nurse needs to examine periodically how well the expectations of his or her role match the actual performance.

INFORMATION SOURCES

Because individuals in management positions must be informed of all actual and potential problems that might have an impact on the delivery of patient care, staff nurses must be skilled in prioritizing and effectively communicating large amounts of information. This communication must take place within the norms of the organization, because all health care institutions have unwritten rules concerning communication between staff members. In one institution, for example, a nurse can send a memo to the chief of radiology without sending copies to her head nurse and assistant director. In another institution this would not be allowed because only the nurse executive communicates directly with the department chief.

A new nurse must learn quickly the nuances of the communication structure within the institution. A mentor or supervisor who is willing to take the time to discuss the institution's communication structure and to provide guidance and feedback can be an invaluable ally in this learning process.

CONFLICT RESOLUTION

Conflict is inevitable in most working relationships. As a part of professional development, the staff nurse must learn to handle situations involving a disagreement with staff members or the immediate supervisor. As with communication patterns, methods for conflict resolution vary among institutions. Generally, the nurse must explore all possibilities for compromise before taking the conflict to a higher level within the organization. If a resolution cannot be found, the nurse may request a meeting with a person higher in the chain of command.

It is seldom appropriate for a staff nurse to circumvent his or her immediate supervisor by taking the problem to the next level. To do so places the supervisor in a difficult position that may escalate the existing problem. It is appropriate, however, for the nurse to inform the supervisor of the desire to take the matter to the superior and to seek support.

Conflict management is a critical and difficult skill for any nurse to learn. It is difficult because conflict is surrounded by a learned defensiveness that protects us from exposing our reasoning and possibly being proved wrong. Being proved wrong is then equated with losing the battle. It is this type of "win or lose" atmosphere that limits our ability to resolve conflict and to learn by being open to new ways of viewing the situation. A preferred method would be one in which individuals are encouraged to reflect on their assumptions and to inquire into each other's thinking in an atmosphere that promotes team learning rather than winning or losing.

DELEGATION

Another difficult skill to learn is delegation. Throughout nursing school, nurses are taught that they are ultimately responsible for everything related to patient care. They are often taught that they cannot depend on anyone else for help. In reality, this is not true. In today's cost-conscious health care system, it is imperative that nurses learn to deliver care through others. This requires skills in appropriate and effective delegation and in the development of monitoring systems to ensure the proper completion of tasks.

Delegation is most effective when it includes clear directions, a time frame for the completion of the task, coaching, and appropriate monitoring. Effective delegation also involves knowing the strengths and weaknesses of each person on the nursing staff and matching tasks to the capabilities of the person. Attention to all these facets of delegation ensures that nursing time is used effectively.

SUPPORT OUTSIDE THE NURSING DEPARTMENT

Nurses must interact with a variety of staff members whose responsibilities directly or indirectly influence patient care. The successful nurse is able to use a systems approach in analyzing the interdependence of roles within a hospital. Acknowledging this interdependence and working effectively with many other departments is critical to the delivery of quality patient care.

The most effective work groups are those that have a "shared vision." This occurs when members from various departments within a system have a similar view of the goals of the organization and are committed to making them a reality. Within a hospital system, these goals are focused on the delivery of cost-conscious quality care for all patients.

The nurse plays a key role in maintaining positive interpersonal relationships among his or her staff members and among the staff members from other hospital departments. The nurse has the opportunity to foster group cohesion and to keep the focus on the common goal of quality patient care.

INSTITUTIONAL MISSION

Once you have reviewed the hospital and nursing department structure, review the hospital mission statement and its short-term and long-term goals. Obtain policy and procedure manuals and hospital publications from the personnel department, and review these to gain a sense of the direction in which the institution is heading and how it plans to reach its goals. Compare these goals with those of the nursing department and assess their similarities and differences. You should be able to identify a shared vision and a common commitment toward the achievement of the overall mission, from top management to the individual nursing unit. A lack of congruence between the two suggests organizational uncertainty and may lead to communication difficulties.

A nurse may find that her philosophy does not match that of an institution. This poor "job fit" between the nurse and the institution may result in managerial disagreements and low productivity. In such cases, the nurse has the option of changing her philosophy, working toward the institutional policies, or finding another institution with a philosophy that is more compatible. The most important point to remember is that delivering excellent patient care depends on the coordination of many persons and the synthesis of many personalities. The nurse must be focused on analyzing these accurately so that the positive synergy within the institution can be directed toward quality care.

As a professional, you should be alert to opportunities within the organization to participate in institutional decision making. By reviewing the committee structures, activities, and reporting relationships, you will gain an understanding of how information is transmitted through the organization to the nursing department and hospital administration.

Another factor to consider is how the organization values it employees. Is the institution unionized? If so, is it an open or closed shop? Has the institution conducted employee satisfaction surveys? Are continuing education programs available to employees at all levels? Is there a clinical ladder in the nursing department? How much importance does the institution place on nursing education and research?

You should become familiar with the ways in which the institution resolves conflicts. Do the supervisors resolve conflicts unilaterally, or is team decision making involved? How often do management and supervisory positions change in the institution?

Organizations that are committed to their employees have mechanisms in place for rewarding outstanding performance, seniority, and low absenteeism. Employee recognition programs such as employee of the month and merit increases based on performance are evidence that employees are valued and recognized for their contributions.

Evaluating these types of issues will help you evaluate the fit between you and the institution, and determine your opportunities for professional growth.

ADDITIONAL RESOURCES

Within any institution there are many resources available to nurses. These include managers, clinical specialists, and educators who offer expertise on specific patient care problems. Advanced level nurses have invaluable expertise and knowledge about the organization culture and patient care. Nurses who are willing to act as mentors can help newer nurses improve their performance and further their career goals. A mentoring relationship, formal or informal, can provide counsel and support that is invaluable in developing professional competence.

SUMMARY

Nursing is a complicated and rewarding profession that involves far more than direct, hands-on patient care. Competency in nursing requires technical expertise, an understanding of systems theory, and a high level of management skill to provide cost-effective, quality patient care. Mastery of these skills has many rewards for patients and the nurses who care for them.

DISCUSSION QUESTIONS

1. Describe an interview process in which you would assess five major organizational characteristics.
2. Discuss ways you will know if an organizational "fit" exists between you and a specific opportunity.
3. Study an organizational chart and decide what responsibilities are centralized and decentralized and what the span of control is for each manager.
4. Develop a set of five expectations for your role as a staff nurse related to decision making, clinical practice, and team learning.

REFERENCES

Argyris, C. (1972). *The applicability of organization sociology.* New York: Cambridge University Press.
Argyris, C. (1985). *Strategy, change and defensive routines.* Boston: Pittman.
McGregor, D. (1960). *The human side of enterprise.* New York: McGraw-Hill.
Senge, P. M. (1990). *The fifth discipline: The art and practice of the learning organization.* New York: Doubleday.
Weber, M. (1947). *The theory of social and economic organization.* Henderson, A.M., Parsons, T. (Trans., ed.) New York: Oxford University Press.

SUGGESTED READING

Althaus, J. N., Hardyck, N.M., Rodgers, M.S., & Pierce, P.B. (1981). *Nursing decentralization: The El Camino experience.* Rockville, MD: Aspen Systems.

Argyris, C., Putnam, R., & Smith, D. (1985). *Action science: Concepts, methods and skills for research and intervention.* San Francisco, CA: Jossey-Bass.

Blau, P. M. (1970). A formal theory of differentiation in organizations. *American Sociology Review,* April.

Champion, D. J. (1973). *The sociology of organizations* (2nd ed.). New York: John Wiley & Sons.

Coch, L., & French J. R. P. (1948). Overcoming resistance to change. *Human Relations, 1,* 512–532.

Connor, P. E., & Lake, L. K. (1988). *Managing organizational change.* New York: Praeger.

deLodzia, G., & Greenhalgh, L. (1973). Creative conflict management in a nursing environment. *Supervisory Nurse, 4,* 33–41.

Deutsch, M. (1973). *The resolution of conflict.* New Haven: Yale University Press.

Dickelmann, N. L., & Broadwell, M. M. (1977). How to get the job done . . . by someone else. *Nurse, 77,* 110–116.

Dieneman, J. (1992). *Continuous quality improvement in nursing.* Kansas City: American Nurses Publishing.

Doona, M. D. (1977). A nursing unit as a political system. *Journal of Nursing Administration, 7,* 28–32.

Douglas, L. M., & Bevis, E. O. (1979). Predictive principles for delegating authority. In Douglas, L. M. (Ed.), *Nursing management and leadership in action* (3rd ed.). St. Louis: CV Mosby.

Drucker, P. F. (1954). *The practice of management.* New York: Harper & Brothers.

Heimann, C. G. (1976). Four theories of leadership. *Journal of Nursing Administration, 6,* 18.

Kast, F.E., & Rosenweig, J. E. (1979). *Organization and management.* New York: McGraw-Hill.

Landy, F., & Trumbo, D. (1976). *Psychology of work behavior.* Homewood, IL: The Dorsey Press.

Lawler, E. E. (1973). *Motivation in work organizations.* Monterey, CA: Brooks/Cole Publishing.

Lewis, J. H. (1976). Conflict management. *Journal of Nursing Administration, 6*(10), 18.

Likert, R., & Likert, J. G. (1976). *New ways of managing conflict.* New York: McGraw-Hill.

Litterer, J. A. (1973). *The analysis of organizations* (2nd ed.). New York: John Wiley & Sons.

Lowin, A. (1968). Participative decision making: A model, literature critique and prescriptions for research. In *Organizational behavior and human performance* (Vol. 3, pp. 68–106). New York: John Wiley & Sons.

March, J. G., & Simon, H. A. (1958). *Organizations.* New York: John Wiley & Sons.

Marriner, A. (1980). Decentralization versus centralization. In R. Hanson (Ed.), *Management systems for nursing service staffing* (pp. 45–53). Rockville, MD: Aspen Systems.

McClure, M. (1985). Managing the professional nurse (Part 1). *Journal of Nursing Administration, 16,* 83–86.

McConnel, E. A. (1979). Delegation—myth or reality? *Supervisory Nurse 10*(10), 20.

Mouton, J. S., & Blake, R. R. (1984). *Synergogy: A new strategy for education, training and development.* San Francisco, CA: Jossey-Bass.

Peterson, M. D., & Allen, D. G. (1986). Shared governance: A strategy for transforming organizations (Part 2). *Journal of Nursing Administration, 16*(2), 11–16.

Peterson, M. E., & Allen, D. G. (1986). Shared governance: A strategy for transforming organizations (Part 1). *Journal of Nursing Administration, 16*(1), 9–12.

Porter-O'Grady, T. (1984). *Shared governance for nursing: A creative approach to professional accountability.* Rockville, MD: Aspen Systems.

Pfeffer, J. (1982). *Organizations and organizational theory.* Cambridge, MA: Ballinger.

Richardson, G. (1990). *Feedback thought in social science and systems theory.* Philadelphia: University of Pennsylvania Press.

Rotkovitch, R. (1985). The head nurse as a first-line manager. *Health Care Supervisor,* 1(4), 14–17.

Shoemaker, H., & El-Ahraf, A. (1983). Decentralization of nursing service management and its impact on job satisfaction. *Nursing Administration Quarterly,* Winter, 69–76.

Stagnitto, M. R. E. B. (1979). Nursing supervision: Leadership or police work? *Supervisory Nurse,* 10(1), 17–18.

Sullivan, E., & Decker, P. (1985). *Effective management in nursing.* Menlo Park, CA: Addison-Wesley.

Taylor, F. W. (1947). *Principles of scientific management.* New York: Harper & Brothers.

Vroom, V. H. (1964). *Work and motivation.* New York: John Wiley & Sons.

Weber, M. (1941). *The theory of social and economic organization* (A. M. Henderson, & T. Parsons, Eds. and Trans.). New York: Oxford University Press.

Whyte, W. F. (1955). *Money and motivation: An analysis of incentives in industry.* New York: Harper & Brothers.

Models of Patient Care Delivery

Karlene Kerfoot

LEARNING OBJECTIVES

This chapter will enable you to:

1. Describe the most common patient care delivery systems.
2. Determine how these systems differ from each other.
3. Describe what goes into the choice of a delivery system model.
4. Differentiate the skills needed by the nurse in each of the models.

Vestal, K.W. Nursing Management:
Concepts and Issues, 2 ed.
© 1995 J.B. Lippincott Company

There are many different ways of organizing and delivering nursing care. In schools of nursing, students are exposed to information about patient care delivery systems, but they rarely have the opportunity to work in several different models of patient care delivery before graduating. Therefore, it is important for new nurses to be familiar with the different models of nursing care that are available and to select carefully the facility that best fits their perceptions of how nursing care should be delivered. Two of the tasks for the new nurse to accomplish during the orientation period is to fully understand the delivery system and to achieve competence within the system.

Throughout our history, nursing has developed many approaches to the delivery of care. However, we have not always developed the theory and research to distinguish the outcomes of these models of delivering care. With the many changes coming to pass with managed care and health care reform, we should see new systems that will better meet the needs of patients for care and the needs of society for care at affordable prices.

A common model in the past has been that of functional nursing, which was based on the assembly-line concept found in industry. In this model, the number of tasks on a given unit were itemized and assigned to particular people to do repetitively. Tasks such as hygienic care, medication distribution, treatment administration, bedmaking, or replenishing water pitchers would be assigned to a particular individual to do for all the patients on the unit. Nurses and other staff would be assigned to specific tasks for a group of patients. It was thought that specializing tasks would increase efficiency because staff would become more efficient as they repeated the task many times. Although this model was considered efficient, the patients were confronted with many strangers who performed single tasks for the patient and could not give personalized care because they did not know the patient.

Team nursing evolved after functional nursing and differed in that it modified the depersonalized approach and focused on individual patient care. The team was made up of a registered nurse and other care givers who would provide care to a designated group of patients on a given shift. The registered nurse who functioned as a team leader would ideally plan the care of the patients, delegate the work through an assignment system to the members of the team, and follow up with them to obtain their observations and to evaluate the quality of care provided.

Although this model was called "team" nursing, sometimes this group of people actually worked as a team and sometimes they worked as a collection of individuals rather than a team. Although team nursing has been shown to be a viable model, it does not provide for continuity of care between care givers or between shifts because assignments can change daily and patients are still confronted with many single-function people entering their rooms. In this model, the nurse must be competent in managing a collection of people, assessing and prioritizing patient needs, and creating teamwork among the people assigned to the team.

Another model that evolved was that of total patient care in which the nurse as care giver provided total care to a group of patients for a designated shift. This model has been effective in reducing the number of strangers that care for a patient because the registered nurse attempts to provide as much of the physical, technical, emotional, and nursing care possible directly to a particular patient. However, the model suffers from problems with continuity of care because the plan of care can be different between care givers and shifts. The total patient care model is very expensive because highly paid nurses are providing all aspects of the care that could be delegated to a less expensive staff member. Some nurses prefer this model, whereas others would rather delegate the simpler tasks and concentrate on nursing activities that cannot be delegated, such as sophisticated education to patients and families and surveillance, assessment, diagnostic, and intervention activities.

Marie Manthey (1980) evolved the concept of primary nursing in which a nurse was accountable for planning, evaluating, and directing the care of the patients 24 hours a day throughout their stay. This model was an attempt to provide consistency between shifts and between care givers. In some models, primary nursing took the form of a staff composed entirely of registered nurses. In others it did not. The model was designed to increase the amount of nursing time spent with patients because the registered nurse focused on the patient's entire stay. When the primary nurse was not there, an associate nurse provided that care by following the primary nurse's orders for care of the patient.

Marie Manthey (1992, 1989) has also developed a nurse extender model for primary nursing in which a paired partner is selected and trained by a nurse. This care partner over time learns to be an extension of the nurse and takes on progressively complicated patient tasks. The nurse delegates these tasks as the partner's expertise and knowledge base permits. Clearly, the primary nurse retains the accountability as in primary nursing but works very closely with the primary nurse to provide many of the skills. The primary nurse has sophisticated clinical and managerial skills at his or her fingertips and is able to conceptualize the patient's and family's care not just for an 8-hour period, but for the course of the illness.

More recently, a case management model has evolved to ensure that patients receive care according to a predetermined course. This model involves a nurse overseeing the quality and financial outcomes of patient care. The nurse directs patient care through the course of the hospitalization according to critical paths that are developed from the time before the patient enters the hospital and extend to the time the patient is discharged. A case manager assumes a planning and evaluative role over many different departments with which the patient will interact and takes on the role of a problem solver and a fixer of systems that stand in the way of effective delivery of care. The case manager ensures that the milestones on the critical paths are met. When they are not met, variances from the expected are carefully analyzed to improve the quality of care. In case management, the nurse works collegially with physicians and other health care providers, including payers, to manage patients along an agreed upon clinical pathway (Zander, 1988).

The case manager is a sophisticated clinical nurse with the financial skills necessary to achieve the best quality of patient care at an acceptable cost. This nurse is knowledgeable about the many kinds of health care reimbursement and about which interventions are effective and which are not. Outcomes managers focus not only on what happens to the patient in the hospital but also on the outcomes achieved for the patient after hospitalization. For example, surgery can be successful, but the long-term outcome may be that the patient will have to live in a nursing home. Outcomes managers are beginning to develop data about the success or failure of treatment as measured months after the event.

A recently evolved model is that of patient-centered care. In this model, cross-functional teams consist of groups of professionals and assistive personnel from nursing and other departments who are assigned reporting responsibility to a patient care unit. They work together as a unit-based team to provide care to a given group of patients. Care is designed around the needs of the patient and not the needs of the departments or professionals. People from other departments still report to those departments in some situations but, in other situations, no longer report to individual departments but to the leader of the particular patient care unit. More sophisticated versions of these cross-functional teams are self-managed teams in which the team takes on most of the management responsibilities such as assignment of staff and monitoring quality and provides the care and management necessary for the unit.

In addition to models of patient care that are specific to nursing, there are situations in which nurses and physicians work together in collaborative practice models. Working from the original research on collaborative practice models at Hartford Hospital under the direction of Doris Armstrong (Koerner & Armstrong, 1983), subsequent research, especially in the intensive care units, has demonstrated that mortality is less than expected when collaborative models of nurse–physician interactions are in place (Knaus, Draper, Wagner, & Zimmerman, 1986).

As can be inferred from this brief overview, the models of nursing care delivery systems have evolved from highly technical, industrial based, assembly-line models to more professional, self-managed, cross-functional units. As nurses have moved to accept more professional status and the responsibility of delegating and working through others, they have moved into advanced practice models in which there is less supervision, more opportunity for independent thought and creativity, and more accountability. In many work situations, patient care units within a facility demonstrate varying degrees of professional accountability and autonomy. In some units, technical nursing will be in place because the expertise of the staff is not sufficient for more expanded professional models. In other units, the staff will want to take on more accountability and responsibility and will therefore have evolved into more sophisticated professional models.

Different skill sets are necessary for various models. It is important to understand this fully when interviewing for a job, participating in orientation, and adjusting to the role of the nurse. New nurses will be most successful if they can choose a position that best fits their skill set and philosophy of nursing. However, the world of health care is changing. Although a nurse might be more comfortable in some of the more primitive models in which management supervises and oversees closely what the new nurse does, those opportunities are becoming more scarce. With advanced practice and higher salaries, it is expected that the nurse will move beyond technical nursing into professional nursing and will be able to accept the challenge of overseeing and directing patient care and working through others (eg, paired partners) to get the job done.

In self-managed cross-functional teams, the responsibility becomes even greater because the nurse now accepts accountability to manage people who come from traditionally centralized departments such as housekeeping or dietary departments. New health care models will see nurses managing their work and the work of others, including technical and professional people. Interdisciplinary, cross-functional teams appear to be the health care model of the future. This mandates that the nurse learns and understands that significant managerial activities are expected of professional nurses as they evolve into directing and orchestrating the activities of patient care, not just nursing care.

Although new nurses may not think of themselves as managers, this is indeed the role that will be expected of them in the health care setting as they learn to manage patient care and to work through others who provide care. Staffs composed entirely of registered nurses are very rare and have not proved any quality or cost advantages (McManus & Pearson, 1993). The new nurse will be expected to manage others to deliver patient care.

WHAT DRIVES CHOICE?

There are many reasons why different nursing care delivery systems are chosen. Sometimes delivery systems are chosen with a lot of research and thought. In other situations, unfortunately, a delivery system is chosen without regard to the environment, philosophy, or resources of a particular unit. Sometimes thought has not gone into the choice—the system has just evolved. Because the choice of a nursing care delivery system is so integrally tied to the quality and cost of nursing care that can be delivered, the choice of a nursing care delivery system must be considered carefully. There are basically four motivators that drive the choice of a nursing care delivery system:

1. Mission or goal of the hospital.
2. Desired level of quality.
3. Resources that drive the delivery system (or the lack of resources).
4. Nursing theories.

If one understands the underlying reason for the development of the nursing care delivery system, the outcomes can be easier understood. The mission or philosophy of the health care facility often drives the choice of a nursing care delivery system. For example, in a teaching hospital, the mission might be viewed as using available research and developing new nursing knowledge. Therefore, the nursing care delivery system might be chosen based on a careful literature review and on the ability to research nursing care outcomes. Case management might be chosen in this situation because the clinical pathways would yield to investigating outcomes in relation to interventions. By contrast, a for-profit system might view their mission as providing income to their stockholders. Therefore, they might choose a delivery system that would provide a targeted level of quality at the lowest cost. A not-for-profit hospital that views itself as having a mission of providing community service, might also choose a very cost-effective model so it would have revenue to devote to designated community service options. Some health care facilities see the nurse as the centerpiece and integrator of the health care of patients and would choose a form of primary nursing. Certain models fit with certain missions and philosophies. Once these underlying models are understood, the choice of delivery system is apparent.

Nursing theories can be useful to guide the choice of a nursing care delivery system, and the purpose of a unit can guide the choice of theory. For example, a rehabilitation unit might see their mission as teaching and helping patients and their families develop better self-care skills. Therefore, Orem (1985) might be the likely choice of theorists to guide the practice because of her work on self care. An oncology unit, by contrast, might believe their role is to help patients cope with the diagnosis of cancer; therefore, Roy's adaptation model (Riehl & Roy, 1980) might be chosen. Other theories such as Neuman's, Levine's, Johnson's, Peplau's, or Orlando's could be chosen for other basic purposes of a particular unit.

A nursing department can choose an overall theory around which functions can be organized. In a division of nursing that has a high commitment to quality, the fragmentation of care and the lack of ability to standardize care given by large numbers of care givers would not be considered appropriate. Therefore, these kinds of divisions would probably choose an interdisciplinary team model, a cross-functional self-managed team, or some form of primary nursing and case management. Higher levels of predictability could be maintained because management would focus on following critical paths and protocols and on decreasing the chance of error by decreasing the number of people that come in contact with the patient.

With the reimbursement models in health care changing with capitated payments such as those provided by Medicare, finite and dwindling resources are driving how care is conceptualized. The lack of financial resources is driving a significant change in health care. In this resource-driven environment, the available financial and human resources often determine the choice of nursing care delivery systems. For example, if a sophisticated nursing staff is not available, it would not be realistic to try to implement the more professional models of nursing. If finances are especially difficult because of the particular financial situation of the health care facility or the financial environment of the particular area, the organization might choose a less expensive model for delivering nursing care for the sake of survival, although this would not be their first choice if given other options.

WHY BE CONCERNED?

New nurses should be concerned about the model of delivery in place for several reasons. Adjustment to a new position will be easier if new nurses understand the delivery model and can be assured that the orientation meets their needs for familiarity and competency. Many schools of nursing teach only one model such as primary nursing and do not allow students to practice sufficiently within other models. Therefore, it is imperative that new nurses understand that models drive the care delivery system and that a part of the nurse's role is the management of patient care through different models. Here are some basic principles about selecting among and working within different models of patient care:

1. Different skills are required in different models. For example, the more sophisticated models of interdisciplinary teamwork require sophisticated expertise in conflict resolution and teamwork. Primary nursing with a paired partner demands expertise in delegation skills and supervision.
2. Nursing models should fit with one's beliefs and values about what nursing should be. If one believes that primary nursing affords the nurse the accountability and autonomy desired, it would be difficult for this person to work in a functional system. The new nurse would be competent but would not reach the high level of job satisfaction desired.
3. The new nurse should search for and support models that are best for the patient. Sometimes the model we are familiar with is not the best one for the patient. Certain patient populations have very limited resources, and society as a whole has mandated that health care reduce the costs to society. Therefore, what we as a professional might think is best might not be in the best interest of the patient and of society because of limited resources. We also have to address the question of what quality really is and how we can provide the appropriate level of quality at the lowest cost.
4. Wide variation in quality can occur between nurses, between shifts, and between different days of the week if a care delivery model is not thoughtfully selected and followed. It is confusing to patients to be exposed to several different delivery systems throughout their stay in a facility.
5. Nursing care models are constantly evolving. What we practice in terms of nursing care delivery today will not be what we are practicing 5 years from now. Delivery systems are dynamic and

should be even more dynamic. We should be pushing ourselves to create new and more effective delivery systems to provide our patients and society with the very best delivery systems available to provide the highest level of quality at the lowest cost.

SUMMARY

We, in nursing, must take seriously the mandate from society and from our patients to improve the quality of patient care and to reduce its cost. We are in a position to do that by looking at our delivery systems and asking ourselves if we are managing them in the most effective way. By continually reevaluating and refining our delivery systems, organizations can proactively respond to the increasingly competitive health care market.

DISCUSSION QUESTIONS

Case Study:

When Jack Samuels joined St. James' Hospital as a new RN 6 months ago, he knew the hospital was in fairly good financial shape but that some of the health maintenance organizations (HMO) were threatening to leave because they could get cheaper prices at another hospital in town. After he had been there 6 months, the largest HMO left, decreasing the patients in the hospital by one fourth. To cope with this situation, the hospital closed several units, but Jack was lucky because his oncology unit did not lose many patients. It was merged with a medicine unit since that unit had a significant loss in patient census.

When Jack came to the hospital, he was oriented under a modified primary nursing system that assigned the accountability for a given group of patients to him, and he then delegated some of the care to nursing care assistants. He had mentored under an experienced nurse and felt that he had learned well and was just beginning to feel a measure of competence with his care.

Because the hospital was already on shaky financial grounds and likely to lose other health maintenance organizations unless it could cut costs, the hospital undertook a major cost-cutting program. The hospital structure was reorganized, departments were combined, and certain functional areas such as government relations and public relations were terminated. To get hospital costs down further, it was mandated that nursing care would be delivered by team nursing instead of the modified primary nursing that Jack had just learned. This would involve a larger patient load for him and, because the skill mix was decreased, more assistive personnel to carry out more of the tasks that could be delegated to non-RNs.

Jack felt distressed because he had been comfortable in the modified primary care system and did not feel so with the team nursing system. He thought about leaving the organization but knew that other hospitals in the city were in the same precarious situation. In fact, most hospitals were not hiring. He felt his best option was to stay where he was and determine how to cope with this dramatic change.

1. What kind of a plan could Jack develop so that he could positively cope with this crisis in his professional life?
2. Discuss the kinds of problems with staff morale you can expect when two dramatic changes such as the combining of two different units and a mandated move to a new delivery system take place.
3. What could the nurse manager do to help people like Jack the most in this particular situation?

REFERENCES

Knaus, W., Draper, E., Wagner, D., & Zimmerman, J. (1986). An evaluation of outcome from intensive care in major medical centers. *Annals of Internal Medicine, 104*(3), 410–418.

Koerner, B., & Armstrong, D. (1983). Collaborative practice at Hartford Hospital. *Nursing Administration Quarterly, 17*(4) 72–81.

Manthey, M. (1980). A theoretical framework for primary nursing. *Journal of Nursing Administration, 10*(7), 11–15.

Manthey, M. (1989). Practice partnerships: The newest concept in care delivery. *Journal of Nursing Administration, 19*(2), 33–35.

Manthey, M. (1992). Practice partners: Humanizing healthcare. *Nursing Management, 23*(5), 18–19.

McManus, S., & Pearson, J. (1993). Nursing at a crossroads: Managing without facts. *Health Care Management Review, 18*(1), 79–90.

Orem, D. (1985). *Nursing concepts of practice.* New York: McGraw-Hill.

Riehl, J., & Roy, C. (1980). *Conceptual models for nursing practice* (2nd ed.). New York: Appleton-Century-Crofts.

Take charge of your health! (1993). *American Health, 7*(3), 43–67.

Zander, K. (1988). Nursing care management: Strategic management of cost and quality outcomes. *Journal of Nursing Administration, 18*(5), 23–30.

SUGGESTED READING

Accountability in nursing practice. (1984). *Nursing Management, 15*(11), 72.

Bush, H. (1979). Models for nursing. *Advances in Nursing Science, 1*(2) 13–21.

Campbell, L. (1986). What satisfies . . . and doesn't? *Nursing Management, 17*(8), 78.

Clausen, C. (1984). Staff RN: A discharge planner for every patient. *Nursing Management, 15*(11), 58–61.

Cohen, M., & Ross, M. (1982). Team building: A strategy for unit cohesiveness. *Journal of Nursing Administration, 12*(1), 29–34.

Dayani, E. (1983). Professional and economic self-governance in nursing. *Nursing Economic$, 1*(1), 20–23.

Ehrat, K. (1983). A model for politically astute planning and decision making. *Journal of Nursing Administration, 13*(9), 29–35.

Felton, G. (1975). Increasing the quality of nursing care by introducing the concept of primary nursing: A model project. *Nursing Research, 24*(1), 27–32.

Gleeson, S., Nestor, D., & Riddell, A. (1983). Helping nurses through the management threshold. *Nursing Administration Quarterly, 8*(2), 27–31.

Logan, C. (1985). Praise: The powerhouse of self-esteem. *Nursing Management, 16*(6), 35–38.

McClure, M. (1984). Managing the professional nurse: Part 1. The organizational theories. *Journal of Nursing Administration, 14*(2), 15–21.

McClure, M. (1984). Managing the professional nurse: Part 2. Applying management theory to the challenges. *Journal of Nursing Administration, 14*(3), 11–17.

National Joint Practice Commission. (1981). *Guidelines for establishing joint or collaborative practice in hospitals.* Chicago, IL: Neely Printing.

Shukla, R. (1982). Primary or team nursing? Two conditions determine the choice. *Journal of Nursing Administration, 12*(11), 12–15.

Swansburg, R. (1993). *Introductory management and leadership for clinical nurses: A text-workbook.* Boston, MA: Jones and Bartlett Publishers.

CHAPTER

4

Communication in Complex Organizations

William M. Warfel

LEARNING OBJECTIVES

This chapter will enable you to:

1. Identify the basic elements of the communications process.
2. Identify barriers to effective communication.
3. Identify strategies for effective listening.
4. Become familiar with a variety of nursing activities as they constitute a communications process.

Vestal, K.W. Nursing Management:
Concepts and Issues, 2 ed.
© 1995 J.B. Lippincott Company

With entire degree programs being offered in the field of communications, it may seem futile to attempt to discuss the subject in one short chapter. But in our highly complex society and profession, and in an ever-increasing environment of technological expansion, the need for more effective communication is clear. Nurses in particular must develop effective writing, speaking, and listening skills to perform their jobs effectively in the large, complex organizations in which they work. Being able to clearly convey your thoughts is imperative:

> You can have expert knowledge; but if you cannot communicate your ideas clearly, forcefully, and fluently, you will have little influence. You can have expert skill; but if you cannot demonstrate your skills to others and move them to action, you will have little power.*

As a nurse, there is no aspect of your position that cannot be analyzed, in part, as a communications process. As professionals, nurses are constantly communicating with their environment—their patients, colleagues, managers, and other care team members. According to Lubbers and Roy (1990), good communication is a vital element in the delivery of quality nursing care, whereas poor communication can lead to lawsuits and avoidable patient death. Effective communications can improve your working relationships, which will lead to higher job satisfaction.

The importance of building relationships is one of the most important communication activities that nurses face and is becoming more important with the growing trend of providing quality patient care. Although institutions are striving to establish more compassionate, patient-friendly environments, this goal will not be achieved unless communication among employees continually improves. Effective communications are also vital to establishing and maintaining the desired atmosphere of professional competence. In this age of health care reform, the opportunity for nursing to assume its leadership position is unsurpassed. Our success will largely depend on our ability to communicate effectively.

*LaRoux, R. S. (1981). Communication and influence in nursing. In A. J. Huntsman, & J. L. Binger (Eds.), *Communicating effectively*. Wakefield, MA: Nursing Resources.

THE COMMUNICATIONS PROCESS

If nurses are to improve communications, they must understand communications theory and process. Although many theorists have described models to explain how individuals communicate, it is generally accepted that there are a few elements basic to any communication process. Communication is the exchange of meanings between and among individuals through a shared system of symbols that have the same meaning for both the sender and the receiver of the message. These symbols include both verbal and nonverbal forms of communication.

In the process, the message may be affected by feedback from the receiver to the sender. The channel that carries the message carries the spoken or written word and includes other aspects of communications such as nonverbal gestures and pictures. The message is surrounded by many other variables—the "climate" in which the transmission occurs—including the environment or circumstances under which the communications take place. A particular message may be interpreted differently by the same receiver, depending on the circumstances surrounding the transmission. Moods, weather conditions and temperature, timing, and many other considerations are a part of the climate. If a person initiates a message while under stress, there may be a distortion in the transmission. The same is true of the reception if the receiver is experiencing a stressful situation—the likelihood of hearing the message clearly is affected.

Disturbances in the environment, frequently called "noise," need to be considered seriously for effective communications to take place. Just as atmospheric disturbances can create static in radio or television reception, disturbances in the climate surrounding the message transmission can seriously distort the communications attempt. Many elements of climate may be controlled. For example, hospital visiting hours may not be the time for the nurse to give discharge instructions if the patient is enjoying time with relatives or friends. Because of its numerous distractions and interruptions, the nurses' station may not be the place to talk about a patient's response to nursing interventions. The only way to communicate effectively may be to leave the station and find a quieter spot.

THE FLOW OF COMMUNICATIONS: UPWARD, DOWNWARD, AND LATERAL

Because communications involves the transmission of information from a sender to a receiver, and because the formal structure of an organization has a powerful effect on communication between workers, it is helpful to study the direction in which communications flow in complex organizations. In this context, all communications can be thought of as falling into one of three categories: upward, downward, or lateral to one's subordinates or one's peers. This framework is particularly appropriate for analyzing the transmission of messages within complex organizations.

The directional flow of communications is important because different strategies are required for different segments. The way you communicate with your superior involves considerations that are different from those influencing the way you communicate with a nurse colleague. The same is true when you are communicating with ancillary staff members. Your position in the organization will, to a degree, determine the way in which you communicate.

Downward communication in a line organization consists mostly of command in authoritarian terms to delegate aspects of care to the ancillary staff. Delegating in authoritarian terms may be perceived in a negative manner. Including staff in planning the assignment communicates a more participative approach and promotes a more satisfactory outcome.

Lateral communications tend to be more consultative or coordinative and are delivered in terms of equality. Their effectiveness depends on the degree of trust and respect within the work group.

When you communicate upward in the organization to your nurse manager or to a member of administration, the communication is much more carefully filtered and is often delivered in apologetic or defensive terms. By virtue of your position in the organization, you will be cautious about communicating upward. However, in a properly structured work environment that fosters openness and creativity, a person is more comfortable with upward communications. The choice of a workplace with a climate that values individual contribution is as important as communicating messages clearly.

The nurse–physician relationship raises an interesting question: How do you communicate with doctors—upward, downward, or laterally? There has been a good deal written about collegial relationship between doctors and nurses suggesting that lateral communication relationships can benefit patient care. Yet it takes time to establish your credibility so that these communications are truly lateral. Although some nurses "talk down" to doctors, others view the physician as "above them." Lateral communications based on mutual respect and trust will have the most benefit for you and your patients. It is hard to establish that type of trust, but it is achievable.

THE NURSE'S CREDIBILITY
AS SENDER OF THE MESSAGE

Your ability to communicate a message is related to your credibility as a source for that message. Successful communication is based to a large degree on whether the receiver believes you are knowledgeable, truthful, and reliable. Lack of credibility, on the other hand, will interfere with the receiver's ability to read or hear the message.

This is especially important for nurses, who must communicate the patient's needs to the physician, the goals for nursing care to peers and ancillary staff, and appropriate information to the nurse manager. Those who operate from a base of knowledge and confidence will increase the likelihood of accurate transmission of messages.

One's credibility then rests on what has to be said and how it is stated. Conveying uncertainty (eg, "I'm not sure why but . . .") or making statements that cannot be supported by a good rationale will diminish one's credibility in the eyes of the receiver. Keane (1981) states that one can be more persuasive if:

1. One is perceived to know what he or she is talking about.
2. One believes in what he or she is saying.
3. One presents himself or herself in a convincing manner.

The nurse's credibility can facilitate or hinder positive communications.

LISTENING

A sometimes underplayed and unappreciated aspect of the communications process is that of listening. It is generally accepted that the receiver actually hears or retains only a small part of the message that is sent. The average person spends 70% of his or her time listening, but retains only 33%. Given the inefficiency of our listening skills, coupled with the busy climate in which most nursing communications take place, nurses cannot passively absorb the spoken word but must try to grasp the facts and feelings of what is being said.

To be able to concentrate on what is being communicated is not easy. Yet it is possible to improve one's listening skills through a variety of activities. Munn (1980) has developed the following guidelines for improving one's listening skills.[†]

[†]Munn, H. E., Jr. (1980). *The nurse's communication handbook.* Germantown, MD: Aspen Systems. Reprinted with permission.

GUIDELINES FOR LISTENING

1. You should prepare yourself physically by standing or facing the speaker. Making sure you can hear physically is essential for good listening. You thereby tell the sender that you are ready to listen and are able to hear the verbal messages and also see the nonverbal messages the speaker is sending. This face-to-face attention also shows that you are interested in what is being said. People tend to avoid and look away from people and things in which they are not interested. Attention and interest are synonymous. You pay attention to the things you are interested in, and you are interested in the things you pay attention to.

2. You should learn to watch for the speaker's nonverbal as well as verbal messages. Everyone sends two messages. One message is sent verbally and the other is sent nonverbally through inflection in the voice or through facial expression, bodily action, or gestures. Sixty-eight percent of all messages are sent nonverbally. The nonverbal message conveys the speaker's attitude, sincerity, and genuineness. To miss the nonverbal message is to miss half of what is being said.

3. You should not decide from the speaker's appearance or delivery that what he or she has to say is worthwhile. When you start to focus on the speaker's delivery or appearance, you become distracted from the purpose of communication, receiving the speaker's ideas! You should be more interested in what people have to say than how they say it or what they look like.

4. You should listen for ideas and underlying feelings. Again, the purpose of good communication is to be able to reflect upon and exchange ideas. For example, if I were to meet you on the street and give you a dollar and you gave me a dollar, and you then went your way and I went mine, neither of us would be better off because of the exchange. But if I gave you an idea and you gave me an idea, then both of us would be better off as a result of the exchange.

5. You should try to determine your own biases, if any, and allow for them. Communication gets blamed for many things. Whenever something doesn't go right, you might say you have a communication breakdown. But many times you don't have a communication breakdown at all. In fact, you might have very good communication; you both know what has been said, and there is a common understanding. But you don't like what you have heard. If the nurse, physician, or surgeon could learn to recognize such differences, better relationships would be

formed. You will not always agree with everyone. The trauma in such situations develops when you discover you are no longer talking about the issues, but about each other.

6. You should attempt to keep your mind on what the speaker is saying. Don't allow yourself to become distracted. Too many times people fake attention and like the little dog in the back of the car window just keep nodding their heads up and down without hearing a word of what is being said.

7. You should not interrupt immediately if you hear a statement that you feel is wrong. Indeed, if you listen closely, you may be persuaded that the statement is right. Sometimes you may fail to listen just because of this fear of something different, of the possibility that you may have to forsake some sacred position you have held for years.

8. You should try to see the situation from the other person's point of view. This doesn't mean that you always have to agree. However, there is no way that you can change other people's perceptions until you can see how they have formulated those perceptions.

9. You should not try to have the last word. Listen to what is being said and then think about it. This reflection may take some time, but you need time to think before you communicate. Sometimes, in order to solve problems, you have to walk away from the problem for a while and think about it from different points of view, and about the advantages and disadvantages of possible solutions.

10. You should make a conscientious effort to evaluate the logic and credibility of what you hear. Our mind functions at some 500 words a minute, but we normally speak at 125 words a minute. In other words, we can think four times faster than we can speak. Rather than letting our minds become bored, we can take advantage of this time differential between thinking and speaking. We can attempt to anticipate the speaker's next point, attempt to identify and evaluate supporting material, and mentally summarize what the speaker has said: What has thus far been said that I can use?

The average nurse spends more time listening than he or she spends speaking or writing. Nurses who are able to improve their listening skills will begin to realize how important active listening is as part of the communication process. When you begin to realize how much information can be gleaned through active listening, it will become apparent that it deserves considerable attention.

NURSING ACTIVITIES AS COMMUNICATION PROCESSES

The remainder of this chapter focuses on communication activities in which nurses commonly engage. By viewing these activities as communication processes, you can improve the information exchanged and the outcomes achieved during the activity.

CHANGE-OF-SHIFT COMMUNICATIONS

In this age of patient-focused care, it is essential to communicate patient needs clearly. Yet nurses frequently and ritualistically do little more than report on the patient using the care plan, work sheets, or a tape recorder. Instead of repeating this easily accessible information, why read the patient information to one another? It is far more productive to spend this relatively brief time observing the patient and communicating about the patient's condition and response to nursing. For example, an excellent way to maximize the exchange of information is by initiating "walking rounds." Actual observation of the patient can assist in focusing on what the patient's needs are and the patient's response to the plan of care. By looking critically at what kinds of information are most beneficial, you can make the change-of-shift report an integral part of the nursing process.

INTERVIEWING AS A COMMUNICATION PROCESS

Interviewing is something that nurses do over and over again. You interview patients, families, physicians, and coworkers. You spend a large part of your day interacting with others for the purpose of gathering information. Interviewing is purposeful communication. It focuses on a specific subject and is one of the most controlled or structured communication experiences. Because it is so planned, it would seem that the information obtained would be accurate. In reality, however, even formal interviews are subject to opportunities for miscommunication.

Nurses may go on job interviews, which offer opportunities to apply principles of communication to achieve a favorable outcome. The employment interview is mostly a verbal communications effort with decisions made on the basis of the information exchanged. The important point is that the interview is two-sided—both parties attempt to gather as much information as possible to make an informed decision.

Assume you are in a job interview. Are you the interviewer or the interviewee? Well, that all depends! If you presume that you are there to be interviewed, you have assumed a passive position and will not obtain the information you need to make a decision. You may be able to assess the environment to a degree by the nature of the questions you are asked, but you will not receive the necessary clarification to accept or reject an offer.

If you assume a more active approach, you too will have a set of questions you need answered. In this way, the communications flow both ways. At any point, you may be the interviewer or the interviewee. Although you should not attempt to "take over" the interview, you have an obligation to yourself to obtain the information you need to make your decision.

There are two ways to ask questions during an interview based on the views of the two theorists who have most influenced the way questions are phrased—B. F. Skinner and Carl Rogers. Skinner, the well-known behaviorist, believed that behavior that is rewarded tends to be repeated. In the interviewing process, this could include listening as a form of positive feedback, looking interested, even nodding approvingly. The Skinnerian line of questioning is directive and provides the opportunity for you to answer a question honestly and factually.

Rogerian questioning assumes a contrasting viewpoint, one in which the questions are open-ended or nondirective. These types of questions allow creative and intellectual expression and are more thought provoking.

Your employment interview is likely to include both types of questions. When the opportunity arises to address some of your concerns, tailor your questioning according to the information you desire. For example, questions about job responsibilities can be direct, whereas questions about philosophy of care may be best approached through a series of indirect inquiries.

There are many ways to maximize this communication opportunity. Consider the nonverbal communications that go on if you are late, if you are not neatly dressed, or if you are chewing gum. The same nonverbal communication goes on with your patients—they expect you to appear and behave in a certain way, and when you fail to meet these expectations, communications are hampered.

In interviewing, many other positive considerations enhance the information imparted. These principles also are applicable in other situations, such as nurse–patient interactions.

1. Avoid being too formal or aloof. Conveying a warm, friendly demeanor will encourage positive communication.

2. Avoid distractions. Communication is an active process that requires focusing on the questioning and giving attention to the interview. Minimize environmental distractions with adequate space, quiet, and comfort.
3. Avoid "yes" and "no" responses. Although appropriate in a very directive line of questioning, such responses discourage further communication.
4. Do not monopolize the conversation. Although "yes" and "no" answers leave a negative impression, so does the interviewee who digresses and fails to respond to the specific question. Answers should be succinct; lengthy answers will be viewed unfavorably.
5. Avoid expressing your personal biases. Successful communications require that information exchanged is objective and factual. Subjectivity may impact the quality of the interaction and interfere with the results or outcome of the process.

The well-planned interview in which these principles are properly applied affords the nurse the opportunity to maximize the communication process. Understanding the dynamics of this process can enhance the opportunity for a favorable outcome.

COMPUTER COMMUNICATIONS

The application of computers to the health care industry and clinical information systems is growing rapidly. The need for better data management systems has hastened the installation of terminals and printers, and the nurse has become one of the "users." The need to communicate by computer is a reality that every nurse faces. Computers enable the nurse to handle an increasing volume of information in forms that can be readily applied to practical patient care or management problems.

Take, for example, patient scheduling systems. Without automation, it is not unusual to have conflicting therapies and tests scheduled for the same patient at the same time. Automated scheduling discourages such conflicts and even prints a work order that informs you of the appropriate patient preparation. Automated patient information systems in which medical records are filed in computer memory and information is added on a real-time basis are becoming more practical.

The communications opportunities that computers afford are both exciting and intimidating. Although nurses will be able to reduce uncertainty in decision making and ensure more timely and effective care delivery, traditionally, they have not been schooled in such technologies. Resistance to automation is, in large part, a result of fear, which is quickly overcome when nurses begin to use computer hardware and software. They find that much of the mystique surrounding computers is more imagination than fact.

The goal for computer systems is the elimination of planning and documentation as we know them and movement toward a "paperless" system. These changes will have dramatic implications for the ways in which nurses communicate with patients and other members of the health care team. The challenge is clear. Nurses will need to acquire new skills to communicate successfully in the near future.

CONFIDENTIAL COMMUNICATIONS

Patients who come into a health care institution place their confidence and trust in that institution's employees. Nurses walk a delicate line between what is appropriate to communicate and what is not, and they often face the danger of divulging confidential information to the wrong person. Infrequently, they are challenged for disclosing personal information they learned about a patient during the provision of care. Nurses often face the dilemma of determining *who* needs *what* information.

Suppose Ms. Smith from another floor informs you in the cafeteria that her neighbor, Mrs. Gomez, is a patient on your floor and then asks you "What's she in for?" Presuming you know the answer, would you stop to think twice about responding? Is it a violation of Mrs. Gomez's confidence for you to answer Ms. Smith? The answer is clearly yes. The appropriate way to answer Ms. Smith is to tell her that she will "have to ask Mrs. Gomez."

Ms. Smith's desire to know why Mrs. Gomez is in the hospital is not a single issue. The fact is, nurses are continually exposed to confidential, sensitive information. As a nurse, you will frequently be in situations in which you are trying to decide what and what not to communicate. There is a fine line between these two extremes. The mistake nurses make is presuming that information they have about a patient is common knowledge that other team members share the right and need to know.

Why not give Ms. Smith the answer to her question? You give the same information to other nurses who are working on the unit. The decision should be based on who has the need for the information to provide Mrs. Gomez with the care she needs during her hospital stay. These are not always easy decisions. But the realization that certain information you have is confidential will help you be aware there is the potential for a violation of a patient's right if you communicate that information. Your employing agency should also have a policy on confidentiality. Familiarize yourself with these guidelines. Like many others, they will not tell you specifically what you may and may not communicate, but they will provide you with the framework to make reasonable decisions. Remember, the patient's right comes first, and the patient can expect that only necessary information will be shared.

COMMUNICATING THROUGH TOUCH

The use of human touch in nurse–patient interactions has received a fair amount of attention in the nursing literature. It is generally accepted that touch may have a beneficial response for patients in developing nurse–patient relationships and in their recovery. But have nurses really viewed touch as a major form of nonverbal communications? Most publications focus on whether or not touching makes a difference in establishing relationships or in promoting recovery. If we begin to view touch within the framework of communication forms, then it follows that the principles of effective communications apply.

A knowledge of when touch can be therapeutic and when it may actually be a barrier is important. Research by Witcher and Fisher (1979) illustrates how touch may and may not be a good form of communications. Specifically, they assessed the effects of nurses touching patients during preoperative teaching. Their results suggest that touch led to positive effects for female patients but had a reverse effect for male patients.

For women, touch resulted in lower anxiety, more positive behavior preoperatively, and more favorable postoperative physiologic responses. The experimenters' results support a sex difference hypothesis. Their rationale is that in American society men are acculturated to be more uncomfortable with dependency situations than are women. Therefore, nurse–patient touch is perceived by male patients as a threatening gesture that communicates inferiority and asserting dominance.

Nurses need to be sensitive to the messages they transmit by touching the patient. The same principles of effective communications apply. For example, the barrier to effective touch communications may be male and female acculturation. However, the response to touching may be improved through considerations for timing, the environment, and so forth. Like other forms of communication, whether touch is experienced positively or negatively depends on the meaning that the patient ascribes to it. Touching can transmit positive messages such as concern or empathy or negative messages such as dominance or a desire for intimacy. Touch messages may be expected to have a negative response to the degree that they overstep the boundaries the patient has defined as appropriate. They will be received positively to the extent that they are appropriate to the situation.

DOCUMENTATION AS A FORM OF COMMUNICATIONS

Documentation, one of the most frequently used forms of nursing communications, validates the care you deliver, offers a means of communicating care between health care providers, and creates a permanent record of that care.

Despite the increased emphasis on good documentation, nurses frequently assign it a low priority, assuming that the time spent documenting patient care takes away from the precious time they have to deliver that care. Yet there is truth to the statement that "if it isn't documented, it wasn't done." The only way to verify patient care is through a record of process and outcomes. The written communication form is a necessary part of the professional nurse's role.

The patient's record is the most obvious example of documentation. It is full of entries that attempt to establish the assessment of and plan for the patient. But few really seize the opportunity to use the record for the intended purpose of communicating among various members of the health team by sharing observations, concerns, plans, and findings.

The patient's record will effectively communicate patient care when those who record entries seize the opportunity. Some of the rules for communicating through documentation include clear and concise messages that are legibly written and properly endorsed. Nurses need to follow hospital policy, such as using only those abbreviations that are on the approved agency list. Health care providers are notorious for formulating new abbreviations. Effective communication requires that we speak the same language. Creating your own language through unapproved abbreviations is not acceptable.

Accuracy and truth in documenting is a must. Legally speaking, you should put the whole truth and nothing but the truth on the medical records. Purposely omitting information or making inaccurate entries can result in legal penalties or loss of license. The courts consider lack of truthful documentation as strong evidence that proper care was not given (Bernzweig, 1985). The importance of medical records as evidence in a court of law cannot be overemphasized. The accuracy and completeness of nurses' entries have received increased attention as the number of malpractice issues increases and nursing becomes increasingly recognized as a profession accountable for its own practice. Following are established, accepted procedures for altering an entry in the medical record that can protect you. All entries, including changes, should include the date, your name, and your title.

The same concerns apply to other forms of nursing documentation. The nurse's plan of care is a permanent part of the patient's needs or problems and nursing interventions. One of the issues that surfaces in nursing documentation is that communication may not be effective because nursing has not sufficiently developed its own language. Although still a long way from standardization, the nursing diagnosis may serve as a common vocabulary for the professions, because it identifies precisely what nurses do. The development of a common vocabulary is essential to improved communications.

Another problem that frequently occurs in documentation is the lack of consistency in format within a particular agency. For example, the problem-oriented approach to documentation is favored by some and discouraged by others. It would be nice to think that the opportunity for creativity and self-expression occurs when nurses are allowed individual ways of approaching the matter. Unfortunately, nurses do not always communicate effectively because they do not speak the same language. It is imperative that all providers decide which format they will use to ensure proper communications concerning patients.

Effective communication is vital to integrated progress notes. All providers are expected to use the same progress note—a positive step toward improved communications. Unfortunately, some physicians are offended when others make entries on "their" progress notes. They argue that there may be conflict between nurses' entries and their entries. How sad this argument is! If nurses were to use the integrated notes approach, the possibility of eliminating such conflicts would be increased through better communications. Nurses can help the system move in the right direction by continually improving documentation, regardless of what approach is used. Clear, concise documentation of patient assessments and responses to nursing interventions eventually leads to improved communications in the medical record.

NURSE–PHYSICIAN COMMUNICATIONS

Considerable attention has been given to nurse–physician relationships, and there seems to be agreement that there is room for improvement. The many articles and research papers on nurse–physician relationships could have been entitled "nurse–physician communications." There has been a breakdown in communications between the two groups that may be attributed to a variety of social, economic, and political changes.

Changing scopes of practice and redefining relationships frequently have led to what are perceived to be competitive rather than collaborative postures. This agenda will not serve to benefit patient care. According to Prescott and Bowen (1985), "when physicians and nurses work together optimally, relationships are positive, disagreements are collaboratively resolved to the benefit of the patient and patient care flows smoothly and efficiently." What exists appears to be a communications breakdown that is manifested by attitudinal responses. Although harder to correct semantic disorders, communication failures due to poor attitudes can be improved through training and effort.

The establishment of collaborative practice models, patient-focused care models, case management models, and nurse–physician forums are attempts, in part, to establish mechanisms that promote improved communications. Because nurses provide complex care for acutely ill patients, there is no room for the errors that can result from poor communications. Doctors comment that "the nurse never makes rounds with me anymore." Nurses respond that "I'm too busy." The patient suffers. The need for effective teamwork that fully uses the potential contribution of *all* care givers is apparent. Teamwork is really all about communicating effectively to the patient's advantage.

NURSE–PATIENT COMMUNICATIONS

No other area affords the nurse so much opportunity to use effective communication as does interaction with patients. Most of the time nurses are engaged in some form of nurse–patient interaction. This interaction represents the most significant part of nursing and is actually a form of continuous communications between you and your patients. Every word and every gesture give the nurse and the patient more and more information about each other. The frequency with which you interact, the tone of your voice, and how you appear all transmit messages that are perceived differently by different patients depending on a variety of influencing variables—the patient's age, sex, race, religion, and many other environmental considerations.

Excellent nurse–patient communications require sensitivity to the patient's needs and a well-developed and carefully thought-out plan to meet those needs. Perhaps your plan includes visiting the patient briefly at least once an hour because your assessment concludes that the patient is lonely. What message are you communicating to the patient? That depends. You may be communicating what you intended.

On the other hand, the patient may become concerned with the frequency of your visits and believe they are due to a serious condition.

One message nurses frequently give patients is that they do not have time to listen. This may be transmitted nonverbally by standing near the doorway when talking to the patient or by confiding to the patient how busy they may be. The unique environments in which health care is practiced today make patient–nurse communication even more difficult. Consider, for example, the difficulty in establishing effective communications with patients in complete isolation. Patients may feel inadequate and estranged. Verbal communications, filtered through the mask you are wearing, may sound strange. In this age of "universal precautions," you bathe the patient while wearing rubber gloves that serve as a physical barrier to tactile communication. The ritualistic way you need to handle linen and fomites further reinforces the patient's sense of alienation. Indeed, most of what you must do to protect yourself and the patient communicates to the patient that he or she is "dirty" or at extreme risk of becoming infected.

If it is accepted that effective nurse–patient communications can positively affect outcomes, then the corollary should be considered. Ineffective communications may have a deleterious effect. Because blood pressure and heart rate are significantly affected while speaking (Thomas, 1984), nurses need to consider the cardiovascular response they invoke when communicating with patients. A nurse who approaches a patient in a brusque manner may elicit higher blood pressure measurements, an undesirable physiologic response to the patient's psychological state.

The most important realization is that communication between nurses and their patients is the essence of nursing practice. Through your understanding of the communication process and the barriers to effective communications, you will have the skill to look beneath the surface of nurse–patient communications for meanings and implications. Among the techniques available to you are interviewing, reading, and consulting with others in developing your plan of care, including nurse specialists, doctors, and the patient's family. You have the opportunity to help educate patients and their families. The nurse is the one who is best prepared to assess and respond to patient needs. Effective communications are synonymous with effective nurse–patient interactions.

SUMMARY

Communication is the core of all elements of nursing practice. Nurses practice in complex organizations in which networks of communication are established. Organizational structures may facilitate effective communications or provide barriers that inhibit communications. Nurses' understanding of the dynamics involved can increase their effectiveness in communicating.

When communicating, nurses send or receive information. The sender-receiver channel is influenced by many variables that determine the climate in which the interaction occurs. The feedback loop further influences the form of the communications. Generally, the sender should be aware that the way the message is interpreted by the receiver is largely determined by the receiver's systems of thought. If the message is to be understood clearly, it must be stated precisely, sent under the appropriate circumstances, and recognized by the receiver as valid to the situation. The receiver has the responsibility for working actively to understand and interpret the content of the message.

Although communicating is a complex process, with many variables that influence the transmission of the message, there are a variety of opportunities for nurses to increase their ability to communicate effectively.

DISCUSSION QUESTIONS

1. Discuss the nurse's role in communicating care plans to the patient and family.
2. Give examples of ineffective communications you have had with patients and discuss ways those communications could have been inproved.
3. Cite several techniques you can use to ensure your listening skills are working.
4. Develop several approaches to nurse–physician communication that will give you confidence in relating important clinical information.

REFERENCES

Bernzweig, E. P. (1985). Go on record with nothing but the truth. *RN, 4,* 63–64.

Keane, C. B. (1981). *Management essentials in nursing.* Reston, VA: Reston Publishing.

Lubbers, C. A., & Roy, S. (1990). Communication skills for continuing education in nursing. *The Journal of Continuing Education in Nursing, 21*(3), 109–112.

Munn, H. E., Jr. (1980). *The nurse's communication handbook.* Germantown, MD: Aspen Systems.

Prescott, P. A., & Bowen, S. A. (1985). Nurse–physician relationships. *Annals of Internal Medicine, 7,* 103–110, 127–133.

Thomas, S. A., Friedmann, E., Lottes, L. S., Gresty, S., Miller, C., & Lynch, J.J. (1984). Changes in nurses' blood pressure and heart rate while communicating. *Research in Nursing and Health, 6,* 7–2, 119–126.

Witcher, S. J., & Fisher, J. D. (1979). Multidimensional reaction to therapeutic touch in a hospital setting. *Journal of Personality and Social Psychology, 1,* 37–1, 87–96.

SUGGESTED READING

Gillies, D. A. (1994). *Nursing management: A systems approach.* Philadelphia: WB Saunders.

Osborne, W. L., & Courts, N. F. (1991). Better communications make more compassionate hospitals. *Nursing Management, 22,* 8, 31–32.

Leadership
and Management

Beth Tamplet Ulrich

LEARNING OBJECTIVES

This chapter will enable you to:

1. Understand the roles of leaders and managers.
2. Compare and contrast leadership and management.
3. Define the sources of power.
4. Compare and contrast motivation concepts.
5. Understand how teams develop and the team leader's role at each stage of development.

Vestal, K.W. Nursing Management:
Concepts and Issues, 2 ed.
© 1995 J.B. Lippincott Company

Leadership and management, often thought to be a function only of those in supervisory positions, are, in fact, necessary abilities for every nurse. If your position includes the responsibilities of team leader, charge nurse, or staff nurse on a unit with licensed vocational (practical) nurses, nursing assistants, unit secretaries, or other ancillary and support personnel, you need to understand how to lead and manage other people. As a professional nurse, you will be managing not only people but the complex processes that enable people to get the work done and move patients through the continuum of care.

LEADERSHIP AND MANAGEMENT

The essence of leadership is the relationship between an individual and either another individual or a group of individuals. For every leader, there must be those who are willing to follow. This relationship develops over time and results in one person (the leader) having influence over others (the followers).

Having followers is one thing, and being an effective leader is quite another. Although the terms are often used interchangeably, leading is different from managing or supervising. Zalenik (1981) offers several distinctions. Managers, he says, are problem solvers who tend to be reactive. Managerial goals arise out of necessity rather than desire, with the manager viewing work as an enabling process. The manager is a negotiator, continually coordinating and balancing to maintain the existing order. Leaders, on the other hand, are risk takers with an active approach to problem solving and goal setting. They look for new ways to solve problems and create excitement in others. Leaders work in organizations but never totally belong to them. Warren Bennis (1989), a long-standing expert on leadership, also differentiates leadership and management, saying that management is about systems, controls, procedures, policies, and structure, whereas leadership is about trust and people. He believes that leaders look at the horizons and managers at the bottom line. Leaders know what the people they lead want and need even before the people do, and then express those unspoken dreams in everything they say and do.

Think of the leaders in nursing. Florence Nightingale certainly chose a new and unique path for a woman of her time, as did Lillian Wald, Mary Mahoney, Virginia Henderson, and many others. Since then, nursing leaders have developed the art and the science of nursing by taking risks and opening new territories for professional nursing.

68

Although it is certainly possible to be both a good manager and a good leader, good managers are not always good leaders and good leaders not always good managers. Likewise, not every good manager or leader matches the descriptions given by Zalenik or Bennis. As you progress through your nursing career, try to determine the difference between managers and leaders. Then look at yourself. What characteristics do you have that would enable you to manage or lead effectively? What abilities do you need to develop? The challenge as you progress through your career is to find a match between what you enjoy doing and what your abilities will enable you to do. There is and will continue to be a need in nursing and health care for both managers and leaders. You need only choose a path.

WHAT MAKES LEADERS AND MANAGERS?

The challenge of defining what makes a leader has plagued researchers since the early 1900s. The question has not yet been answered conclusively, but many concepts have been proposed.

Trait Concept

The trait or "great man" concept was popular in the 1930s and 1940s. It assumed that there was a finite number of identifiable traits that differentiated between successful and unsuccessful leaders. Originally, believers in the trait concept thought the traits were inherited. This gave rise to a term still used today, the "born leader." Later, however, popularity shifted to the theory that traits could be obtained through learning and experience. The traits identified most often were intelligence, attitudes, and personality measures. But study results were not consistent, and no pattern could be identified that accurately predicted leaders.

Behavioral Concepts

Because inconclusive data were obtained in researching the trait concept, investigators began to focus on analyzing just what a leader does and how the leadership function is carried out. Behavior was most often seen as a continuum, ranging from autocratic to democratic or from production-centered to employee-centered. The move to behaviorism was accompanied by an increasing concentration on management rather than leadership. Production-centered versus employee-centered management distinguishes between task-oriented and employee-oriented, or, sometimes in nursing, patient-oriented management. This is also known as the structure-consideration concept. Each aspect or structure-consideration is regarded independently. Attention to both can be high or low at the same time, or high to one and low to the other. This concept paved the way for the contingency leadership concepts that followed.

Contingency Concepts

An alternative to the belief that the effectiveness of a leader is based solely on traits or behaviors, the contingency approach holds that leader effectiveness is contingent on some combination of traits, behavior, and situation. A number of contingency models have been proposed. The most popular is the situational leadership (or situational management) approach, which holds that the effectiveness of a leader or manager is based on the task to be performed, the person or persons performing the task, the degree to which the leader is perceived to have influence, and the style of leadership. Under this concept, there is no one right way of doing things in every situation.

Nowhere is that clearer than in health care. A participative approach may work well, for example, when the staff is developing patient education programs, but it does not work well in the middle of an emergency procedure such as a cardiac arrest, when one person must be in charge. Conflict between a manager or leader and employees (followers) occurs most often when the roles and decision-making authority are unclear. It does little good to request participation in decision making if employees feel the decision has already been made. One should only invite participation when contribution to the decision can really be made. It must be clear whether the participants are being asked to contribute their input and advice only, or whether they are being asked to help make (and therefore to assume responsibility for) the decision. If you have the most information and knowledge about a subject and if you are ultimately responsible for the decision, it is reasonable for you to make the decision and to let others know that you are doing so. People generally accept the manager's right to make decisions and to direct behavior. What they don't like is being given orders in a manner that implies that they or their abilities are not respected. For example, in some patient care situations, you as the registered nurse should make decisions because your education and experience make you the expert when compared with nonprofessional health care workers. In other situations, such as when you are the case manager or primary nurse for a patient, it may be very beneficial to hold a patient-care conference to collect information and establish the plan of care as a team.

Whatever style you use or participate in at any given time, it is more effective if everyone involved knows their roles ahead of time.

From a Follower's Perspective

Kouzes and Posner (1990) studied more than 7500 workers to determine what followers look for or admire in a leader. The four crucial attributes that appeared most often were honesty, competence, a forward-looking approach, and the ability to inspire others. Honesty was the most selected attribute and was measured by the leader's behavior, not by what he or she said. It is also important that the leader display a trust of others. To followers, competence means being capable and effective, with an ability to challenge, inspire, enable, and encourage. A forward-looking approach in a leader includes having a sense of direction and a concern for the future of the organization as a whole. Finally, followers want a leader to be inspiring, enthusiastic, energetic, positive, and able to communicate a vision. Demonstrated consistently, these attributes lead to credibility.

Leaders are, at times, followers. In fact, most good leaders know how to follow and are good role models for others. Kelley (1988) describes the main qualities of effective followers as self-management (eg, thinking for themselves, able to work independently), commitment, competence, focus, courage, honesty, and credibility. As you can see, these characteristics are very similar to those that followers profess to admire in a leader. For a team to be successful, there is a need for both effective followers and effective leaders.

MANAGEMENT STYLES

Management style is the way in which a manager goes about accomplishing his or her goals and those of the organization. There are numerous ways of classifying styles, most of which rely on some continuum of behavior patterns. Although it is unusual today to see a manager who practices only one style, it is important to recognize the styles and the situations in which each style is most effective.

The most common classification of management styles is the continuum that ranges from autocratic to democratic to laissez-faire. Autocratic or authoritarian management is a style in which the manager makes the decisions and the employees carry them out. Little input is requested or received from the employees. Autocratic management is effective in a crisis, but it encourages dependency. In democratic management, everyone contributes information and input into the decision-making process and everyone has a say in the decision. It is a very people-oriented process. Democratic management often increases employee morale, but it can decrease efficiency.

Autocratic management often has been viewed as undesirable, whereas democratic management has been favored and hailed as a sign of enlightenment. The difference between the two is the degree to which the decision-making function is shared.

Participative management is an outgrowth of democratic management. Participative management is a matter of degree rather than the all-or-nothing approach often seen in the past. Employees participate in problem-solving activities and some decision making, but not to the degree seen in democratic management. In laissez-faire management, the opposite of authoritative or autocratic management, the manager takes a "hands off" approach and lets the employees make decisions and implement plans. Although some people protest that laissez-faire management is no management at all, others note that it can work well when the employees are competent, work well independently, and are committed to the job and the organization.

Likert (1961, 1967) proposed four management styles: exploitive-authoritative, benevolent-authoritative, consultative, and participative. The first two categories are both authoritative but differ in the manager's approach to the employee. In the exploitive-authoritative style, the manager makes the decisions and communicates them in a dictatorial fashion. In the benevolent-authoritative style, the manager occasionally seeks some minor input from employees but does so in a condescending manner. The manager still makes the decisions. Neither of these approaches is likely to result in a commitment by the employees to the organization or to the manager. In the consultative style, as the name implies, the manager consults the employees, and decision making begins to filter into the non-management levels of the organization. Likert is a major supporter of the participative style, in which increased communication and group decision making are the norm. It is interesting to note that Likert originally developed the now widely used scale bearing his name as a means of measuring factors related to management.

Blanchard, Zigmari, and Zigmari (1985) describe the four management styles shown in Figure 5-1: directing, coaching, supporting, and delegating. These four styles are composed of various combinations of two basic behaviors: directive and supportive. In the early development of the situational leadership concept, these behaviors were referred to as task behavior and relationship behavior. Directive behavior involves structure, control, and supervision, whereas supportive behavior involves praise, listening, and facilitation. Blanchard and co-workers note that in deciding which style to employ, the manager must

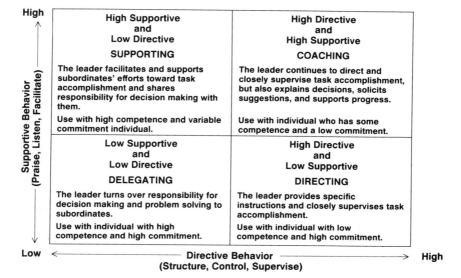

High Supportive and Low Directive	**High Directive and High Supportive**
SUPPORTING	**COACHING**
The leader facilitates and supports subordinates' efforts toward task accomplishment and shares responsibility for decision making with them.	The leader continues to direct and closely supervise task accomplishment, but also explains decisions, solicits suggestions, and supports progress.
Use with high competence and variable commitment individual.	Use with individual who has some competence and a low commitment.
Low Supportive and Low Directive	**High Directive and Low Supportive**
DELEGATING	**DIRECTING**
The leader turns over responsibility for decision making and problem solving to subordinates.	The leader provides specific instructions and closely supervises task accomplishment.
Use with individual with high competence and high commitment.	Use with individual with low competence and high commitment.

High ↑
Supportive Behavior (Praise, Listen, Facilitate)
Low ↓

Low ← Directive Behavior (Structure, Control, Supervise) → High

FIG. 5-1. Four basic leadership styles. (From Blanchard, L., Zigmari, P., & Zigmari, D. [1985]. *Leadership and the one minute manager*, pp. 30, 56. New York: William Morrow & Co.)

assess the competence (knowledge and skills) and commitment (confidence and motivation) of the individual.

Sometimes, you work with an individual in the directive style, telling the person what must be done and how it must be done. This generally occurs with a new employee or when implementing a new procedure or process. As the employee demonstrates proficiency, the manager moves toward a coaching style. This is a scary time for the employee, who may not yet be confident of his or her ability. When the employee is proficient enough to begin to function independently, the manager changes to a supportive style. Finally, if appropriate, the manager may delegate the job to the employee. It is generally easier to go from tight managerial control to loose managerial control rather than the other way around. As a new graduate, it is likely that you will witness, firsthand, your manager moving through these styles as you gain more expertise as a registered nurse. You earn movement through the management styles of your manager by demonstrating competence and commitment.

You will be in a management and leadership position on your first day of work as a professional nurse. The patients see you as a leader and, as a registered nurse, you have management responsibilities for the licensed vocational nurses, the nursing assistants, and other nursing support personnel who by law work under your supervision. Think about the task to be performed, the ability of the person performing it, and the nature of the situation (life-threatening or routine) before you decide what approach to take.

CHOOSING AND WORKING WITH YOUR MANAGER

Although many students pursue job opportunities in a nursing specialty they believe they will enjoy, it is equally important to find a work environment that fits your goals, personality, and style. It is important for you to understand yourself and how you work best. If you are someone who likes to work independently, calling on resource people only when needed, then working with a manager who is very structure-oriented probably would not satisfy either of you. As a new graduate, however, keep in mind that you will need more resources and structure than nurses who have been in practice for a while. When you interview for a position, ask about the management style of the person for whom you will be working and find out what resources are available to assist you in expanding your knowledge and skills. Aim for the best fit between your needs, an organization's culture and needs, and the style of the manager.

Once you have joined an organization, you need to consider not only how your manager works with you, but also how you work with your manager. LeBoeuf (1985) states that individuals own 50% of the relationships with their bosses and are 100% in control of their own behavior. He further states that the way an individual behaves towards a boss teaches the boss how to treat the individual. The first step to successfully work with your manager is learning more about that person. What are his or her strengths and weaknesses, likes and dislikes, pet peeves? At the same time, let your manager know more about you. Act on this knowledge to build on your effectiveness and that of your manager. Your success and your manager's success are intimately related. When you look good, your manager looks good and vice versa.

INFORMAL LEADERSHIP

In addition to the formal management structure, you need to become familiar with the informal leadership of the unit and the organization. Organizational charts do not always paint a clear picture of the real world. On patient care units, there are often informal leaders among the ancillary staff. Their power may be derived from a variety of sources, some of which are described in the following section. Regardless of the source of their power, be it knowledge, skills, length of service, or who they know, it is important for you to recognize who these leaders are. Power is not always used positively and you may not agree with their beliefs. Before you can change beliefs, you must plan, and planning involves obtaining information. An informal leadership structure is usually more evident in units or organizations without strong formal leadership.

POWER

Del Bueno and Freud (1986) note that "organizations are made up of people who are consistently vying with one another for power, status, and prestige." This statement aptly describes health care organizations, especially as resources become increasingly scarce. Power is the ability to impose the will or desires of one person or group of persons on another individual or group of individuals to influence and alter their behavior. In any discussion of power, one must first move beyond the point of seeing all power and those who have it or seek it in a negative way. Power and the balance of power are facts of life. Power itself is neither good nor bad. It is how an individual or group uses or abuses power that ultimately colors its perception. Power is inherent in the ability to lead. How that power is used ultimately determines the effectiveness of the leader. Some power is gained from the position held by an individual and some power is derived from the leader herself. Power is in the eye of the beholder. If you feel that someone has power, then in your relationship with them, they do.

Power is most often classified using descriptions developed by French and Raven (1968) that include reward power, coercive power, legitimate power, referent power, and expert power. As its name implies, reward power is based on the ability to control the administration of incentives. The department manager has reward power when making out the staffing schedule or promoting someone. As a staff nurse, you have reward power over a patient when you control visiting hours or activity levels. The charge nurse has reward power when making assignments. Rewards are most effective when used to reinforce desirable behaviors, not when used to bribe people.

On the other hand, coercive power is based on the ability to control the administration of punishment. The nurse must take care not to use coercive power with patients. "If you don't drink your fluids, we'll have to start another intravenous line," or "If you don't stop pulling at your tube, I'm going to tie your hands down," are misuses of coercive power. In such cases, using reward power is often more effective and, indeed, more morally right.

Legitimate power rests on the authority given to an individual by an organization because of the position held by that individual. The registered nurse, assistant head nurse, department manager, and others all have power based on their positions. The department manager, for example, has the power to reward or discipline staff members based on their performance. This can be done with verbal feedback, formal counseling sessions, merit-based salary increases, promotions, or demotions.

Referent power is power granted to an individual in one area based on the individual's performance, position, or relationships in another area. One example of referent power based on performance would be the nurse who is good clinically and always helps others. This nurse may have more power to influence the unit decisions of the manager than a nurse who constantly complains and offers no support. An example of referent power based on relationships is when you as a staff nurse work for a manager who has a great deal of influence with the director, or a nursing vice president who is well-known nationally. Among nurses, you are bestowed with a certain degree of power within the organization because you work for that manager and outside the organization because of your vice president.

Expert power is based on being recognized as knowledgeable or skillful in a certain area. On every unit, there always seems to be one nurse who is the expert at starting difficult intravenous lines or one nurse who works well with a specific kind of patient. The patient may well (and should be able to) perceive all professional nurses as experts in health care. In doing so, the patient grants the nurse power. The nurse, in turn, must be careful not to abuse that power.

Because power is in the eye of the beholder, you must use it or lose it. A way to increase power is to form coalitions with other persons who have power. As a newcomer to the organization, you need to learn who has power and why, and what resources are valuable enough to contribute to the establishment of a power base. You can then work to increase your own power and work more effectively with the power of others.

MOTIVATION

Think back over your years in school. Do certain courses stand out as especially good? Do you remember feeling like you learned more with a certain professor? The key to your successes was probably motivation in one form or another. Sometimes you were motivated to study because you wanted to pass the course and graduate; other times because you knew a patient would be depending on you to care for him the next day, and still other times because you were really interested in the topic or because you wanted to do well for a certain professor. As a professional nurse, you will need to understand what motivates you and how to motivate other nurses, ancillary personnel, patients, and other health care personnel.

HAWTHORNE STUDY

The emphasis on motivation dates back to the often-quoted Hawthorne study performed in the early 1900s by Harvard researchers at the Hawthorne plant of Western Electric in Chicago. The study investigated the effects of changes of illumination on productivity. Lighting was changed for one group of employees but remained constant for another group. When the lighting was incrementally increased for the first group, the production of both groups increased. When lighting was incrementally decreased for the first group, production continued to rise for both groups until the lights were so low that the first group could not see. The conclusion was that the attention paid to members of each group was the key factor that increased production. For you as the professional nurse, the message is clear. Sometimes, the only thing required to motivate people is to pay attention to them. This applies to patients, peers, and other health care staff.

Additional studies at the same plant revealed the influence of norms set by the work group. As you progress in your career and move into positions of added authority, you will find that norms set by those you supervise are often much more stringent than those you or your manager would set and, at the same time, much more accepted by the group.

MASLOW'S HIERARCHY OF NEEDS

The next major concept in motivation came from Abraham Maslow, a psychologist. Maslow believed that every individual has ever-increasing needs and seeks to meet those needs. He proposed a needs hierarchy consisting of five levels presented in a pyramid diagram (Figure 5-2).

Physiologic needs form the base of the pyramid and the base of the individual's existence. These include the survival needs of food, air, drink, clothing, and shelter. Safety needs form the next level and consist of items such as safe working environment and personal security. Once physiologic and safety needs are met, the individual moves on to

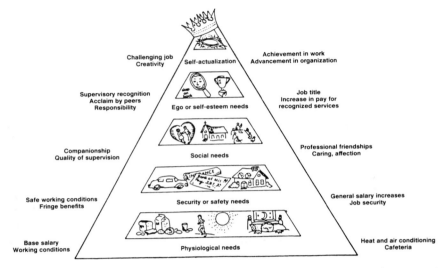

FIG 5-2. Maslow's hierarchy of needs with application to members of an organization. (From Szilagyi, A. [1985]. *Management and performance*. Santa Monica, CA: Goodyear Publishing.)

fill social needs through friendships and group memberships. Ego needs are next and are satisfied by internal feelings of achievement, recognition and personal respect. At the apex of the pyramid is the need for self-actualization.

Maslow's hierarchy of needs underscores the concept of individuality and, therefore, of not trying to motivate everyone in the same way. It underscores the need to work progressively with an individual rather than starting at the top. For example, in dealing with a patient you must first provide reassurance that life will continue before you can move on to other things such as returning to work. In your own case, you are unlikely to be motivated to be a star if you are worried about how to feed and shelter your family. To motivate, based on Maslow's concept, you need first to assess the level of the individual's need, provide motivation at that level, and then progressively move through the hierarchy.

THEORY X–THEORY Y

Douglas McGregor (1960) proposed the Theory X–Theory Y concept. Theory X is based on the traditional assumptions that persons consider work as a job to be done with no pleasure involved, are inherently lazy, are productive only when they fear demotion or termination, do not want to think for themselves, resist change, and must be coerced. Theory Y, which McGregor proposed as a more successful alternative, includes the assumptions that people are inherently good and enjoy work, take personal pride in a job well done, can be self-directed, are constantly striving to grow, and perform well if given the opportunity. Theory Y assumes that if the needs of an individual, as described by Maslow, are met, then the individual will contribute effectively to the organization. Theory X can be regarded as the pessimistic approach, whereas Theory Y is an optimistic one.

HERZBERG'S TWO-FACTOR APPROACH

Frederick Herzberg (1968) took Maslow one step further. He looked at both job satisfaction and dissatisfaction. The result was two lists of factors, one which Herzberg termed motivation and the other hygiene or maintenance. Hygiene factors are those which, if not met or satisfied, will lead to dissatisfaction but whose presence will not create satisfaction. These include money, working conditions, interpersonal relations, degree and quality of supervision, and policies and administration of the organization. Motivation factors, those whose presence leads satisfaction, include achievement, recognition, challenging work, increased responsibility, and growth and development (Figure 5-3).

As you can see, the maintenance factors are generally those from the lower level of Maslow's hierarchy, whereas the motivation factors are found in the higher levels. Herzberg notes that although some persons are maintenance seekers and will concentrate mostly on those factors, most individuals are motivation seekers.

Factors may change with the individual or the environment. Insurance coverage is a good example of something that was once a motivation factor, became a maintenance factor, and is now a motivation factor again. When health insurance first came into being, having it provided as an employment benefit was seen very positively by employees. After a period of time, however, persons grew to expect health insurance. Dental insurance then became the insurance benefit that gained "points" for the organization in the eyes of the employees. In the current economic environment, health care is once again becoming a benefit rather than an expectation, and some persons, especially heads of households, may decide to stay with or leave an organization based on insurance plans.

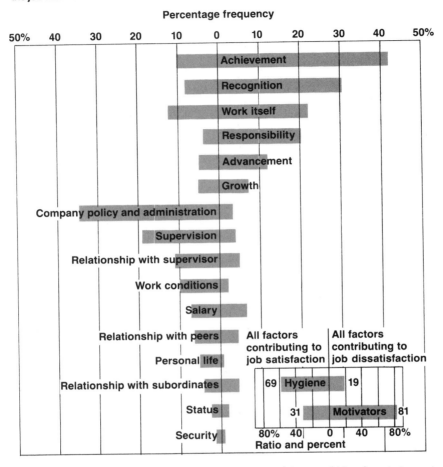

FIG. 5-3. Factors affecting job attitudes as reported in 12 of Herzberg's investigations (From Herzberg, F. [1968]. One more time: How do you motivate employees? *Harvard Business Review 46*, 53–62.)

EXPECTANCY CONCEPTS

Vroom (1964) proposed that the effort a person exhibits is based on the person's expectations that the effort will pay off in performance and the likelihood that performance will pay off in outcomes such as money, a sense of accomplishment, or promotions. Carried one step further, this concept becomes "you get what you expect to get."

In Vroom's model, individuals are seen as rational, intelligent, and capable of pursuing actions based on their beliefs and expectations. Motivation and the resulting performance are based on three dynamic processes: effort-performance expectancy, instrumentality, and valence. In the effort-performance expectancy process, the individual assesses the likelihood that a certain effort will result in a desire performance and whether the individual has the ability to perform that effort. Instrumentality is related to the belief that a certain performance will lead to a certain outcome. Valence refers to the value an individual assigns to the outcome.

Michael LeBoeuf (1985) defines the "greatest management principle in the world" as being that the things that get rewarded are the things that get done. People, he says, do the things that they believe will benefit them the most. LeBoeuf advises managers to look carefully at what they are really rewarding because sometimes they unintentionally reward behavior that they don't want repeated. For example, if the only time the manager pays attention to the employee one-on-one is when the employee does something wrong, the employee may repeat the same negative activity because that's what gets rewarded.

The nurse who puts forth an effort directed toward an outcome that is personally valued will very often reach that outcome. The nurse who puts forth a good deal of effort at advancing in a career usually does. The nurse who has realistic expectations for patients usually sees them materialize. Expectations, however, can work in two directions. The nurse who expects nothing often gets just that.

Individualizing Motivation

Levine (1983) and Fitzgerald (1982) both found that there is no single motivator that works with all individuals. Rather, a unique combination is usually necessary for optimal results. Just as with leadership, motivation must be situational. In this case, the style or technique employed depends on individual's personality, career goals, job and job requirements, age, and so forth.

It is important to understand what motivates you and to convey that information to your peers and your supervisor. Do you have an identified career goal that you are working to reach? Are you motivated or embarrassed by public positive verbal feedback? What do you consider a reward? Until you understand your own motivational needs, it is unfair to expect your supervisor and peers to understand what motivates you and to contribute to that motivation.

Working as a Team

Although one nurse alone can accomplish a lot, a team can very often accomplish a great deal more. As far back as 1881, Florence Nightingale challenged nurses to band together in their efforts: "Let us each and all, realizing the importance of our influence on others—stand shoulder to shoulder—and not alone, in good cause." (Vicinus & Nergaard, 1990) A team, however, rarely starts out as a team. It is generally a group of people brought together to address an issue in which they all either have a stake or can contribute some vital information.

Tuckman and Jensen (1977) have described the phases of team development as forming, storming, norming, performing, and adjourning. In the forming phase, it is important for the manager or leader to provide structure, clarify goals, and refocus as necessary. In this stage, productivity and morale are often low because the group members don't fully know or trust each other and it is too early to see results. In the storming phase, individual team member differences become evident as the real issues begin to surface. The group may break into factions and often begins to challenge the leader. At this point, it is important for the team leader to allow differences, to focus on the problem and not the person, to expect to be challenged, and to keep goals realistic. As the group progresses to the norming phase, members settle in and work begins to get done. At this time, it is important for the leader to clarify roles and responsibilities once again. The performing phase is the most productive. Group members trust each other and are headed in the same direction. The role of the leader in this last phase is to allow flexibility, to work for collaborative decisions, and to let the group manage its own issues. The final stage, adjourning, is sometimes overlooked. Yet it is important for closure to occur on the results of the team's work. The leader should summarize what the team has accomplished both for the team members and other interested parties. Of equal importance in the adjourning phase is acknowledging the work of team members and celebrating the team's success.

As a registered nurse, you will have the opportunity to participate in and to lead many teams. Initially, you will become part of the team of staff on your unit. On a day-to-day basis, you will be part of a patient care team composed of nurses, nursing assistants, other health care professionals, and ancillary personnel, all aiming to optimize patient care while maximizing available resources. When the patient care team is dealing with an individual patient, that patient and any appropriate significant others should be included as part of the team.

As you gain more experience, you will be asked to lead the patient care team. You may be asked to serve on quality improvement teams as either a participant or a leader. These teams are designed to improve the way care is delivered and generally are composed of individuals from many health care disciplines.

Leading and Managing: From Concept to Practice

Throughout this chapter, we have reviewed the concepts related to leadership and motivation. The practical aspects have been well summarized in *The One Minute Manager* by Blanchard and Johnson (1982) and *Leadership and the One Minute Manager* by Blanchard, Zigmari, and Zigmari (1985). The highlights of these books include the following:

"People who feel good about themselves produce good results." Remember the Hawthorne effect discussed earlier? A few positive strokes and a little recognition go a long way. In an international study of factors influencing hospital employee motivation, Alpander (1985) found that the crucial motivational element in hospital employees in the United States is the degree to which a feeling of recognition is experienced.

"Help people reach their full potential. Catch them doing something right." Rather than always telling the licensed vocational nurse or aide what was done wrong or how the job could be done better, try pointing out the things that are done well. At the very least, balance the negative with something positive. One popular management education program has as its first key principle to maintain and enhance self esteem.

"Everyone is a potential winner. Some people are disguised as losers. Don't let their appearance fool you." Sounds like Theory Y, doesn't it? Giving people the benefit of the doubt isn't always easy, especially on typically crisis-oriented patient care units, but it is far more effective in the long run than assuming the worst. The person to whom you give the benefit of the doubt today may be in a position to do the same for you tomorrow.

"When the best leader's work is done, the people say 'we did it ourselves!' " Strong leaders develop the people who work with them and then give credit to those people. When you as a staff nurse do a good job, it reflects on you, your manager, your director, the organization, and nursing in general.

SUMMARY

Leadership and management are a part of professional nursing. Understanding these concepts and learning to put them into practice are necessary parts of your education and of the transition from student to professional. All these concepts can be viewed from two sides.

It is important for the new nurse to see both sides—to recognize needs and responsibilities.

DISCUSSION QUESTIONS

1. How do leaders and managers differ? What are some examples of leadership and management skills you will need as a professional nurse?
2. Compare the various concepts of motivation. Which do you think fits best with your management style?
3. What are the stages of team development? What are the functions of the team leader in each stage?

REFERENCES

Alpander, G. G. (1985). Factors influencing hospital employee motivation: A diagnostic instrument. *Hospital & Health Service Administration, 30*, 67–81.

Bennis, W. (1989). *Why leaders can't lead: The unconscious conspiracy continues.* San Francisco: Jossey-Bass.

Blanchard, K., & Johnson, S. (1982). *The one minute manager.* New York: William Morrow and Co.

Blanchard, K., Zigmari, P., & Zigmari, D. (1985). *Leadership and the one minute manager.* New York: William Morrow and Co.

Del Bueno, D. J., & Freud, C. M. (1986). *Power and politics in nursing administration: A casebook.* Owings Mill, MD: National Health Publishing.

Fitzgerald, P. E. (1982). *Developing the health worker's attitude inventory: A tool for assessing worker/management relations in health care institutions.* Unpublished doctoral dissertation, University of Alabama, Birmingham.

French, J., & Raven, B. (1968). The basis of social power. In D. Cartwright, & A. Zander (Eds.), *Group dynamics, research and theory.* New York: Harper & Row.

Herzberg, F. (1968). One more time: How do you motivate employees? *Harvard Business Review, 46*, 53–62.

Kelley, R. E. (1988). In praise of followers. *Harvard Busines Review, 66*, 142–147.

Kouzes, J. M., & Posner, B. Z. (1990). The credibility factor: What followers expect from their leaders. *Management Review, 79*, 29–33.

LeBoeuf, M. (1985). *The greatest management principle in the world.* New York: GP Putnam's Sons.

Levine, H. A. (1983). Efforts to improve productivity. *Personnel, 60*, 4–10.

Likert R. (1961). *New patterns of management.* New York: McGraw-Hill.

Likert R. (1967). *The human organization.* New York: McGraw-Hill.

McGregor, D. (1960). *The human side of enterprise.* New York: McGraw-Hill.

Tuckman, B.W. & Jensen, M.A. (1977). Stages of small group development revisited. *Group and Organizational Studies, 2*, 419–427.

Vicinus M. & Nergaard, B. (Eds). (1990). *Ever yours, Florence Nightingale: Selected letters.* Cambridge, MA: Harvard University Press (p. 385, May 6, 1981, Address)

Vroom, V. *Work and motivation.* New York: John Wiley & Sons.

Zalenik, A. (1981). Managers and leaders: Are they different? *Journal of Nursing Administration, 11*, 25–31.

SUGGESTED READINGS

Byham, W. C. (1993). *Zapp! Empowerment in health care.* New York: Ballantine Books.

Crosby, P. B. (1984). *Quality without tears: The art of hassle-free management.* New York: New American Library.

Kantner, R. M. (1983). *The changemasters.* New York: Simon & Schuster.

Paulsen, T. L. (1988). *They shoot managers don't they? Managing yourself and leading others in a changing world.* Berkeley: Ten Speed Press.

Peters, T. (1987). *Thriving on chaos.* New York: Alfred A. Knopf.

Walton, M. (1986). *The Deming management method.* New York: Pedigree Books.

Ulrich, B. T. (1992). *Leadership and management according to Florence Nightingale.* Norwalk, CT: Appleton & Lange.

Delegation—The Path to Professional Practice

Carolyn C. Boyle

LEARNING OBJECTIVES

This chapter focuses on the definition of delegation, why it is important in providing nursing care, how it should occur, what requirements are necessary to meet before delegating, and who should delegate and to whom. This chapter will enable you to:

1. Describe delegation and discuss why it often fails.
2. Discuss the foundation for effective delegation.
3. Identify the guidelines for effective delegation for professional nurses.
4. Discuss the barriers to effective delegation.
5. Demonstrate the interconnection of leadership skills with effective delegation.
6. Provide sufficient information to support the professional nurse to use delegation in managing care.

Vestal, K.W. Nursing Management:
Concepts and Issues, 2 ed.
© 1995 J.B. Lippincott Company

Today's managed care environment challenges every nursing division to reduce costs, decrease nursing service intensity, and deliver the highest quality care. The goal is to ensure the maximal benefit to patients in the shortest possible stay. This challenge clearly calls for fundamental changes in the way we organize and deliver nursing care. The key to a successful nursing model in today's managed care environment is effective delegation skills.

A care management approach incorporates support personnel into the nursing care delivery model so that professional nurses can manage and direct all patient care. The role of the professional nurse is to guide patients through the shortest possible hospital stay, ensuring maximal benefit from needed care.

Directing and delegating patient care can be difficult for nurses because both functions represent giving orders to other people. Most nurses practicing in today's changing environment did not learn delegation skills. They entered the job market at a time when total and primary care were the accepted nursing models. These models did not require delegation skills but, instead, stressed equality in roles, care loads, and communications. Many RNs practicing in the total or primary care models believe they can effectively delegate care. However, they often find that delegated care is not successfully completed. This may be, in part, due to a lack of trust in those to whom tasks are delegated. Individuals who cannot bear to depend on the words and work of others consequently find themselves doing all the work themselves.

INEFFECTIVE DELEGATION EXAMPLE

The following example comes from a surgical step-down unit historically staffed with all RNs. On a particular day, the unit was short-staffed and a technician from the emergency room was floated to assist with care. The technician was assigned to assist an RN with her heavy assignment.

The RN delegated a patient's hourly output measurement to the technician and asked him to inform her if the urine output dropped below 50 cc an hour. After 4 hours of no communication, the RN asked the technician if there were any problems. He replied, "Her hourly output is fine but there is a great deal of blood in the bag." The RN became exasperated with the technician because he had not told her about the blood. When she questioned his failure to report the blood he said, "You said to let you know if her output dropped below 50 cc's an hour.

You didn't say anything about looking for blood, so I assumed that you knew that there was blood in her urine."

This scenario is quite common. The actual delegated task may be different but the results are the same. The RN in this example had little experience with delegation. She truly believed that she had communicated the patient care needs to this technician. If questioned about the outcome of this assigned task, she would probably have said, "You see, this is why we can't use technicians in this unit . . . the patients are too sick."

In reality, this incident is the result of ineffective delegation. It is insufficient merely to make assignments and wait for results. The RN did not adequately explain the priorities of care for this patient. She merely assigned the technician a task. If the RN had communicated the patient's condition to the technician and enumerated the priorities of care, this scenario may have ended with a more positive outcome for the patient.

The RN should have explained that the patient had undergone a genitourinary procedure and that blood in the urine (as well as decreased urine output) was a possible complication for which to be alert. The technician would have then known that there was no history of blood in the urine. He would have reported this change to the RN before the blood loss became significant.

DELEGATION IS NOT MERELY DISTRIBUTING CARE

Delegation does not mean distributing all nursing care among the various staff members as was done in the old team model. Effective delegation is a more sophisticated process requiring professional skills. Delegation involves matching aspects of work required to carry out the prescribed nursing orders (and to accomplish patient outcomes) with the most appropriate personnel, while maintaining professional standards of care. Most people have the capacity to handle additional work, especially if it provides opportunities to prove that they are capable of more demanding jobs.

There are **three major reasons why attempted delegation fails** to produce desired results:

First, nurses fail to recognize and incorporate the principles of effective delegation. Basic nursing education has not included the skill of delegation for almost 2 decades. Nurses will have to go back into the classroom to learn and practice this important skill. Primary nursing textbooks did discuss effective delegation of responsibility to primary nurses (Volante, 1974). It seems, however, that concepts such as defining the task to be done, relaying your definition of the task, and establishing controls, checkpoints, and dialogues were lost in the more focused efforts of one-to-one care assignments.

Second, nurses don't recognize that habits ingrained from old practice patterns prevent improvement in delegation skills. Total care practice patterns actually encourage solitary practice by professional nurses. Nurses do not acquire delegation skills through experience or value delegation skills as a practice enhancement. Nurses are used to making decisions and then immediately carrying out care without communicating the process to anyone else. This type of care perpetuates an isolation of nursing from other team members. As nursing became more focused in this solitary practice, the coordination of all aspects of care became fragmented and lacked clear leadership, thrusting the patient advocacy role to a designated, centralized patient advocate.

Third, nurses are unwilling or unable to view delegation from the perspective of the delegatee. Stimulating a group of people to achieve a goal is vastly different from achieving a goal yourself. Power motivation, or concern for having an impact on others, requires an outlook and actions considerably different from those needed for making an individual contribution. It must be assumed that a given organization, department, or section has a number of competent, willing, and responsible individuals employed. A staff that is not used effectively because of an RN's failure to delegate is a major loss to an organization. It is a waste of human resources.

THE FOUNDATION FOR DELEGATION

Delegation depends on a balance of responsibility, accountability, and authority (Figure 6-1).

> **Responsibility** is the condition of accepting important duties or obligations.
> **Accountability** is the condition of being answerable.
> **Authority** is the right and power to determine, influence, or evaluate.

There are five basic concepts that build the foundation for effective delegation:

1. **Delegation is not a system that reduces responsibility. It is a way to make responsibility meaningful.** An RN manages and directs patient care much the way a nurse manager delegates the responsibility for bedside care to appropriate staff. The RN, like

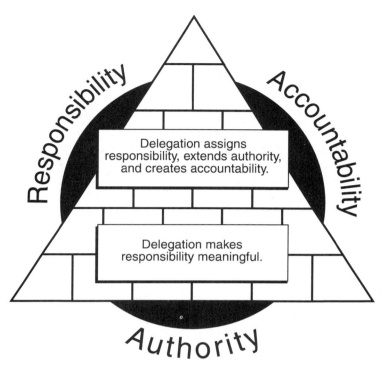

FIG. 6-1. Foundation for delegation.

the nurse manager, retains the overall responsibility for patient care. By effectively delegating, the RN simultaneously gives the resource staff the responsibility and authority to carry out nursing orders to achieve patient outcomes. It is important for RNs to be involved in the decisions regarding the assignment, use, and supervision of assisting personnel. They need to understand the clinical and financial rationales for staffing strategy.

2. **Responsibility and authority must be delegated equally!** The RN establishes patient care outcomes. Responsibility to accomplish selected outcomes is delegated to appropriate members of the resource group. The RN sets the limits within which the appropriate staff can work to accomplish the patient outcomes and *then allows the care giver to decide how to achieve the goals.* If the outcome has been delegated along with the latitude to decide, the RN has delegated responsibility and authority equally. This process assumes that a framework has been established within each clinical setting for the use of assisting personnel and should include:

- An assessment of patient needs
- Identification of tasks that can be performed by assisting personnel, with frequency and opportunity to perform as important considerations
- Education and training so that the task is performed safely and competently
- A process for determining competency of assisting personnel
- Availability of appropriate supervision by the RN
- A process for ongoing evaluation of the assisting personnel
- A process of communication of patient information between the RN and the assisting personnel.

3. **The process of delegation allows RNs to assign responsibility, extend authority, and create accountability within the resource group.** Successful RNs systematically plan delegation by determining (1) what kind of care is required; (2) who is ready and appropriate to assume additional work; (3) what assistance is needed; and (4) what outcomes are expected.

   The RN assigns responsibility by delegating specific outcomes to appropriate care givers, extends authority by authorizing care, and creates accountability by following up on delegated care to ensure that it is accomplished in an effective and timely manner.

4. **The concept of empowerment applies to all members of the resource group.** Empowerment requires assertiveness. The RN should review patient care results—not methods. After a clear delegation of care (eg, outcomes, latitude to decide care methods and expectations), the RN must show trust by allowing experienced, credentialed nursing staff to carry out the delegated aspects of patient care alone. When problems or issues arise, the experienced RN will always ask the resource group, "What do you think we ought to do?" Empowerment involves giving people important work to do on critical issues; giving people discretion and autonomy over their tasks and resources; providing visibility to others and recognition for their efforts; and building relationships for others.

   Trust is the central issue in human relationships both inside and outside the care environment. Trust is an essential element of effectiveness as well. You demonstrate your trust in others through your actions—the extent to which you check and control their work, delegate work, and allow people to participate.

5. **The care giver must take an active role in accepting the delegated patient care.** To take the initiative, care givers must exercise the authority delegated to them and act. An active role opens the

channels of communications between assisting personnel and RNs. Assisting personnel should neither have to wait until told to do something nor should they have to ask. They should practice the completion of assigned tasks. By keeping the responsibility where it belongs, the RN will increase discretionary time to truly manage the care of assigned patients and still handle system-imposed tasks. Assisting personnel should be made aware of the confidence placed in them. You can demonstrate this confidence by indicating that personnel can handle the assigned tasks and allowing them the option of determining how the task can best be accomplished. This action tells them that you are assured of their skills and encourages them to do the best job possible.

These five basic concepts of delegation build a foundation for all care communications. RNs achieve full and effective delegation through mutually interactive communication among all of the members of the resource group. Figure 6-2 illustrates how an RN can use all five of the basic delegation concepts to integrate responsibility, authority, and accountability into the practice of delegation. The RN and the entire resource group become focused on achieving patient care outcomes.

Delegating patient outcomes makes responsibility meaningful. Involving the resource group in deciding how to achieve patient outcomes extends authority as well as responsibility. Setting reporting expectations transfers accountability to the resource group, completes communications, and results in true empowerment.

EFFECTIVE DELEGATION: GUIDELINES FOR PROFESSIONAL NURSES

Delegation begins with a solid information base. Every nurse should be aware that full delegation of patient care is impossible until the preliminary and fundamental steps of managing care are completed. These preliminary steps result in an information base that guides others in delegated care and makes care expectations clear to the resource group. The RN provides:

1. Specific Outcomes
   Clear and specific outcomes based on objective physical and psychosocial parameters must be established for all patients for whom the resource group is responsible. **What outcomes would**

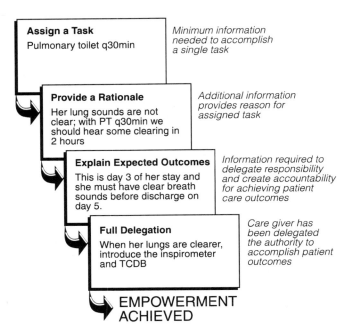

FIG. 6-2. Five basic concepts lead to full, effective delegation.

you expect for patients on a geriatric unit in which assisting personnel have specific responsibilities?

2. Target Dates

The RN must set specific target dates measured by day of stay for each parameter. This is often simplified by case management plans that define the diagnosis and the care to be provided by the day of stay and not necessarily by daily tasks. **Does the case management model exist in any medical center where you have worked? Discuss how it supports a clarification of outcomes.**

3. Nursing Orders

The RN must identify and order nursing interventions that are appropriate to a patient's needs and that will result in measurable progress toward patient care outcomes. This assumes the appropriate use of nursing assessment and independent decision making regarding the actions that will meet the patient's nursing care needs. **Discuss some examples of nursing assessment and intervention in which you have been involved.**

When this three-part information base is complete and available, the expectations for results of care are clear to all who will participate in its delivery.

GUIDELINES FOR DELEGATION

Nurses who are learning to delegate may find it helpful to use some simple guidelines.

- **Describe the task to be accomplished.** Give a clear description of what you want the care giver to accomplish with the patient.
- **Explain why the task is necessary to achieve an established outcome.** Through nursing orders, describe the overall background (patient status and a brief history) as necessary to explain the scope of the current care.
- **Discuss the degree of responsibility and authority that is required to carry out the delegated assignment.** There must be a mutual understanding of the degree of responsibility and authority that the assignment entails. The RN must give the staff member the authority to accomplish the outcome, and the staff member must accept the responsibility and accountability for completing the assignment. The RN, however, is still ultimately responsible. If the staff member doesn't exercise the responsibility properly, the RN can always withdraw the authority. Delegation without control is abdication.
- **Summarize the delegated care and assignment as a whole to ensure mutual understanding.** Ask the staff member to summarize the main points of the care that has been delegated. Answer any questions or clarify details as necessary. If, in our earlier example, the RN in the surgical step-down unit had used these guidelines when delegating care to the emergency room technician, the outcome for that patient may have been different. Both the RN and the technician would have had a more positive experience working together with the common goal of achieving specific patient care outcomes.

In most situations, key phrases simplify the delegation process and clarify the expectations. The following represent some suggested approaches.

> "I expect that . . ."
> —I expect that Mrs. Stein's skin integrity will remain intact and that you will report any redness or signs of breakdown.

"You are responsible for . . ."

—You are responsible for turning Mrs. Stein from her left side to her right side every 2 hours. She prefers not to be on her back or abdomen.

"Do you have any questions?"

—Would you please tell me your understanding of Mrs. Stein's care?

"Report back to me at . . ."

—Report back to me after you have completed hygiene and skin on Mrs. Stein. At that time we will discuss any further skin care that may be necessary later in the shift. **Have you worked with experienced delegators who use other phrases to clarify expectations? What are they?**

PRINCIPLES FOR SUCCESSFUL DELEGATION

Delegation improves the ability of the nursing staff and the performance of the RN. When assisting personnel are delegated authority and responsibility for a job, they are given an opportunity to apply what the RN has taught. Certainly they will make mistakes, but you should be able to turn these mistakes into learning experiences. Through delegation, they should steadily increase their skills and their confidence to deal with problems.

Employee motivation and job satisfaction increase with effective delegation. If your staff is typical, they want the opportunity to handle new problems and increase their skills. Through delegation, you provide them with such an opportunity. To delegate effectively and successfully, you must follow these principles:

1. **Communicate clearly and completely.** The way an assignment is communicated can determine how successfully it is completed. Inadequate communication is the most frequent reason that delegated care is not completed as expected.

2. **Make your availability clear to the resource group.** If the RN expects staff members to report patient progress, then the RN must be available. If there are periods of time when the RN cannot be available, then clear alternative reporting lines must be communicated to the staff.

3. **Retain control.** The RN gives the resource group the necessary freedom to think and act. However, if there is a particular patient who is of concern, do not assume that "no news is good news." Follow up with the resource group.

4. **Expect progress reports.** As an RN, you set the expectations for reporting and updates. Ask for and expect regular updates. Then follow up on changes.

COMMON BARRIERS TO EFFECTIVE DELEGATION

The value of delegation for continuous quality improvement cannot be overstated. Yet often nurses who are learning the leadership expectations of a professional nursing role are reluctant to delegate. There are many barriers to effective delegation built into our current delivery methods.

The most common barriers are those reflected in the following statements made by RNs who have participated in action planning for care management:

"I can do it better myself."

Many nurses believe the hands-on performance of even basic tasks (such as bathing patients, making beds, and taking routine vital signs) is the essence of nursing practice. We cannot continue to hold this belief and at the same effectively delegate aspects of patient care.

Nurses must recognize that credentialed nursing assistants can give some types of patient care at a higher quality level than many RNs. Patients appreciate uninterrupted hygiene and basic care. Often RNs are interrupted by other care priorities and unit-related matters. Nursing assistants can devote time and attention to basic details that result in greater patient comfort and satisfaction. What is ideally needed is a method of care that will help RNs concentrate on what is expected of a professional RN managing care while delegating those activities that members of the resource group are qualified to perform.

"It takes too much time."

Nurses have commented that in the time it takes to delegate care effectively, they could have completed half the care themselves. Although this is an overstatement, we must acknowledge that delegation communications do take time. However, the actual time saving is realized in the future. Delegation ultimately provides time for those aspects of professional practice that often are not carried out because there is "no time" left after the tasks are completed.

"I don't know what they are allowed to do."

For many years, RNs have worked only with other RNs and with LPNs. Many nurses feel unsure of the limited scope of practice of assisting personnel. But the scope of practice is not really the issue. Nursing assistants and LPNs carry out a wide variety of functions and tasks that contribute to quality patient care. Assisting personnel have only one limitation: they cannot engage in professional practice.

Managing care effectively should define and use the skills and talents of all members of the multi-level resource team. RNs must learn to rely on position descriptions, policies, and procedures that clarify the roles and functions of assisting personnel. An effective care manager recognizes the strengths and capabilities of the staff and uses those talents appropriately to maximize the benefit for patients.

"I am concerned about supervising assisting personnel."

Many RNs who have practiced in the total care model have had little experience with supervising staff. Therefore, many RNs do not realize that a major component of supervision is leadership. Supervision and leadership are skills that require effective communication and a knowledge of group dynamics (See Chapter 5). RNs are leaders and must become comfortable with being recognized as having the authority to carry out the leadership role. One of the more significant benefits of delegation is its value as a development tool for the staff. RNs can provide the opportunity and atmosphere for staff to continue to develop skills.

SUMMARY

Delegation is the path to and a significant success factor for professional practice. The new health care delivery systems of the 1990s demand more from all health care providers. To meet the increasing demands for nursing care, professional nurses will have to plan and manage care differently. Rather than maintain the "nurses can do it all" philosophy of the past, professional nurses will come to value their care management skills. The key to successful nursing care in this new environment is the skill of delegation. Professional nursing practice must embrace all aspects of delegation including:

- Why nurses must delegate aspects of care
- How to take the first steps
- The basic concepts of delegation

- The communications of delegation
- Role playing and follow-up

Those who have practiced in primary and total care models will find that some patient care will have to be delegated with the increasing patient care loads experienced with managed care programs. A well-planned and thoughtful approach to the use of assisting personnel will ensure that these care givers can make a valuable and important contribution to quality nursing care.

DISCUSSION QUESTIONS

1. Describe a patient care team you have worked with that had multiple needs for the RN to delegate activities and responsibilities.
2. Cite an example of delegation of work that did not result in a good outcome. Why not, and what could have improved the outcome?
3. How will you prevent yourself from falling into the traps that prevent effective delegation?
4. As a nurse, when activities are delegated to you, how will you clarify expectations and measure and report results?

REFERENCE

Volante, E. (1974). Mastering the managerial skill of delegation. *Journal of Nursing Administration, 4*(1), 21–23.

SUGGESTED READINGS

Arthur, D. (1979). Guidelines for effective delegation. *Supervisory Management, 24*(10), 9–13.
A supervisor asks: "Delegation's downside." (1991). *Health Care Supervisor, 10*(2), 78–82.
Branat, M., & Craig, R. (1985). Follow the leader: A learning exercise. *Journal of Nursing Education, 24*(4), 139–142.
Byham, W., & Zapp, W. C. (1988). *Zapp! The lightning of empowerment.* New York: Fawcett Columbine.
Byham, W., & Zapp, W. C. (1992). *The heightening of empowerment.* New York: Harmony Books.
Caruth, D. & Middlebrook, B. (1983). How to delegate successfully. *Supervisory Management, 28*(2), 36–42.
Cavey, S. R. (1989). *The seven habits of highly effective people.* New York: Simon & Schuster.
Conger, J. (1992). *Learning to lead.* San Francisco: Jossey-Bass.

Davidhizar, R., & Kuipars, J. (1988). Delegation, the art of letting go. *AORN Journal, 47*(1), 172–175.

Gross, K. (1992). *Intercare: Care management systems for nursing, 2*(8).

Herbin, R. (1990). Practicing effective delegation. *Pediatric Nursing, 16,* 91–92.

Hirschhorn, L. (1991). *Managing in the new team environment.* New York: Addison-Wesley.

Kouzes, J. M., & Posner, B. Z. (1987). *The leadership challenge.* San Francisco: Jossey-Bass.

Lane, A. J. (1990). Nurse extenders: Refocusing on the art of delegation. *Journal of Nursing Administration, 20*(5).

Manshe, F. A., Jr. (1987). *Secrets of effective leadership.* Germantown, TN: Leadership Education and Development, Inc.

McAlvanah, M. (1989). A guide to delegation. *Pediatric Nurse, 15*(4), 379.

Montana, P., & Nast, D. (1981). Delegation: The art of managing. *Personnel Journal, 60*(10), 784–787.

Parker, G. (1990). *Team players and team work.* San Francisco: Jossey-Bass, 1990

Porter-O'Grady, T., & Finnigan, S. (1984). *Shared governance for nursing: A creative approach to professional accountability.* Rockville, MD: Aspen Systems.

Saccardi, T. A. (1985). Delegation: A revelation. *Hospital Health Services Administration, 30*(6), 128–133.

Stone, S., et al. (1984). *Management for nurses.* St. Louis: CV Mosby.

Taylor, H. (1984). *Delegate.* New York: Time Warner.

Yura, H., Ozimek, D., & Walsh, M. B. (1976). *Nursing leadership—Theory and process.* New York: Appleton, Century, Crofts.

Zander, K. S. (1980). *Primary nursing: Development and management.* Rockville, MD: Aspen Systems.

Decision Making

Eula Das
Linda Myers

LEARNING OBJECTIVES

This chapter will enable you to:

1. Establish the rationale for professional nurses to participate actively as decision makers in a variety of organizational processes.
2. Establish a decision-making process for a variety of situations.
3. Appreciate the complexity of decision making required by the professional nurse.

Vestal, K.W. Nursing Management:
Concepts and Issues, 2 ed.
© 1995 J.B. Lippincott Company

Health care is undergoing a paradigm shift from a medical model to a customer-oriented model. Customers are becoming more knowledgeable about health care and more sophisticated in selecting health care options. They expect providers to allow them to become involved in decision making. Nurses are responding to customer needs by advocating high-quality care that meets the customer's expectations. This shift in paradigm provides a golden opportunity for nurses to advance their professional practice but requires a foundation of sound decision making.

RATIONALE FOR PROCESS

Creativity is an element of the decision-making process. The generation of possible strategies is a major step in planning decisions. Creative thinking can produce solutions that are not at first apparent but that are practical and effective. Outcomes predicted creatively will reveal advantages and disadvantages of the various strategies, thus helping to prevent mistakes.

In today's environment, decision makers are challenged to plan innovative and creative ways to provide high-quality patient care and to maximize available resources. These challenges require one to be knowledgeable and astute in the basics of the decision-making process. Using decision-making skills can be a contributing variable to improving patient care, enriching job satisfaction, decreasing liability, and promoting cost-containment.

Professionals must gain control over decisions that affect them and their patients. Decision-making autonomy, the freedom to act on what you know, is frequently equated with nursing professionalism. It includes not only the freedom to act and succeed but also the freedom to act and fail. If autonomy itself is to succeed, the climate must support these freedoms, allowing both accountability and authority.

Hospitals that specify and clarify responsibility and decision-making authority allow staff nurses to be more effective and efficient in their areas of expertise. If the nurse has the knowledge and the skills to initiate and carry out actions and to answer for the results, the nurse is practicing autonomously.

Systematic decisions can be analyzed if you have followed specific steps that can be scrutinized. The decision can be evaluated to determine the need for revision.

FAMILIAR DECISIONS

Driving a car is a familiar situation that, moment by moment, requires decisions. A cardboard box tumbling onto the road in front of the car, for example, requires an immediate decision. The proficient driver and the new driver will differ in the way they make their decisions.

Using critical thinking skills, the experienced driver constantly maintains a running assessment of the road conditions, positions of other cars, speed, car performance, sound of the engine and wheels, feel of the road surface, and the car's motion. These observations may be made half-consciously, but they are, nonetheless, monitored constantly and form a continuous baseline of data. Maintaining the flow of observations, expert drivers are open to unexpected cues and can make decisions accordingly.

The novice driver, on the other hand, has a narrower view. With attention focused on the basic elements of driving—clutching the steering wheel, pressing the gas pedal, and watching the road ahead, the novice probably will not comprehend the situation involving the box as soon as the proficient driver. The novice may have more preconceptions than the experienced driver, such as believing the road to be safe and clear. Therefore, the novice may not be prepared to anticipate changes.

Once both drivers see the box, they will assess it differently. The proficient driver will ask many questions. From what direction did it come? Did another car hit it? How did the box move? Did it roll heavily as if something were inside it, did it bounce, or did it skim over the road as if it were empty? How wide and how tall is the box? Is there anything in the car that could fly around and hurt passengers after a sudden stop or swerve?

The novice will ask questions that the proficient driver has been mentally processing all along. Is the road slick or dry? How fast is the car moving? Are there cars behind or in the left, right, or oncoming lanes? Is there a shoulder, a ditch, or a guard rail? How good are the car's brakes and steering?

After they assess the situation, the proficient driver and the new driver may differ in their planning. Having a narrower view of the situation, the new driver may see only the option of stopping or not stopping. However, the proficient driver will take all the information and generate the options of stopping, going around, running over the box, or slowing down to let it blow out of the way.

The proficient driver will also hypothesize the numerous consequences of potential strategies. A car swerving on the slick street may not be controllable. Coming to a complete stop may result in a rear-end collision with the car behind. The novice driver may see only limited consequences of the action. The box will be avoided if the car is stopped. If the car does not stop, the box will be hit.

The proficient driver will weigh the risks of each of the alternatives, gauging the effect each will have on the driver, the passengers, and other drivers. The novice may not be able to weigh such risks.

Based on critical thinking skills, the strategies and predictions of their outcomes, and weighing of risks, the proficient driver will choose the best action. The novice may react impulsively and, therefore, select a less acceptable alternative.

THE PROCESS

Decision making is a process of choosing between alternatives. The decision maker must:

1. Assess the situation.
   Define the situation that has given rise to the opportunities for decision making.
2. Plan the process.
   Set the criteria for the decision to satisfy personal, professional, and institutional values.
   Determine who can make the decision.
   Recognize possible strategies and screen them for acceptability.
   Predict the possible outcomes of strategies and the positive and negative impact of each.
   Weigh the risk involved.
   Select the most satisfactory strategy.
3. Implement the decision.
4. Evaluate the outcome of the decision.

This process applies to any decision-making situation, whether professional or personal. At each step of the assessment, planning, implementation, and evaluation, a decision should be justifiable and effective.

A decision-making process leads you to assess the situation thoroughly. The process should help you consider most factors that will affect your decision. You can prove that a choice was made only after the relevant data were considered, yet, because the system allows for orderly grouping of pertinent information, you can avoid wasting time with inconsequential details. To help you acquire the ability to make effective decisions, a decision tree is provided in Figure 7-1. By following this step-by-step approach to decision making, you will be more likely to select the best strategy to achieve the desired outcomes.

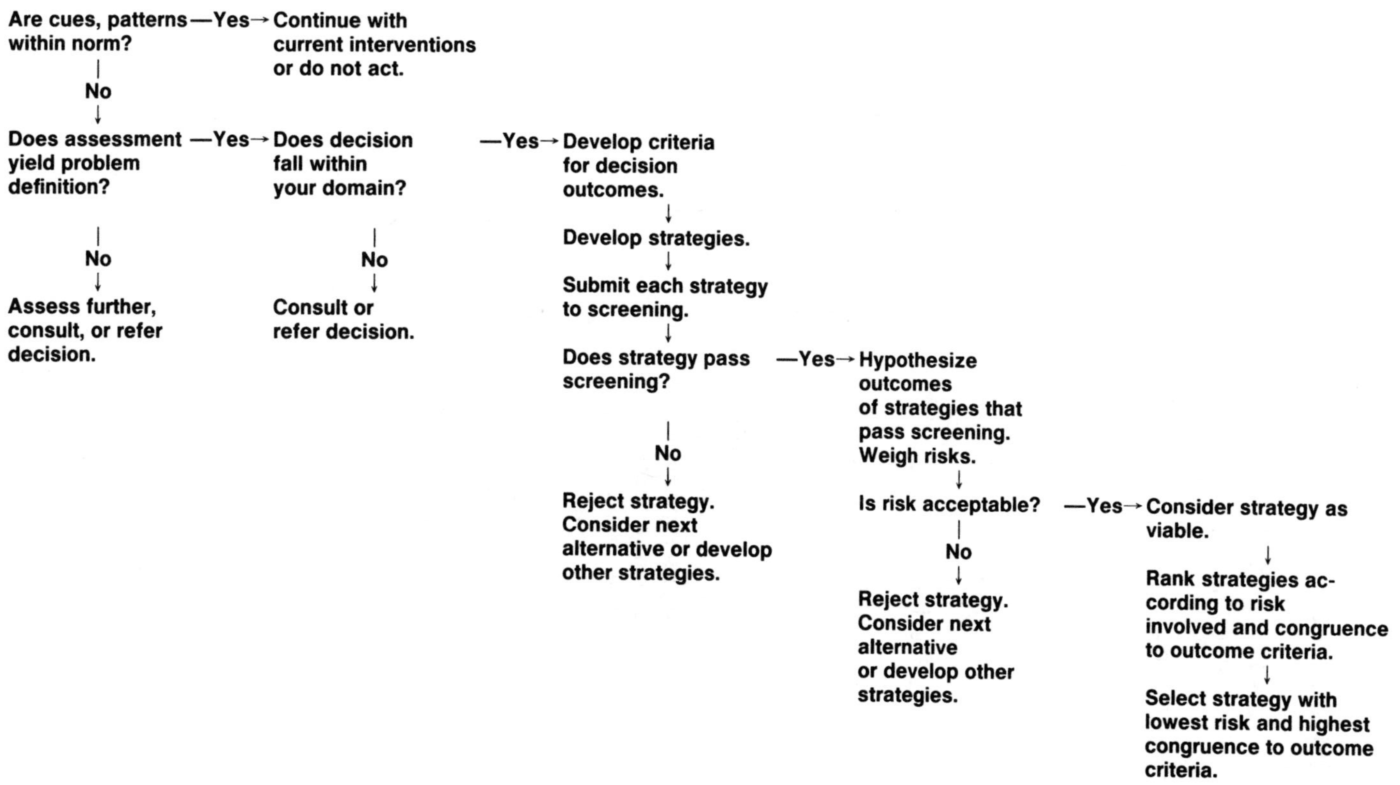

Are cues, patterns within norm? —Yes→ Continue with current interventions or do not act.

No ↓

Does assessment yield problem definition? —Yes→ Does decision fall within your domain? —Yes→ Develop criteria for decision outcomes.

No ↓   No ↓

Assess further, consult, or refer decision.   Consult or refer decision.

Develop strategies.

Submit each strategy to screening.

Does strategy pass screening? —Yes→ Hypothesize outcomes of strategies that pass screening. Weigh risks.

No ↓

Reject strategy. Consider next alternative or develop other strategies.

Is risk acceptable? —Yes→ Consider strategy as viable.

No ↓

Reject strategy. Consider next alternative or develop other strategies.

Rank strategies according to risk involved and congruence to outcome criteria.

Select strategy with lowest risk and highest congruence to outcome criteria.

FIG. 7-1. Diagram of the decision-making process.

NURSING DECISIONS

The process that nurses use to make decisions has the same elements as that of making any other decision. The steps of assessment, planning, implementation, and evaluation determine the way you view a situation and lead you to your decision.

ASSESSMENT

Assessment is the collection of data about a situation. It involves maintaining baseline data and defining the problem.

Maintaining Baseline Data

Assessment is done continuously. It is often carried out unconsciously because it has many sources. Through the senses of sight, hearing, touch, and smell, nurses assess constantly. They see skin color, drainage, and nonverbal behavior such as restlessness. By hearing heart and breath sounds and listening to the patient's concerns, they assess other areas of health status. Signs such as skin turgor, warmth, and pulse quality are assessed by touch. The smells of urine, breath, and wounds yield other information. Other sources of information include the patient's history, the physical, sociologic, economic, cultural, and psychological assessment, diagnostic data, and reports from other members of the health care team.

From all these sources, nurses form a running assessment of patient status. This baseline of knowledge is the foundation for comparing information obtained in future assessments. These pieces of gathered information are signs indicating whether something is within or outside the norm. When related and categorized, these signs or cues may form patterns indicative of the situation's status. You need to accumulate cues and cue patterns to determine if the situation is congruent with the norm or if a discrepancy exists.

Standards of practice for nursing actions are established by the institution's policies and procedures, by professional theory, and by literature on the subject. The standards of care expected by patients are influenced by the values and expectations of the nurse, patient, significant others, and managers or other superiors. When cues or cue patterns are within the set standard or norm, the decision can be made either to continue with current interventions or not to act. Identifying a discrepancy between the situation and the standard also signals the beginning of the decision-making process.

Defining the Problem

If the baseline assessment meets the standard (ie, there are no new relevant cues) and future assessments yield no deviation from the standard, then the decision to continue with present interventions or to start no new interventions may be made. However, if the presenting cues indicate a discrepancy between the present situation and the desired situation, you must decide what, if anything, needs to be done.

The first step in making a decision is additional assessment to define the situation or to state clearly the problem needing resolution. A single cue often is not enough to determine whether action is needed. Go back and assess the situation further. Find other cues and determine their relevance to the situation. Then group or cluster them into categories to form possible diagnoses. You may find several explanations, and cues may fit into more than one grouping. Gather sufficient information to define the problems.

This critical thinking process is referred to as *clinical judgment* and is a necessary component of nursing practice. Simply stated, it is the selection of nursing interventions based on a diagnosis that is arrived at through a decision-making process.

The following example illustrates the use of critical thinking skills to formulate a clinical judgment.

> A patient, Mrs. Jones, calls on the intercom: "My arm with the IV hurts." Maria B., RN, replies that she will come and check it. As Maria walks down the hall, she mentally reviews what she already knows about Mrs. Jones and her IV:
>
> The IV has been in for 48 hours.
> I checked it within the last 4 hours.
> It met standards for a patent IV site in that the site was not tender or edematous and the skin color around the site was undifferentiated from surrounding tissue.
> Mrs. Jones was admitted for electrolyte imbalance and dehydration.
> Her condition is listed as good.
> Her veins are small and venipuncture is difficult.
> Mrs. Jones is "very afraid of needles" and becomes distraught during venipunctures.
> She is receiving potassium, 40 mEq in 1000 mL D5NS at 125 mL/hour.
> Maria has started the assessment process even before she enters Mrs. Jones' room. She is reviewing her baseline data (ie, what she already knows about the situation). She will then begin collecting new data.

Although, in assessing a situation, you identify and group cues, it is important not to be burdened with preconceptions and to remain open to additional information. Prematurely or haphazardly making a decision could have a negative outcome. Make sure that the problem producing this set of cues is identified correctly. The differentiation between the cause and the symptoms is critical to making a decision. For example, Mrs. Jones may be experiencing vein irritation, phlebitis, or infiltration of the IV site. She could, however, be uncomfortable in her strange surroundings or be lying in a position that has decreased circulation in that arm. Because she is anxious about having an IV, she may dismiss such a simple explanation and call the nurse. When Maria arrives, she finds Mrs. Jones lying in a comfortable position that should allow good circulation. Examining the site, Maria notes the area around and above the site to be red, tender, edematous, and without return blood flow into the tubing. Maria groups the subjective and objective data into related clusters and compares them to standards for IV sites. Now Maria has identified the discrepancy between "what is" and "what should be." From the cues, her knowledge of theory, and her experience, Maria defines the problem as "infiltrated, phlebitic IV site."

Many conclusions related to nursing observations are not the result of slow, deliberate, and conscious thought processes like those described in the above example. These cognitive processes often occur so rapidly that they bypass conscious awareness. By making this process deliberate and conscious, however, you can organize your approach and recognize the variables influencing the situation.

PLANNING

Once you have defined the problem, the next step in decision making is planning how to solve it. This includes establishing criteria for the outcomes of the decision, classifying the decision according to domain, identifying individuals who can make the decision, identifying possible strategies and screening them for acceptability, hypothesizing outcomes, and weighing risks of strategies.

Planning should include examining your resources. Technology and computerization, for example, can often help hospital staff make the best and most timely use of their valuable knowledge, skills, and expertise. Systems may be designed with nursing standards and nursing priorities built into them. Using a bedside terminal, for example, Maria may access Mrs. Jones' serum potassium level, the date the IV was started, the time the current bottle was hung, her intake and output, her weight, and the last IV site assessment. With this data, she may determine that, due to the patient's low serum potassium, decreased intake, and weight loss, the IV should be started immediately. Using

the computer, she can then send a message to the blood bank requesting a STAT IV restart.

Establish Criteria for Decision Outcome

Define the outcomes or effects your decision must have, regardless
of what the decision is. Desired outcomes may be derived from standards such as the ones previously discussed. For example, Maria wants
to relieve Mrs. Jones' pain, avoid inflicting more pain, maintain the patient's fluid balance, keep a line open for administering fluids and medications, and prevent inflammation and infection at the IV site. The
standards for these desired outcomes are derived from institutional
policies and procedures, nurse–patient expectations, pathophysiologic
theory, and personal values. Any action Maria decides to take must satisfy these criteria as closely as possible. Comparison of the desired outcomes, standards, and actual results is the basis for evaluation of
decisions.

Classify According to Domain

Classify the problem by determining who has the authority to
make the decision, that is, within whose domain of responsibility the
decision lies. Your nursing license, hospital policies and procedures,
and job description define your domain of decision-making authority.
Depending on the domain of the decision, you can make it yourself, share
the decision, or refer it to someone else. In our example, Maria must determine if the decision to discontinue and restart the IV is within her
domain.

Discerning if the decision lies within your domain may be easy. If
you have the legal, institutional, and moral sanctions to make it, and
the resources to carry it out, proceed. In Maria's case, her nursing license and the policies and procedures of her hospital allow her to
discontinue the IV and to prepare for restarting it.

At other times, however, the domain of responsibility may be quite
vague. Situations will occur in which nursing action is sanctioned by
legal and institutional guidelines, but the means necessary to carry out
the decision are lacking. Situations that require decisions to be shared
or referred to someone else include the following:

1. The nurse recognizes the discrepancy but cannot define the
   problem.
   Example: A patient becomes increasingly restless. The nurse recognizes the single cue of restlessness but is unable to recognize

other cues to establish a label. As a result, she does not know the etiology and cannot intervene.

2. The nurse recognizes the discrepancy and can label it, but the required interventions or the desired outcomes are not known.
   Example: The nurse observes bright red blood spurting from a tracheostomy. The desired outcome is to stop the bleeding and maintain a patent airway, but the nurse does not know what to do.

3. The nurse lacks the necessary resources—skills, knowledge, equipment, or time—to make or carry out the decision.
   Example: The nurse is unable to palpate a pedal pulse and does not have access to a Doppler. The action may be to collaborate with others to borrow the necessary equipment or to delegate the task of obtaining it.

4. The nurse lacks the legal, moral, or institutional sanction to intervene.
   Example: The nurse finds a patient in acute respiratory distress. There is an urgent need for intubation and mechanical support, but the nurse is not sanctioned by the institution and the state law to perform that procedure.
   Example: A nurse may believe strongly that life support should be initiated in a case of terminal illness, but the patient has an advanced directive that forbids life-sustaining procedures.

Identify Strategies for Problem Resolution

The next step in effective decision making is identifying possible strategies for solving the problem. This is where creativity enters the picture. Try not to make a decision until you have considered several strategies for handling the situation. Devising several strategies increases the likelihood that the decision will yield the best results. Possible courses of action include direct and indirect intervention, purposeful inaction, delegation, collaboration, and referral.

Direct Intervention. In direct intervention, you carry out physical or verbal activities. Discontinuing or restarting an IV, counseling subordinates, and teaching patients and colleagues are examples of direct intervention.

Indirect Intervention. As a nurse at the center of the communications and operations network of the health care setting, you may intervene indirectly with interpersonal skills. In the example above, if the IV was not infiltrated, allaying Mrs. Jones' fears might have been an appropriate indirect intervention. Negotiation, conflict resolution, persuasion, and confrontation are examples of indirect intervention.

Delegation. You may delegate certain responsibilities to others who are available, capable, and allowed to take action. Delegation is preferable when that individual can better accomplish the desired outcome. For example, in assessing potential sites for restarting the IV, Mary finds that a suitable vein cannot be located. In this instance, she may elect to delegate this task to someone with venipuncture expertise, such as the IV team.

Purposeful Inaction. A conscious decision not to act is advantageous in some instances. For example, a patient with Borderline Personality Disorder questions your authority relating to the enforcement of unit rules and regulations. The patient is noncompliant, and anger escalates into threats and intimidation. The appropriate inaction would be for you to allow the patient to ventilate, while you remain calm and supportive. Other action may be required if the limits are exceeded. If a decision is not yours to make alone, your options include interdisciplinary teamwork, collaboration, and referral.

Interdisciplinary Team. To be effective, interdisciplinary team decision making must include a clear definition of the problem and an understanding of membership roles in the decision-making process. As with independent decision making, there must be relevant data available to generate options. Interdisciplinary team efforts succeed best in an environment that respects contributions and expertise, offers constructive feedback, and shares the responsibility for the outcome.

When the decision-making process is inadequately managed within the team, decision error and obstruction may result. Factors contributing to ineffective team process include lack of clarity regarding the problem or the expectations of members, lack of sufficient data, and selecting the first option as the best. When these factors surface, team members become frustrated and disinterested and return to autonomous practices.

Collaboration. Registered nurses use the nursing process most effectively when they practice the professional role collaboratively both within the nursing staff and with other clinical disciplines (eg, physicians, therapists, and pharmacists). The expert knowledge shared within these groups improves the nurse's ability to make more effective decisions about patient care needs.

Collaborative practice is frequently done on a case-by-case basis and can occur informally over coffee or in scheduled meetings.

Referral. When the decision lies totally outside your domain, refer it to someone who is willing and mandated to intervene. This may result in a referral to a supervisor, a physician, a minister, or members of other disciplines.

Screen Strategies for Acceptability

Once you have identified strategies, you must screen them for acceptability. To be considered seriously, a strategy must be scientifically sound, legal, and consistent with personal and organizational value systems. Ask these questions about each strategy:

1. Do related scientific principles, research evidence or findings, and professional literature support it?
2. Is it legal?
3. Does the decision fit into your value system?
4. Would your organizational structure and your managerial and supervisory environment condone the strategy?
5. Are there unit culture and environmental constraints on the strategy?

If the strategy passes this screening, it is eligible for further consideration. In the IV example, Maria can restart the IV herself or she can summon the IV team to perform the venipuncture. Both strategies pass the screening.

Hypothesize Outcomes and Weigh Risks

After you have screened the strategies, you must hypothesize their outcomes. This will help you recognize and consider the advantages and disadvantages of each. Imagine each strategy in operation and list the problems that could arise. What are the potential risks? Think in terms of yourself and others involved, including the patient, your co-workers, and the organization.

For example, Maria imagines two strategies—restarting the IV herself or calling the IV team. Maria knows that Mrs. Jones has small deep veins. Maria's experiences with difficult venipunctures is limited. She considers the outcomes of her strategies:

A. Restart the IV herself
   1. Unsuccessful venipuncture attempts resulting in excessive pain and anxiety for the patient and multiple venipuncture sites
   2. Damaging veins through unsuccessful venipuncture, making a restart more difficult for an experienced venipuncturist
   3. Increased anxiety for Maria in light of Mrs. Jones' fear of venipuncture
   4. Loss of time in attempting a difficult venipuncture
B. IV team restarts the IV
   1. Successful venipuncture with fewer attempts
   2. Less anxiety and pain for patient and fewer venipuncture sites
   3. Less anxiety to Maria
   4. Time saved for Maria
   5. Higher costs for the patient and hospital

To be viable, a strategy must be associated with an acceptable risk factor. When you are considering each strategy, ask the following questions about risks, and then rank the strategies based on your answers.

1. How much effort is required for yourself or other parties involved?
2. Which alternative gives the greatest results with the least effort?
3. How much change would each alternative require?
4. Which alternative takes the best advantage of your resources?
5. How will employees be affected by the alternative and what will their reactions be?
6. How will patients be affected by the alternative and what will their reactions be?
7. What past failures or successes have you or others had with the alternatives?

Of all the viable strategies, select the one most desirable based on the lowest risk. Asking these questions about both her strategies, Maria decides to request assistance from the IV team. The risk associated with that strategy is lower to the patient, Maria herself, and the organization.

IMPLEMENTATION

To implement your decision, gather the necessary resources and carry out the action. This may be a fairly straightforward operation when you make the decision alone, implement it yourself, use resources at your disposal, and perform the action immediately.

The issue becomes more complicated, however, if other persons are involved. Communication or negotiation become very important. When you share responsibility for a decision, delegate a task, borrow equipment or supplies, ask for assistance, or delay performance, other people are affected. They must be informed and included in the process. Negotiating with them to accept or share the responsibility for implementation makes success more likely. In Maria's situation communication is done through the bedside computer terminal. After accessing the computer, Maria documents her assessment. She notes that the IV site in the patient's left lower arm is red, tender, edematous, and without return blood flow into the tubing. Maria recalls that the patient's serum potassium is low, her weight is still 5 pounds below her "normal" weight, and her IV is at 125 mL/hour to alleviate dehydration and to supplement potassium needs. Maria then sends a message to the IV team requesting a STAT IV restart.

Decision making is based on a body of expert knowledge. Whether the decision is made autonomously or interdependently, the nursing process must be documented in the patient's medical record.

EVALUATION

Evaluation is based on the degree of congruence between the desired outcome, the standard, and the actual outcome. By comparing these elements, you can evaluate the effectiveness of your decision. Dissatisfaction with the outcome leads you to reenter the process of assessment, planning, and implementation and, ultimately, to a more satisfactory strategy.

Your judgment of a decision's effectiveness, however, can be colored by other factors. Time may be needed to determine whether a decision achieves the outcome desired. You must consider both the long-term and short-term effects in evaluating the success of some decisions.

Your values also determine how you evaluate a decision. If you value consistency and following hospital rules, you may decide to adhere to the hospital's policy of not permitting visitors under 12 years of age. However, if in some circumstances the needs of an individual supersede hospital rules, you may decide to allow a child to visit a relative.

In the delivery of health care, you will be confronted constantly with decisions that involve conflicting values. You may question the usefulness of some decisions or even disagree with them. Decisions about the allocation of limited resources such as funds, space, equipment, and services are laden with value. Patient care entails value judgments, such as patients' rights regarding advance directive and your charge to protect patients against themselves.

Often decisions are compromises with which no one is completely satisfied. If a patient is having severe pain 2 hours before he is scheduled to have more medication, you may decide to reposition him. The outcome is less effective than medication, and neither you nor the patient are satisfied. However, because the risk associated with medication is high, the decision is a good one.

DECISIONS ABOUT PRIORITIES

Management of a patient assignment depends heavily on setting priorities—deciding what to do and when to do it. The novice nurse tends to focus on one problem at a time rather than seeing the whole picture.

Even the nurse attending to only one patient must prioritize the needs of that patient. For example, if a patient has been subject to hourly vital signs checks that are consistently stable, and the doctor's order states that vital signs are to be checked hourly until stable, the nurse may decide to check less frequently. The cues that lead to the nurse's decision to decrease the frequency of vital signs checks are as follows:

1. The vital signs have been consistently stable.
2. The patient has been deprived of rest because of frequent vital signs checks.

The first standard to be met is that of patient stability. Hourly assessment of vital signs reveals that this standard has been met. The nurse then focuses on the cue that reveals rest deprivation. The standard is that sufficient rest is necessary for health maintenance. The cue deviates from this standard. The discrepancy between the cue and the standard leads the nurse to decide to decrease the frequency of vital signs checks. The nurse continues to monitor the patient to ensure that the first standard of patient stability is maintained.

The nurse accountable for more than one patient must be able to prioritize a number of pressing needs of different degrees of complexity, as in the following example:

> At 3:10 PM, Brian C., RN, finishes receiving the following reports on his assigned patients for the 3:00 to 11:00 PM shift:

Patient A—Diagnosis: Pneumonia. NG tube not draining. Complains of shortness of breath.
Patient B—Diagnosis: Possible appendicitis. In OR. Returning to floor at 3:30 p.m.
Patient C—Diagnosis: Abdominal pain. To OR for exploratory laparotomy at 3:30 p.m.
Patient D—Diagnosis: Metastatic CA. Chest tubes. Confused. Asking for pain medication and doctor has ordered stat lab. When Brian leaves the report area, Dr. Smith arrives on the unit and asks him to make rounds on her patients with her.

Brian is aware that all four patients and the physician need intervention. To determine which needs must be addressed first, he must select the actions that would be best for each need presented. He must prioritize meeting the needs of individual patients, while prioritizing those needs in relation to his total workload. Brian can choose to intervene directly or indirectly with some needs, delegate some responsibilities, or delay some actions until later. He also has the option of consulting with others or referring decisions to them.

COMPLEXITY OF DECISIONS

By now you can see that even as a beginning nurse you are continually making decisions, some simple and others complex. Simple decisions have a single cue or familiar or congruent cue patterns that lead to definition of a problem. The domain of the simple decision is clear. The choices of strategies are established by standards, and the outcomes of these strategies are predictable. Examples of simple decisions are giving acetaminophen for fever above 101°F or calling the physician for abnormal laboratory results.

Complex decisions involve unfamiliar, multiple, or conflicting cues or cue patterns that do not present definable problems. The choices of strategies are not clear, are not covered by standards, or do not have known outcomes. For example, a patient whose diagnosis is unknown and who is febrile and complaining of pain may present the need for a more complex decision than the patient who has a urinary tract infection and has expressed the same symptoms. Risk factors are greater in complex decisions because the outcome may alleviate one set of cues while aggravating another set. Weighing the outcomes and risks is particularly important in complex situations.

The nurse's ability to identify the degree of a decision's complexity will influence his or her ability to select an appropriate strategy. Knowledge and experience can influence the perception of the complexity of the decision. For proficient clinicians, some complex decisions have become simple. Their decision making has become almost automatic due to expert critical thinking skills.

On the other hand, a situation that appears simple to a novice nurse may be considered complex by a more experienced nurse due to the experienced nurse's ability to assess numerous cues simultaneously. Having the ability to predict the impact of a decision in terms of the whole picture can change the assessment, the strategies considered and, consequently, the action taken. Novice nurses can be very alarmed to realize that decisions they thought were simple and clear-cut are actually very complex and can have a major impact on the entire organization.

New situations present more complex levels of decision making. You must be conscious of the situation and environment and be willing to use a structured process. You must draw upon knowledge, theories, and experience instead of making decisions automatically. Experienced nurses who move into management or other clinical specialties, for example, may find themselves less proficient in making decisions. Using the structured process may clarify such situations.

Use of Process in Other Decision-Making Situations

Until now, the decision-making process has been related primarily to patient care. The same process, however, applies in other situations. For example, you may be involved in making a decision to initiate a new nursing procedure. Assessment is done during committee meetings, personal interactions, and observation of staff performance. Once your assessment has led you to define the problem, you will plan your actions by setting criteria for outcomes and discerning who holds responsibility for making the decision. If the responsibility is not yours, you will refer the decision to someone else. If the responsibility is yours or yours and that of others, you will develop strategies for resolving the problem and then hypothesize their outcomes. Your strategy will change if the decision is made collaboratively or by an interdisciplinary team. Based on an assessment of risks, you will choose a strategy. Using resources at hand or negotiating for others, you will implement your decision and evaluate its outcomes.

SUMMARY

As health care becomes increasingly customer oriented, nurses are responding by establishing close patient care advocate relationships. Sound decision making is the foundation needed to advance professional practice.

The decision-making process outlined in Figure 7-1 offers a step-by-step approach to decision making. By following this process, you should be able to make rational, justifiable, and effective decisions. Using resources such as computers and clinical experts makes the process more efficient. The quality of your decision making will be further enhanced by using a collaborative, interdisciplinary approach. Proficient decision-making skills are an essential part of providing high-quality, cost-effective patient care. By repeatedly applying the process, you will integrate it into your nursing practice and can, with time, become a proficient decision maker.

DISCUSSION QUESTIONS

1. List the four components of the decision-making process.
2. Define autonomy as it is related to accountability of the clinical nurse.
3. Describe how cross-functional, interdisciplinary teams support a total quality environment.
4. Discuss potential outcomes of haphazard decision efforts.

SUGGESTED READING

Baggs, J., Phelps, C., & Johnson, J. (1992). The association between interdisciplinary collaboration and patient outcomes in a medical intensive care unit. *Heart and Lung, 21*(1), 18–24.

Banner, P. (1984). *From novice to expert: Excellence and power in clinical nursing practice.* Menlo Park, CA: Addison-Wesley.

Caruso, L., & Foster, D. (1990). Collaborative management: A nursing practice model. *Journal of Nursing Administration, 20*(12), 28–32.

Collins, S., & Henderson, M. (1991). Autonomy: Part of the nursing role? *Nursing Forum, 26*(2), 23–29.

Del Bueno, D., Weeks, L., & Brown-Stewart, P. (1987). Clinical assessment centers: A cost-effective alternative for competency development. *Nursing Economic$, 5*(1), 21–26.

Dwyer, D., Schwartz, R., & Fox, M. (1992). Decision-making autonomy in nursing. *Journal of Nursing Administration, 22*(2), 17–23.

Gilliland, M. (1991). Productivity: Electronics saves steps and builds networks. *Nursing Management, 22*(7), 56–69.

Ivey S., Brown, K. S., Teske, Y., & Silverman, D. (1988). A model for teaching about interdisciplinary practice in health care setting. *Journal of Allied Health, 17*(3), 189–195.

Kerrigan, K. (1991). Decision making in today's complex environment. *Nursing Administration Quarterly, 4*(15), 1–5.

Kramer, M., & Schmalenberg, C. (1988). Magnet hospitals: Institutions of excellence (Part 1). *Journal of Nursing Administration, 18*(1), 13–24.

Leming, T. (1991). Quality customer service: Nursing's new challenge. *Nursing Administration Quarterly, 4*(15), 6–11.

Mariano, C. (1989). The case for interdisciplinary collaboration. *Nursing Outlook, 37*(6), 285–288.

Matteson, P., & Hawkins, J. (1990). Concept analysis of decision making. *Nursing Forum, 25*(2), 4–10.

Mundinger, M. (1980). *Autonomy in nursing.* Germantown, MD: Aspen Systems.

Patterson, C. (1991). New joint commission standards for 1991 require R.N. decision making. *Nursing Administration Quarterly, 4*(15), 65–68.

Simpson, R. (1991). How to avoid system obsolescence. *Nursing Management, 22*(7), 20–21.

Strasen, L. (1989). Self concept: Improving the image of nursing. *Journal of Nursing Administration, 19*(1), 4–6.

Wiens, A. G. (1990). Expanded nurse autonomy: Models for small rural hospitals. *Journal of Nursing Administration, 20*(12), 15–22.

Financial Management

Nannette L. Goddard

LEARNING OBJECTIVES

This chapter will enable you to:

1. Explain the general trends related to financial issues in nursing.
2. Describe the link between clinical nursing practice and financial management functions.
3. List strategies for assuming accountability for cost-effective nursing practice.
4. Discuss ideas for improving clinical productivity.

Vestal, K.W. Nursing Management:
Concepts and Issues, 2 ed.
© 1995 J.B. Lippincott Company

In educating the nursing professional, much time is spent familiarizing the student with the clinical functions and departments of the health care institution. As the on-the-spot clinician who oversees the total needs of the patient, the staff nurse interacts most frequently with clinically focused hospital employees who work in diagnostic and treatment departments (eg, laboratory, central supply, pharmacy, and radiology) and in other nursing units. There is little call for the individual nurse to be involved with the personnel of the business office or financial planning department on a day-to-day basis. Yet the role of the staff nurse is vital to the financial health of the institution.

This chapter will explain general trends in health care costs, hospital financial performance, and the functioning of the nursing unit. The link between individual staff nurse clinical practice or behavior and the financial implications of clinical team work patterns will be established. Some specific strategies for developing fiscal awareness and responsibility will be introduced, along with ideas that the staff nurse might implement to improve the productivity and job satisfaction of the entire unit staff.

HEALTH CARE COSTS AND ISSUES

The nurse manager or administrator may function as an intermediary between the personnel or payroll department and the staff in matters regarding wages and paychecks. Traditionally, the nurse manager or assistant nurse manager is responsible for the business communications representing the nursing unit's staffing and budgetary needs. In today's more decentralized management structures, staff nurses may find themselves communicating routinely with the admitting or business department on matters of patient placement, transfer, and discharge. Given a hospital's need to control costs, all staff may take part in decision making about shift-by-shift workload fluctuations and staffing coverage alternatives.

HOSPITALS ARE BUSINESSES TOO

The trend in many health care centers around the country is to define the role of the unit nurse manager as a department head position requiring a combination of clinical expertise and business management skills. With the continuing changes in governmental regulation and reimbursement methods, hospitals must place even more emphasis on evaluating each phase of their operations. All managers have been required to gain skills in financial analysis and productivity monitoring; costs need to be reduced and practice patterns need to be streamlined. Increasingly, it is essential for each clinical practitioner to recognize the economic pressures faced by hospitals and to understand that the institution must be run as a business if its doors are to remain open.

"The hospital as a business" may be a difficult concept for some persons. In the United States, people tend to regard access to health care as an inalienable right, not as a privilege or luxury. Society has been oriented to expect that the appropriate amount of the best care will be provided to any individual, regardless of his or her ability to pay or the extent of the illness or injury. From the critically ill neonate to the multiorgan transplant candidate, past focus has been on providing the highest quality inpatient care—frequently to the exclusion of cost considerations. The laws of the land have provided for many disabled, indigent, or elderly sectors of the population to be served through federal, state, or locally supported programs. Hospitals, therefore, have been perceived as benevolent organizations from which society expects excellent care and services.

Walking through the corridors of the modern hospital, one is impressed by the abundance of equipment, supplies, and professionals. It is easy to think that the hospital has much to give from its seemingly "limitless resources." It is more difficult to fathom the costs of such a mammoth operation and the size of the institution's bills—even for such basics as water, electricity, and waste disposal. When the amount of research and technological development involved in medical science and health care is considered, the ultimate cost in time and dollars becomes staggering. Progress made over the last few decades, including radically new surgical techniques, complex space-age equipment, new treatments, and lifesaving drugs, underscores the need for reconciling the amount that hospitals must charge for these services and the amount that society, in turn, is willing to pay.

SOCIAL POLICY AND ECONOMIC DECISIONS

In the last 30 years, the nation's budget allocation for health care expenditures has grown at an alarming rate and has developed into a major issue in the country's legislative bodies, where tax rates must ultimately be adjusted to fund much of the increase. Laws were passed that mandated or supported programs such as health systems agencies, certificate of need applications, professional standards review organizations, and the expansion of health maintenance organizations—all in what now seems a vain attempt to curtail the rapid growth in spending (Schwartz & Mendelson, 1991). The call for true health care reform has become an economic battle cry for private citizens, the federal government, and big business.

In addition to social programs for the needy, Americans came to expect that employee benefits packages would provide health insurance covering the payment of hospital bills. Many citizens lost track of how much their families' health care really cost because someone else was paying the bill. The relatively small deductible paid by the individual worker was much easier to swallow when the insurer or employer picked up the bulk of the payment required by the health care institution. The insured employee did not actually see the money change hands and found it easy to ignore the specifics of how much each x-ray or blood test or room charge actually cost the employee benefit system.

In truth, costs are skyrocketing so dramatically that employers have begun to balk at paying the increased insurance premiums. Most employed Americans are now paying higher copayments or deductibles for employer-provided coverage. Many businesses are redefining their role in the funding of health care for retired workers, with the resulting limits or withdrawals of benefits angering pensioners on fixed incomes.

Many small businesses cannot afford to provide health care insurance for their workers. At the same time, economic conditions have forced other companies out of the marketplace, and their workers have become the unemployed uninsured. American industry has been compelled to join forces with various governmental bodies, labor representatives, and community groups to investigate innovations in health care that could hold the line on costs to employers and taxpayers.

The detailed history and specifics of the Medicaid, Medicare, and other entitlement programs are beyond the scope of this text and have been well documented in other sources. Statistics related to cost escalations in the public and private sector are available in other publications that the reader may choose to explore. (See the reference list at the end of this chapter.)

The increased participation of American industry and the recent upsurge of concern in governmental circles have sparked an overall direction of change in health care economic and social policy. Decisions are being made more in response to business issues than in response to clinical concerns. The United States is experiencing the emergence of a revised health care system. Staff nurses must be aware of new trends that require the hospital's concentration on financial stability to survive.

The New Direction in Reimbursement

Ten years ago, a major trend in health care reimbursement policy was engineered by the Health Care Financing Administration during President Ronald Reagan's first term in office (Jones, 1989). Payments made to hospitals on behalf of Medicare recipients were no longer based on retrospectively reimbursing the hospital for its "allowable costs" relating to the specific services and number of days of care provided to each individual patient. By categorizing the patients into diagnostic related groups and assigning an expected flat rate dollar payment to each diagnostic related group, the government attempted to dictate how much money the hospital would receive for care of a specific patient, regardless of how many services or days of care the hospital provided.

In addition, by analyzing the normal case mix of the numbers of patients in each diagnostic related group for which the hospital usually supplies care, the government could provide the institution with lump sum payments prospectively. Therefore, the hospital was supposed to receive a predetermined, fixed amount of money for its Medicare patients and then to provide care to those clients, while not exceeding the budgetary allotment it had already received from the federal government.

Under the former cost-based reimbursement plan, hospitals paid little penalty for being inefficient and were, to some extent, rewarded for the amount of money they spent. This led to increasing the services offered and prolonging the days of care provided. Now hospitals are trying to minimize the amount of services and days of care, in an attempt to spend the least amount of money possible and to live within the dollars Medicare promises up front. In this way, the government has built in significant incentives for efficiency. The major insurance companies have followed in the footsteps of Medicare and have adapted similar prospective pricing and payment systems, thus allowing them to set flat fees for their coverage plans and to supply some relief to the employers and individuals who pay for benefits. Insurers and employers have responded by initiating managed care plans, requiring second opinions before surgery and negotiating group contracts on a capitation ("per head") basis.

The Shift Away From Acute Care

The health care industry has been forced to decrease its concentration on acute care inpatient services and to focus instead on developing alternative and cheaper methods of delivering care through outpatient care, home care, ambulatory care, same-day admission surgery, rehabilitation, long-term care, and health maintenance services. In many respects, the only patients who remain hospitalized in the system are those who are the sickest and who cannot be treated in or transferred to other facilities. One prediction is that by the year 2000 the only surgical patients in hospitals will be those who are having major organ transplants or recuperating from life-threatening traumas.

There may be fewer persons hospitalized less frequently and for shorter lengths of stay, but patient acuity levels and the need for more intense medical and nursing care may be higher today than in the average hospital census of the past. Nurses employed in these acute care settings will be challenged to gain additional skills in the organization and management of patient caseloads and in the clinical performance of the nursing process.

The changes of the last several years have emphasized hospital competition, redesigned care delivery systems, and marketing of health care services. Competing hospitals in a given community want to outdo each other by offering the highest quality of care for the lowest possible price. Competent and speedy services delivered in a caring atmosphere will be the marketing strategy that hospitals use to attract consumers and the employing industries who represent large groups of customers.

If the acute care setting sees fewer total inpatients, then the percentage of total market share attained by the individual institution will be a vital statistic tracked in the boardroom and the executive suite. Many institutions have already established satellite referral centers in surrounding communities and are attempting to build their reputations to attract clients from other states and countries. Hospitals have extended their business structures to include freestanding clinics, home care divisions, outpatient surgery centers, and other ambulatory services that focus on preventive or rehabilitative health care (Lee & Clarke, 1992). The business acumen, financial savvy, marketing ability, and negotiating skill of the administrator and the hospital staff member will be of even greater importance to the survival of the fittest institutions.

MINIMIZING LOSSES RELATED TO UNIT FUNCTIONING

The basic revenue/cost center of the nursing department is usually the individual nursing unit. The nursing unit normally houses groups of patients who have similar or complementary diagnoses, treatment plans, and needs for nursing care. The nursing revenue/cost center is the common denominator of the nursing budget; in most cases, the supplies, expenses, personnel time and dollars, and capital equipment requests are tracked and allocated according to the individual nursing unit.

As the staff attempts to render the best care possible in the amount of time available, the staff nurse is often asked to police cost containment carefully and to use the hospital resources wisely. The hospital worker may be asked to conserve water, use supplies sparingly, and turn off electricity when lights or pieces of equipment are not in use. These are things that any household consumer might do to minimize costs at home.

RISK MANAGEMENT AND INSURANCE COSTS

Most hospital staff are taught to be concerned about the safety of the environment—for the sake of both staff and clients alike. Safety campaigns and posters caution about potential electrical hazards, various types of spills on the floor, improper disposal of used needles, and the dangers of cumulative exposure to radiation. Any homeowner or licensed driver learns quickly about safety issues, the costs of accidents or repairs, and the advisability of insurance policies. Similarly, most businesses attempt to cover themselves with the correct types of insurance that will protect them against major claims and losses.

The costs of insurance policies are usually based on a calculation involving the historic average number and types of claims processed and the average expected dollar payments needed to pay the insured or beneficiary for any loss. For example, an automobile driver who has a good driving record is, often times, eligible for discounted insurance rates based on a history of an uneventful experience on the road and the likelihood of that pattern continuing. Rates are higher for younger drivers and those who own high-powered, sporty vehicles. The insurance industry has compiled detailed customer and claims surveys to document that these types of drivers historically have represented a higher risk and expense to the insuring company.

Given the high-risk nature and complex environment of the acute health care setting, it is not surprising that insurance rates and premiums represent costly items in the hospital budget. In addition to the normal business coverage for accidents, theft, and natural disasters, hospitals must insure themselves and their employees or representatives against malpractice and negligence claims. Currently, the United States is in the midst of a review of the "insurance crisis" that parallels and dovetails with the movement toward health care reform.

Liability coverage for many businesses and professionals has become more difficult to find and to fund. Many state legislatures are considering limitations on the amount of cash awards that jurors would be allowed to grant in malpractice or negligence cases.

Clinical care givers may on occasion exercise poor judgment and be responsible for errors or omissions in care (or in the documentation of care). These workers may inadvertently expose the patient to potential harm and the health care institution to costly lawsuits, damaging press coverage in the news media, and escalating insurance fees. The American society is a litigious one, and consumer activism is a potent force in the marketplace.

Physicians and nurses are guided by codes of ethics, standards of practice, hospital policies, published procedures, and recommendations from their professional bodies, not to mention government statutes and rulings from other regulatory agencies. The beginning practitioner in any clinical discipline has the responsibility of understanding the skill level expected by the employer and of knowing when to seek advice and counsel from more experienced colleagues. Validating an opinion or discussing a planned course of action with a supervisor or clinical specialist may turn out to be the most timesaving and moneysaving approach in the long run; every institution has its unique methods of operation and recordkeeping that the novice nurse must learn. The staff nurse will function more cost effectively over an entire career by establishing good practice habits, recording facts and assessments accurately, and safeguarding against errors and omissions in care.

ABSENTEEISM

Risk managers, administrative supervisors, and personnel representatives are vitally interested in the safety and security of the organization's employees. Employees who value their jobs and their health are motivated to follow appropriate procedures when operating equipment or working with critically ill and potentially contagious patient populations; it is a matter of protecting oneself from injury or physical complications. Benefit time for illness and worker's compensation coverage are usually available for full-time or regular part-time employees who are injured while on duty. However, it is best for everyone to stay healthy and avoid having to use such sick time and injury coverage so that staff members remain productive and on the job.

There are many direct and indirect costs that the institution may incur due to the absence of a regular employee. Direct costs include the outlay of funds for benefit days or worker's compensation and the additional payroll dollars (which may have to be paid at overtime) required to replace the individual who is absent. Like any other employer providing health care benefits, the hospital must pay its promised share of health insurance premiums or payments. Most health care centers fund and staff an employee health office that monitors the health care needs of the organization's employees and certifies when sick or injured employees are restored to health and may therefore return to work.

The level of functioning of the nursing unit suffers when one of its regular staff is absent and that person is replaced with someone who may not know the unit's routine or its patients. The productivity of the staff may be undermined if other members of the same unit are asked to work excessive amounts of overtime and then become mentally or physically strained by the additional workload. A vicious circle of fatigue, more illness, and more overtime coverage can become a demoralizing work experience for a unit staff and an expensive drain on the institution. Eventually, the staff's stress may affect its ability to work at peak performance. Errors and omissions in care are more apt to occur under these circumstances.

In some settings, a nurse manager may feel compelled to take a full clinical assignment and thereby cover the temporary vacancy left by a staff nurse who is ill. This is one solution to the immediate need for staff coverage, but if the head nurse performs this replacement function repeatedly, the management work of the unit may not be accomplished in a timely fashion. This, in turn, may cause the unit to function less cost effectively. If supply orders are not processed, the next round of time schedules left uncompleted, and other management planning functions ignored, the unit and its staff can suddenly find themselves lacking basic supports and in need of immediate crisis management.

PRODUCTIVITY OF THE STAFF AS A UNIT

The individual staff nurse may spend many years refining skills and applying a wealth of knowledge to gain competence in professional nursing practice. However, the delivery of nursing care is almost exclusively a "group sport" (Zander, 1979) rather than an individual endeavor. The nursing unit staff is composed of many individuals with differing education and experience who are expected to work together to further the institution's goals and meet the needs of its patients. In some hospital environments, multi-skilled workers and cross-educated staff from other departments are intricately involved in the broader patient care process. Hospitals of the future will include more robot workers to whom nurses will assign elements of the patient care and support services. It is feasible that human practitioners will work side-by-side with entities similar to the Star Wars characters known as C3PO and R2D2.

Nursing staff members must rely on each other to communicate, follow through, and substitute for one another. Even in a primary nursing, case management, or primary care setting, clients may require nursing care when the assigned principal care giver is off duty or at lunch. Another nurse may need to act on behalf of the absent nurse and provide care for the patient. During a cardiac arrest or other emergency situation, a multi-disciplinary group is often called on to function with the rhythm of a well-rehearsed orchestra.

From a financial viewpoint, the staff's ability to work well as a team and to provide competent care for a group of patients while using an appropriate amount of hospital resources is measured by the staff's productivity. The institution's resources include labor, supplies, buildings, equipment, and other assets. Jelinek (1979), in an important contribution to the management engineering literature, described some key terms:

> . . . production is defined as the output of the hospital operation. The output measures, in order to be meaningful, must not only reflect the quantity produced by the hospital but also must reflect the quality of these outputs. Productivity is defined as the ratio of output to input. Thus, productivity relates the output to the resources being expended (input) to produce that output.

In the case of an inpatient nursing unit, the inputs are primarily staff time, supplies, and equipment; the output is patient care, usually expressed in terms of hours or days of care delivered (sometimes adjusted for patient acuity levels, as explained later in this chapter).

Quantity of care and quality of care must be considered in any discussion of productivity. The radiology department could set a world's record in speed of performing chest x-rays and complete more chest films per hour than ever before, but the films would be of no diagnostic use if their quality were so poor as to render them useless.

Efficiency and effectiveness are related but by no means interchangeable concepts. The original hospital industrial engineering text by Smalley and Freeman (1966) explains the difference as follows: "Effectiveness is the degree of achievement of objectives, while efficiency [like productivity] is the relation between achievement of objectives and the consumption of resources." Edwardson (1985) explained effectiveness in health care by referencing the work of the Applied Management Sciences, Inc., in a Department of Health and Human Services publication on productivity and health:

> Effectiveness refers to the safety, appropriateness, and excellence of care. An acceptable output specifies the minimum level of patient outcome, patient satisfaction, and change in health status approved by decision makers.

Therefore, in establishing its productivity goals according to its projected workload and standards of care, an organization provides a criterion for measuring the actual versus the expected performance of the staff involved in the "production" of each department. The nursing unit staff that meets the institution's productivity goals will be using the expected level of resources to deliver the projected workload (amount of care for a number of patients) within the budgeted dollars of that fiscal period. The unit staff that uses more than the recommended amount of supplies or more than the allocated level of staff to deliver the projected amount of care may cause the institution to spend more resources or dollars than planned, thereby diminishing the productivity of the department. If the staff is highly efficient, delivers care effectively, and uses fewer resources than expected per unit of care delivered, the department will exceed its productivity and quality objectives and may present a more positive financial picture.

Long-term survival of health care organizations—like any other competitive business—may depend on achieving a certain level of productivity relative to competitors. Skillful implementation of an objective productivity and cost-monitoring system is a key step in establishing and maintaining a high degree of productivity and other significant operational benefits. Young (1992) explained that enlightened management must rely on a variety of productivity measurement approaches. The role of nursing and the expected accomplishments of the nursing staff are negotiated at the uppermost administrative level in the organization. Professional bodies and regulatory agencies may publish recommended standards of practice for use in health care settings, but subtle nuances of interpretation, variations in leadership styles, and philosophical differences may cause one institution to function quite unlike another in the same community.

Part of the task of setting realistic productivity goals for the nursing unit staff may revolve around the geographic design of the work setting itself. Some nursing units are designed for better visibility of patients, efficient work flow, and less congested traffic patterns. Long corridors can mean more nursing staff footsteps to reach patients, supplies, charts, telephones, medications, computer support, and other personnel. The placement of patient rooms or care areas in relation to supply closets, utility rooms, medication stores, and even laundry shoots is a science and architectural art in itself.

Arranging for ancillary or support staff to deliver the most frequently used items to the patient's bedside may increase the productivity of the nursing staff by eliminating many unnecessary footsteps. Today's emphasis on patient-focused care has spawned a decentralization and redistribution of patient care equipment and staff (Watson, 1991).

Depending on the labor force employed by the organization and the priority with which patient needs are addressed, the amount and function of ancillary personnel may vary considerably. The staff nurse is wise to evaluate the institution's performance expectations of the individual nurse and of the entire unit's nursing staff before joining an organization, to determine whether practice according to one's philosophy and nursing standards is feasible.

Relating to Other Departments

Swenson, Wolfe, and Schroeder (1984) cited two studies that highlight the importance of effectively employing support services as a method of increasing the productivity of nursing personnel:

> A well-organized materials management department can cut an average of 1.5 nursing hours per patient day. That means, for a hospital with a daily census of 150 patients, a savings of 39.5 full-time equivalent personnel. With support service instead of nursing personnel performing logistics and transportation activities, potential salary savings can run $118,500 annually if the salary difference between the two personnel groups averages only $3,000. . .

> In a suburban hospital with an average daily census of 200 patients, 46 nursing service hours per day were devoted to transport: 26 in "unnecessary" patient transport and 20 in the transport of supplies, equipment and papers—clearly not nursing tasks, although necessary in providing patient care. About three-fourths of the trips, none requiring nursing participation, had been made by registered nurses, including head nurses and supervisors.

Almost 10 years after these studies, nursing managers are still documenting the same issues. Biuso, Lalor, and Mueller (1992) identified more than one dozen tasks (none of which required professional nursing skill or judgment) typically performed by registered nurses in their critical care division. These time-consuming contributions to patient care could have been handled by 2.8 full-time equivalent support staff members, in lieu of professional or licensed staff. The costs incurred by the hospital were estimated to be $45,427 more than required—because nurses were being paid to perform these jobs instead of ancillary personnel.

Support services personnel, ancillary staff, and other professionals are not on the payroll for the convenience or whim of the individual nurse staff member; neither are nurses on the payroll to "pick up the slack" or substitute routinely for other workers. Role definitions and primary job functions must be established according to licensure laws and standards of practice and in line with the financial resources of the institution and the labor force available within a community. On the other hand, overly strict delineation of task assignment can manifest itself as a collection of turf or kingdom battles; this outcome is detrimental to the smooth delivery of services and is equally costly in time delays and care interruptions. It is essential to negotiate these issues carefully with all parties involved.

If the general goals of all related departments within the health care setting are focused on the provision of care and services to the consumers, who are patients within the system, the stage is set for cooperative relationships between the departmental personnel who interact on a daily basis. Employee understanding of the basic institutional mission and the importance of patient satisfaction may help each staff group to view its daily tasks more in terms of "the needs of the patient or family" rather than "the needs of my department." Beyond the global raison d'être, the employee needs to understand the fit of each job within the structure of a department and the accepted intra- and interdepartmental communications required to accomplish that job.

The solutions to care delivery problems involving other staff members (whether across departments or across tours of duty) are discovered and negotiated more easily when the patient is the focus of everyone's problem-solving abilities. Delays in care are costly to the institution and inconvenient, if not detrimental, to patients. If vital information in a written request for diagnostic testing has been omitted by a staff nurse, an employee in another department may be forced to postpone a scheduled test until the appropriate information is supplied. If the patient has not been prepared for a diagnostic imaging procedure according to the standard or prescribed protocol, a full 24 hours or more may be required before another appropriate opportunity for testing may be arranged.

Similarly, the nurse may be hampered in the performance of patient care responsibilities if medications are not ordered correctly, dispensed accurately, and delivered to the patient care area on time. When assigned staff do not respond to patients' requests or needs within a reasonable amount of time, it is primarily the nursing staff that must deal with patients' questions, anger, or resultant complications in physical status.

There will always be a potential for human error in a system such as health care that functions with so much human involvement. Although human error and personality affect the delivery of care, most care delivery problems stem from flaws in the design of delivery systems and in the work flow and communications across the departments within a system. Continuous quality management programs may identify some issues related to patient care; it may take additional support from management engineers, internal auditors, and task forces of staff members to attack and solve the nagging and repetitive problems that disrupt the smooth operations and communications within and across departments.

PRODUCTIVITY OF THE INDIVIDUAL NURSE

Even when the nursing unit staff's collective productivity appears to be meeting the department's goals, attention to the practice of the individual within that work group is essential. Patient care provided by the individual staff nurse is a relatively intangible product. The professional component of the job greatly complicates the measurement of the individual's productivity by standard industrial engineering techniques such as time and motion study or work sampling. How does one account for the "think time" involved in patient care? How does one measure the amount of assessment or reevaluation performed at every contact with the patient?

Benner (1984) provided the groundbreaking research to document that the proficient and expert levels of practice are more difficult to explain and describe:

> The expert nurse, with her/his enormous background of experience, has an intuitive grasp of the situation and zeros in on the accurate region of the problem without wasteful consideration of a large range of unfruitful possible problem situations. It is very frustrating to try to capture verbal descriptions of expert performance because the expert operates from a deep understanding of the situation, much like the chess master who, when asked why he made a particularly masterful move, will say, "Because it felt right. It looked good."

The consideration of individual productivity must have its foundations both in the degree to which the individual approaches expert practice and in the philosophy by which one practices the profession. If productivity is the ratio of output per unit of input, then one must have a sense of one's output—in relation to outcomes, appropriateness of function, actual versus potential achievement, feedback from peers, and individual accountability.

A more wide-ranging look at the output of the individual staff nurse may incorporate the level of a nurse's contributions to the work environment and work systems. Does the staff nurse actively support fellow nurses and other personnel in the workplace? Is the individual advancing ideas to improve systems, ethics, and methods of care? Is the staff nurse participating diplomatically within the institution in such a way as to promote its philosophy and the highest standards of care? Is there a willingness to work fairly and forthrightly within the system to help bring about changes that may be beneficial to everyone involved?

Streamlined charting systems, flow sheet documentation tools, innovative plans of care, bedside computer support, group teaching and counseling, and packaged patient information programs are just some of the timesaving techniques being introduced around the country. These are all attempts to lead the individual staff nurse toward more efficient ways of meeting patient and family care needs. The staff nurse must be willing to experiment with these and other changes in the practice setting and to learn quickly and well those lessons that foster personal growth and professional expertise.

SUPPLY COSTS AND MATERIALS MANAGEMENT

The health care institution stocks myriad supply items, medications, and pieces of equipment. Its storerooms house the bulk of these items, with mini-storage areas set up in appropriate work stations or major departments throughout the organization. Some supplies must be packaged together to provide the convenience of correct assembly for use in a particular procedure. Many supplies must be sterilized for use in areas such as the delivery room, operating room, postanesthesia recovery, emergency department, intensive care units, and other specialty areas.

The availability and integrity of supply items is crucial to the delivery of patient care. The nurse must be confident that medications have not reached their expiration dates, that equipment is in good working order, and that supplies have not been damaged or contaminated in storage. A good materials management system may save money through standardization of products, purchasing products through group consortium arrangements, centralizing purchasing activities, establishing outsourcing agreements with vendors, and controlling inventories (Becker, 1989).

Staff nurses handle supplies and medications on a daily basis. As the professionals with the most consistent and constant patient contact and as the care givers responsible for carrying out the bulk of the treatment plan, nurses serve as the final link between the patient and most supply items (Myers, 1990). The nurse who exercises appropriate judgment in assessing and intervening with patients will use supplies and administer medications in a cost-effective manner.

Staff nurses should be involved in determining which supplies to purchase and stock in the institution. Many health care settings have established ongoing, multi-disciplinary committees to review the institution's supply needs. Once the purchasing decisions are made and the selected items arrive at the institution, the procedures for stocking and delivering the routine or requested items to patient care areas are set in motion. Determining realistic numbers of items to be stored at certain standard or par levels on the nursing unit may be accomplished by periodic surveys of what supplies are used and at what frequency.

Backup procedures for obtaining additional items or special requests must be designed to meet emergency situations or unusual fluctuations in workload. Stockpiling, overstocking, or hoarding supplies or medications may result in items becoming misplaced, damaged, or out-of-date. The costs of spoilage, obsolescence, and maintaining too much inventory must be minimized. Storing too many items in unsecured areas, where the general public may have access to them, can contribute to losses due to theft. Stealing by employees and others is estimated to cost the industry thousands of dollars per hospital bed per year (Wilkinson, 1986).

Recording the items used by individual patients during their hospital stays or visits is an extension of the exacting system of accounting that documents the costs or charges according to the care provided each patient. Good documentation on the patient record helps to substantiate the appropriateness of care administered (based on the individual needs of the patient) and offers rationales for the use of certain supplies and medications. Inadequate nursing charting or recordkeeping can lead to lost charges, which will not appear on the patient's bill, or charges that will be disallowed by insurance companies or other third-party payers who perform audits of patients' hospital bills. Beyond the direct cost of the item that will not be reimbursed to the hospital, there are other indirect charges for handling, storing, dispensing, and packaging supplies and medications for which the institution will not be paid.

THE NURSING CARE DELIVERY SYSTEM AND THE REQUIRED HUMAN RESOURCES

DECISIONS REGARDING MODALITY OF CARE

The choice of a nursing care delivery system (eg, case management, team nursing, patient-focused care, or primary nursing) is based on many factors. The administrative staff may evaluate the success of practice patterns used previously and of systems currently in use and in vogue in other community institutions. Executives may be forced to consider the available labor pool in the community and the institution's track record in recruitment and retention of qualified staff. Leadership styles and political factors may cause the institution's management team to choose a system that is not their ideal but is the only feasible alternative at the time. (Evaluation of various delivery systems is beyond the scope of this chapter and has been addressed in the nursing literature since Nightingale's time. See Chapter 3, Models of Patient Care Delivery, for further information on the choice of a nursing care delivery system.)

PLANNING FOR APPROPRIATE STAFFING

Once the basic modality of care has been chosen, a host of management decisions about the staffing of the nursing department must be addressed. The three most popular guidelines that managers use to determine the amount of total staff to supply care for a given group of patients are (1) nurse:patient ratios, (2) the target nursing hours of care per patient day, and (3) a patient acuity classification system. Other considerations focus on the skill mix of the staff—some combination of unlicensed, licensed, or professional personnel—and the distribution of the total staff over several tours of duty to provide care around-the-clock or whenever the department is open to clients.

The simplest option for determining the desired amount of staff may be the nurse:patient ratio. The types of patients commonly housed on a given nursing unit are reviewed to discover their usual nursing care needs and the estimated workload they place on the nursing personnel. A reasonable nurse:patient ratio or staff:patient ratio that will support the particular care delivery system is determined for each tour of duty and becomes the basis for daily assignment patterns on the unit.

Another method of planning for the total amount of staff establishes a standard of the average amount of nursing care a patient will receive in a 24-hour period. This is expressed in a numerical value of nursing care hours per patient day (HPPD). The expression of a daily HPPD figure is calculated using the following formula:

$$HPPD = \frac{total\ number\ of\ shifts\ worked/day \times hours\ of\ care/shift}{average\ number\ of\ patients/day\ (census)}$$

For example, if everyone worked an 8-hour tour of duty, and the staff supplied to a given unit in a 24-hour period broke down to 6 staff on day shift, 4 staff on evening shift, and 3 staff on night shift, then the total of 13 staff would have worked a total of 104 hours. If, during that same 24-hour period, the staff cared for 24 patients, then the 104 hours of care supplied to a total of 24 patients would have resulted in an average amount of care per patient of 4.33 HPPD. Fitting the numbers into the formula results in the following solution:

$$HPPD = \frac{13\ shifts\ worked/day \times 8\ hours\ of\ care/shift\ worked}{24\ patients/day}$$

$$= \frac{13 \times 8\ hours\ of\ care/day}{24\ patients/day}$$

$$= \frac{104\ hours\ of\ care}{24\ patients}$$

$$HPPD = 4.33\ average\ hours\ of\ care\ per\ patient$$

Although this formula is a classic in the health care industry, problems are encountered when managers attempt to compare their HPPD statistics with those of other units or hospitals. There may be subtle differences in identification of the formula's elements.

First, who is counted in the number of total staff? Some institutions include the nurse manager, unit secretaries, and everyone assigned to the unit; other departments may count only those staff members who are involved in the direct, hands-on care of patients.

Second, can we expect any staff member to be fully productive during the entire tour of duty for which the nurse or aide is being paid? Most hospitals acknowledge that the employee needs a periodic rest break in addition to a meal break, and many institutions' personnel policies identify two 15-minute breaks per tour of duty as the normal expectation. That allowance would automatically reduce the expected work time from 8 full hours to 7.5 hours. Beyond the scheduled break times, industrial and management engineers often acknowledge an additional "personal fatigue and delay" factor that should be considered in conjunction with mentally, emotionally, or physically taxing work.

The third component of the standard formula—"average census"—can also be questioned. Does the institution use a midnight, afternoon, or morning census figure? What about those patients who may be transferred in or out of the unit during the normal course of the day? With the fluctuations in occupancy rates experienced in many settings and the number of transfers logged in some nursing units, it is difficult to understand how the simple census or patient day figure can be used as a measure of nursing workload. Finally and probably most important, the number of beds occupied does not depict any variations in care needs of those patients.

Some of the most extensive research done in an attempt to compare nursing hour figures across hospitals was performed by the National Association of Children's Hospitals and Related Institutions (NACHRI). To view data consistently and make more appropriate comparisons between units, the NACHRI Nurse-Staffing Data Program collected detailed information for a hospital profile and an individual patient care unit profile. However, Gorman and Borovies (1985) found that even with this sophisticated approach there were astounding variations in nursing HPPD standards among like units caring for like patients:

> The total hospital median or worked nursing hours per patient day was 11.8 hours. Individual hospital values ranged from 8.2 to 14 hours. The median of worked hours per patient day for the medical–surgical units was 9.3, with the intensive care units recording a median value of 22.6 hours. The ranges in worked hours per patient day for the medical–surgical units and intensive care units were 5.9 to 14.7 hours and 16.2 to 30 hours, respectively

Patient classification systems are a third method for assisting administrators in assigning the total number of staff. These systems were developed in an attempt to project the nursing workload from assessment of the acuity level (or level of illness) of the patients in question. In the course of their clinical experience, nurses learn very quickly that the number of patients housed on a given unit may not be as significant as the types of patients counted in that department's census. As clinicians, nurses appreciate that medical and nursing diagnoses are only basic factors that may provide some inkling of the amount of nursing care needed by an individual patient. The patient's age, anxiety level, dependency needs, intellectual capacities, and cultural background will have impact on the individualized plan of care. Underlying diseases, past health history, previous hospital experiences, amount of family support, language barriers, psychological trauma, emotional stability, or relationships with other health care team members will also influence the priority level of the nurse's involvement with that client.

In her classic work on this subject, Giovannetti (1979) supplied the pertinent definitions related to this complex topic:

> In nursing, the term patient classification means the categorization of patients according to some assessment of their nursing care requirements over a specified period of time. The most common purpose has been for determination and assignment of nursing care personnel . . . To encompass both the definition and the purpose, the term patient classification system is commonly used. It refers to the identification and classification of patients into care groups or categories, and to the quantification of these categories as a measure of the nursing effort required.

There are a multitude of patient classification schemes in use today, employing varying levels of sophistication, background research, reliability and validity studies, and philosophical approaches (Kelleher, 1992; McHugh & Dwyer, 1992). Moreover, the actual use of classification systems varies from a token use during accreditation visits to daily use for the purposes of variable staffing decisions and, in a few settings, variable patient billing (Nagaprasanna, 1988; Prescott, 1991).

In an institution that takes patient classification systems seriously and applies the data to management decision making, the accuracy and reliability of the periodic classification results may be of paramount importance. The data may serve as a guideline for annual staffing budgets, shift-to-shift assignment of staff across nursing units, and intradepartmental assignments of individual staff nurses to specific caseloads of patients. In these settings, staff nurses on the same unit and the same tour of duty would not necessarily be assigned equal numbers of patients; their patient caseloads might vary according to the acuity information and such management parameters as the expertise of the individual staff member or other duties assigned.

Giovannetti (1979) reminds the industry that "patient classification systems are based on a unidimensional and partial assessment of patient requirements for care." It would be impossible to document every iota of care required by every individual patient; an attempt to do so would result in tools far too cumbersome for the staff to use in periodic assessment. Moreover, most patient classification schemes focus on the quantification of care supplied through the existing practice of nursing on a given unit, not necessarily the ideal practice (Giovanetti and Mayer, 1984). Accounting for this potentially major difference would require separate quality monitoring systems or performance evaluation mechanisms to evaluate the quality of the outcomes of care.

The final issue likely to affect staffing plans and their budgetary impact is the specific collection of personnel policies and scheduling practices unique to each setting. The distribution of staff around the 24-hour time frame may be influenced by the amount of shift differential, if any, that is promised and paid to employees. Weekend and holiday scheduling patterns, some of which may involve bonus pay, must be taken into account. Policies related to sick, vacation, and holiday time, and which employees are eligible for how much, may influence the number of part-time workers the organization will attempt to hire. The availability (or lack of availability) of supplemental staff who might fill in temporarily during periods of high census and acuity might influence the administration to employ fewer (or more) full-time staff in a given unit.

Staffing and scheduling decisions represent a major effort in the budgeting process of the organization. Executive financial negotiations often center around the number of part-time, full-time, permanent, temporary, per diem, or float staff that will be approved for the next fiscal year for each department. The staff nurse needs to understand as much as possible the specific institutional process of these decisions and contribute to the accurate collection of pertinent data that may influence key decision and policy makers.

HIDDEN HUMAN RESOURCES COSTS

Finally, there are other related personnel costs incurred by the institution that are not as obvious as the salaries and benefits received by the employees. Hoffman (1985) identified the top four costs:

- Advertising and recruiting
- Hiring
- Orientation and training
- Turnover

Advertising and recruiting costs include everything from the salaries of recruiters and the cost of classified advertisements in professional journals to attendance at school career days and special externship programs that hire senior nursing students. Hiring involves interviewing time, the processing of applications, many types of correspondence, and the payment of moving expenses for some workers. Hoffman's list of several major costs related to orientation and training includes the salaries of the educational staff, costs of supplies, the overhead on the building space used in education, and the preceptor time of the experienced staff who provide orientation for new employees. When an employee leaves the organization, personnel policies may dictate that the individual be compensated for some amount of accrued benefit time that had not been taken. If the vacated position is not filled in a timely manner, the institution may be forced to pay hundreds of dollars in replacement staff costs for temporary workers or in overtime to regular staff who work extra duty.

THE NEW NURSE'S ROLE IN HEALTH CARE FINANCIAL MANAGEMENT

UNDERSTANDING THE NEW ORIENTATION OF HEALTH CARE

For a variety of complex economic reasons, the hospital industry is experiencing the most challenging period in its history. Nurses will need to understand the meaning of and accept the use of the terms *profit* and *productivity* as part of their everyday language. Clinical professionals must be aware of the business side and the new trends of health care financing. It is important to be an educated consumer and an educated provider of health services. If the industry's new directions are recognized, it is easier to accept the expanded role now required of the staff nurse.

Just after the advent of the 1983 prospective payment structure, one prominent nurse executive realized that nurses and physicians may control up to 80% of the resources used in patient care (Twyon, 1985). Her nursing staff, already adept at primary nursing practice, rallied to the concepts of case management and more collaborative practice patterns with physicians. The staff nurse, as a case manager in this system, has been "accountable for meeting outcomes within (1) an appropriate length of stay, (2) the effective use of resources and (3) established standards" (Zander, 1985). This model for addressing the new orientation of health care has stood the test of time and has been implemented successfully in many hospital settings around the country.

UNDERSTANDING THE MARKETING ASPECTS
OF THE NURSE'S JOB

Patients' perceptions of the quality of care are critically important to the marketing of the institution's services—even if those perceptions are not consistent with carefully developed nursing definitions of quality. Although the latter may have a greater effect on patient outcomes, in this competitive environment, the former may have a greater effect on hospital outcomes (or survival).

Patients expect competence from health care professionals. Through customer relations programs and other promotions, hospitals are becoming more attentive to the impressions that employees may leave with the patient. Nurses often are in the best vantage point to discover what patients want from their health care providers and to generate ideas for new and appropriate services that will increase the attractiveness of the institution in the local community. If physicians, as individuals or in groups, still hold the key to large numbers of admissions, the nursing staff plays a pivotal role in advising the administration on the best strategies for approaching those physicians. The kind of care supplied by the nursing staff and the creative ideas of the clinical care givers that come to fruition may develop into the strongest draw for physicians and consumers alike (Okorafor, 1983).

UNDERSTANDING CHANGES BROUGHT ABOUT
BY ECONOMIC REALITIES

The health care industry is experiencing a form of "reality shock" all its own—and on a national scale. The political climate may change under each new presidential administration, but health care philosophy and economics will undoubtedly continue to evolve as society faces difficult funding and access decisions (Rooks, 1990). In addressing the issue of paying for health care, other countries have opted for socialized medical systems and variations on that theme (Southby & Rakich, 1991). The United States economy, however, is based on capitalistic beliefs and the principles of an open market. Some aspects of this free market system are now being used to regulate the health care industry.

An organization's economic "accountability to society" is measured in part by its profit and its ability to deliver goods or services at a quality and cost that society can embrace. How "embraceable" will the health care industry become, and how much change will those involved have to endure (or enjoy)? The understated response is that the changes are happening fast and that the system is evolving slowly.

SUMMARY

Nursing practice patterns and behaviors have a profound impact on the financial picture of the health care agency. To understand the pressures now coming to bear on the entire system and on the role of the nurse, the staff nurse must keep abreast of changes in the political arena, the marketplace, and the work setting. Change is inevitable, and economic realities will drive the change. With the proper understanding and skills, we in nursing can participate in and contribute to this evolutionary and revolutionary process.

DISCUSSION QUESTIONS

1. Within the context of health care reform, financial issues in nursing will change professional practice. Describe five major trends that you will need to consider when delivering care to patients.
2. Make a list of common nursing practices that must be accomplished in increasingly cost-effective ways. How will you ensure cost-effective practices?
3. Study a clinical setting in which you have delivered care, and describe at least three ways that productivity of the staff could be improved.

REFERENCES

Becker, E. G. (1989). Formal plan for major equipment purchases saves money. *Healthcare Financial Management, 43*(8), 26–32.

Benner, P. (1984). *From novice to expert.* Reading, MA: Addison-Wesley.

Biuso, J., Lalor, L., & Mueller, L. (1992). Non-nursing task: Do they make "cents"? *Nursing Management, 23*(9), 128L–128P.

Edwardson, S. R. (1985). Measuring nursing productivity. *Nursing Economic$, 3*(1), 9–14.

Giovannetti, P. (1979). Understanding patient classification systems. *Journal of Nursing Administration, 9*(2), 4–9.

Giovannetti, P., & Mayer, G. G. (1984). Building confidence in patient classification systems. *Nursing Management, 15*(8), 31–34.

Gorman, M., & Borovies, D. L. (1985). Comparative nursing hours in tertiary pediatric facilities. *Nursing Economic$, 3*(5), 146–151.

Hoffman, F. (1985). Cost per RN hired. *Journal of Nursing Administration, 15*(2), 27–29.

Jelinek, R. (1979). The relationship between productivity and cost containment. In B. J. Jaeger (Ed.), *Evaluating Hospital Productivity.* Durham, NC: Department of Health Administration, Duke University.

Jones, K. R. (1989). Evolution of the prospective payment system: Implications for nursing. *Nursing Economic$, 7*(6), 299–305.

Kelleher, C. (1992). Validated indexes: Key to nursing acuity standardization. *Nursing Economic$, 10,* 31–37.

Lee, J. G., & Clarke, R. W. (1992). Restructuring improves hospital competitiveness. *Healthcare Financial Management, 46*(11), 30–37.

McHugh, M. L., & Dwyer, V. L. (1992). Measurement issues in patient acuity classification for prediction of hours in nursing care. *Nursing Administration Quarterly, 16*(4), 20–31.

Myers, S. (1990). Material management: Nurses' involvement. *Nursing Management, 21*(8), 30–32.

Nagaprasanna, B. (1988). Patient classification systems: Strategies for the 1990's. *Nursing Management, 19*(3), 105–112.

Okorafor, H. (1983). Hospital characteristics attractive to physicians and the consumer: Implications for public general hospitals. *Hospital and Health Services Administration, 28*(2), 50–65.

Prescott, P. A. (1991). Nursing intensity: Needed today for more than staffing. *Nursing Economic$, 9,* 409–414.

Rooks, J. P. (1990). Lets admit we ration health care—then set priorities. *American Journal of Nursing, 90*(6), 39–43.

Schwartz, W. B., & Mendelson, D. N. (1991). Hospital cost containment in the 1990s: Hard lessons learned and prospects for the 1990s. *New England Journal of Medicine, 24*(15), 1037–1042.

Smalley H. E., & Freeman J. R. (1966). *Hospital industrial engineering.* New York: Reinhold.

Southby, R. F., & Rakich, J. S. (1991). International healthcare expenditures. *Hospital Topics,* pp 8–13.

Swenson, B., Wolfe, H. B., & Schroeder, R. (1984). Effectively employing support services the key for increasing nursing personnel productivity. *Modern Healthcare, 14*(51), 101–104.

Twyon, S. (1985, August). Fiscal environment 1985. *Network Q Newsletter.* (Available from Massachusetts Organization for Nurse Executives).

Watson, P. M., Lower, M.S., Wells, S.M., Farrah, S.J., & Jarrel, C. (1991). Discovering what nurses do and what it costs. *Nursing Management, 22*(5), 38–45.

Wilkinson, R. (1986). Murders get the press, but theft is the problem. *Hospitals, 60*(7), 97–98.

Young, S. T. (1992). Multiple productivity measurement approaches for management. *Health Care Management Review, 17*(2), 51–58.

Zander, K. (1979, May). Achieving the goals of the primary nursing care. Paper presented at Baptist Hospital of Miami, Florida.

Zander, K. (1985). Defining nursing . . . roots and wings. *Definition, 1*(1), 1, The Center for Nursing Case Management.

SUGGESTED READING

Barrett, M. J. (1989). How nurses can help hospitals achieve financial goals. *Healthcare Financial Management, 43*(6), 64–70.

Barron, J., Hollander, S. F., & Smith, M. (1992). Cost reductions (Part II): An organizational culture perspective. *Nursing Economic$, 10,* 402–405.

Blodgett, T. B. (1989). Why General Mills mixes in health care. *Harvard Business Review, 67*(2) 32–36.

Budd, M. C., Blaufuss, J., & Harada, S. (1988). Nursing: A revenue center, not a cost center. *Computers in Healthcare, 9*(11), 24–26

Campbell, B. (1992). Assessment of attitudes toward cost-containment needs. *Nursing Economic$, 10,* 397–401.

Capuano, T. A., Fox, M. A., & Gresh, B. (1992). Staffing nurses according to episodic census variations. *Nursing Management, 23*(10), 34–37.

Cleverley, W. O., & Harvey, R. K. (1992). Is there a link between hospital profit and quality? *Healthcare Financial Management, 46*(9), 40–45.

Cleverley, W. O. (1992). *Essentials of health care finance* (3rd ed.). Gaithersburg, MD: Aspen.

Deines, E. (1985). Coping with PPS and DRGs: The levels-of-care approach. *Nursing Management, 16*(10), 43–52.

Ethridge, P., & Lamb, G. S. (1989). Professional nursing care management improves quality, access and costs. *Nursing Management, 20*(3), 30–35.

Finkler, S. A. (1992). *Budgeting concepts for nurse managers* (2nd ed.). Philadelphia: W. B. Saunders.

Fisher, R., & Ury, W. (1981). *Getting to yes.* Boston: Houghton Mifflin.

Goddard, N. L. (1985). *The workbook on financial management, staffing and budgeting for nursing.* Houston: Goddard Management Resources.

Hollander, S. F., Smith, M., & Barron, J. (1992). Cost reductions (Part I): An operations improvement process. *Nursing Economic$, 10,* 325–330, 364.

Jones, C. B. (1992). Calculating and updating nursing turnover costs. *Nursing Economic$, 10,* 39–45.

Lipetzky, P. W. (1990). Cost analysis and the clinical nurse specialist. *Nursing Management, 21*(8), 25, 28.

Loevisohn, H. T. (1992). A new perspective on scheduling: Freedom and cost control. *Nursing Management, 23*(7), 56–61.

McDonagh, K. J., & Sorensen, M. A. (1988). Restructuring nursing salaries: A mandate for the future. *Nursing Management, 19*(2), 39–41.

Nelson, B. J., & Blasdell, A. L. (1988). Comparing quality on eight- and twelve-hour shifts. *Nursing Management, 19*(11), 64A–64H.

Oszustowicz, R. J. (1992). Quality of care emerges as a determinant of creditworthiness. *Healthcare Financial Management, 46*(3), 48–58.

Patterson, C. (1992). The economic value of nursing. *Nursing Economic$, 10,* 193–204.

Ringl, K. D., & Dotson, L. (1989). Self-scheduling for professional nurses. *Nursing Management, 20*(2), 42–44.

Sharp, N. (1991). Direct reimbursement for nurses. *Nursing Management, 22*(1), 34–35.

Shepard, R. (1988). 'Cadillac Care': Advances in technology raise cost-control questions. *Healthcare Financial Management, 42*(11), 23–28.

Soule, T. R., & Dobson, J. M. (1992). SEPPD and HPPD: More effective control of nursing care costs. *Nursing Economic$, 10,* 205–209.

Sovie, M. D., Tarcinale, M.A., Van Putee, A.W., & Stunden, A.E. (1993). Amalgam of nursing acuity, DRG's and costs. *Nursing Management, 16*(3), 22–28, 32–34, 38, 40, 42.

St. Morris, K. K. (1992). Criteria for selection of an automated "intelligent" scheduling system. *Nursing Administration Quarterly, 16*(4), 70–77.

Stefan, S., Gillies, D. A., & Biordi, D. (1992). Nursing care costs for a DRG subgroup. *Nursing Economic$, 10,* 277–281.

Stuart, G. W. (1986). An organizational strategy for empowering nursing. *Nursing Economic$, 4*(2), 69–73.

Swansburg, R. C., & Sowell, R. L. (1992). A model for costing and pricing nursing service. *Nursing Management, 23*(2), 33–36.

Vaughan, R. G., & MacLeod, V. (1985). Comparing acuity among hospitals—Who has the sickest patients? *Journal of Nursing Administration, 15*(5), 25–28.

Zachry, B. R., & Gilbert, R. L. (1992). Director of nursing planning and finance: A new role. *Nursing Management, 23*(2), 50–52.

9

Managing Your Work Setting: Positive Work Relationships, Conflict Management, and Negotiations

Susan Roe

LEARNING OBJECTIVES

This chapter will enable you to:

1. Apply strategies necessary to build a positive work climate.
2. Use "power balancing" as a means of developing collegial relationships.
3. Outline the method for building teams using principles of teamwork.
4. Manage conflict using strategies of positive confrontation.
5. Discuss approaches for successful negotiation.

Vestal, K.W. Nursing Management:
Concepts and Issues, 2 ed.
© 1995 J.B. Lippincott Company

Cost-effective avenues for delivering quality health care services, technology management, and the demand for and effective use of human resources are just a few of the concerns of nurses and those who manage the systems in which they work. The health care environment will continue to be complex and turbulent as we approach the 21st century with changing requirements and goals. Intrinsic to the successful management of change in the work setting is the development of a positive work climate, the resolution of organizational and interpersonal conflict, and the successful negotiation for services and resources.

Some health care organizations have survived because they have been able to expand their marketability and services, whereas others have become vulnerable and foundered. Organizations often find that a significant contributor to their demise is the disgruntled or disenfranchised employee who feels alienated from the organization's objectives and the mission of delivering quality care.

Health care organizations that fare well are those committed to a vision and mission and those that provide opportunities for workers to develop skills and become involved in the organization's future. In these organizations, a positive work climate fosters success in the marketplace and promotes effective delivery of quality patient care. A positive work climate is built through an understanding of the organization's vision and mission and the development of cohesive work relationships. Excellence in work relationships requires establishing rapport, developing collegial relationships, and building teams. Effective conflict management and negotiation provides further assistance in facing difficult situations and achieving necessary organizational and departmental goals.

MANAGING WORK SETTINGS

Nurses can manage a work setting effectively if a positive work climate is established. Establishing such a climate is a worthwhile task, although it is difficult to take a large and diverse group of people who have specific roles and ask them to work harmoniously to achieve prescribed objectives. Climbing Mount Everest might seem easier; however, with thoughtful planning, necessary resources and skills, concentrated energy, and commitment, the goal is attainable.

The payoffs for investing in departmental human resources and building a positive work climate are many. Potential outcomes include the satisfaction of using one's individual and teamwork skills to their

148

fullest, greater job satisfaction, and the excitement of experiencing a fully functioning team and organization.

There are three essential components in developing a positive work climate:

- Establishing rapport
- Developing collegial relationships
- Building a team

In addition, the ability to manage conflict and negotiate successfully for particular outcomes and resources ensures a positive environment and enables nurses to achieve organizational and departmental objectives.

Because conflict (eg, informational, perceptual, emotional, or value differences) is a normal occurrence in all work groups, understanding conflict and determining how to bring differences to productive resolution are necessary to ensure continuance of a positive work climate. The ability to negotiate with others for needed resources is imperative to maintain the positive work environment.

If you and those involved in delivering care in your department want to work effectively, feel good about what is done, grow as individuals and professionals, and influence your organization positively, read on. This chapter provides theories, concepts, and techniques to assist you in managing your work setting.

ESTABLISHING RAPPORT

Positive relationships include communication patterns that are built on trust, clarity, common goal orientations, and collaboration. The basis for positive relationships is rapport. When similarities rather than differences are emphasized, rapport is more easily established (Richardson & Margulis, 1981). In nursing settings, rapport is established by setting a tone that is mutually growth producing—by treating each other as allies and maintaining a common goal of enhancing each other's practice.

In *Megatrends 2000,* by Naisbitt and Aburdene (1990), a leader is described as an "individual who builds followership by ethical conduct and by creating an environment where the unique potential of one individual can be actualized." Establishing rapport, then, focuses on what each individual can contribute.

Setting a positive tone in a health care environment requires a work philosophy that focuses on what can be done, rather than on what cannot be done. For example, concentrating on what was accomplished at the end of a shift or workday allows nurses and their colleagues to feel the day was productive. Sometimes just getting through the day is accomplishment enough.

A positive tone means that the underlying perceptual base for communicating is a positive one. The nurse who is able to set a positive tone sees work as "half-full," rather than "half-empty." Assessment of situations and the wording of assessments should focus on strengths. Although not all situations are positive, those areas that are perceived as weaknesses should be seen as learning opportunities. Additionally, nurses must be aware and sensitive to the multicultural diversity among their colleagues.

Giving positive feedback or compliments to others can reinforce strengths. When a nurse notes another's strength, that individual tends to repeat the positive behavior or action. Compliments promote positive feelings about one's work and skills and about others in the work environment. Feedback provides an opportunity for self-growth through the assessment of another's skills. "Compliments beget more compliments."

Despite the potential growth-producing aspects of feedback, most responses to compliments tend to negate compliment giving. More often than not, recipients become embarrassed when positive feedback is given and respond by negating the compliment. Unfortunately, this indicates to compliment givers that they are ineffective evaluators. Consequently, few compliments are given.

To ensure a positive tone that promotes rapport, use the following guidelines for giving and receiving feedback:

1. Give positive feedback on genuine characteristics, qualities, or behaviors. Giving a compliment just for the sake of doing so will be seen as manipulative and suspicious.
2. Use "I" statements when giving positive feedback. The assessment must have the appropriate frame of reference.
3. Be specific about what is shared. Concentrate on what the individual did and describe it in behavioral terms: "I was impressed with the way you handled Mrs. Lane's son. Your willingness to listen to his complaints helped ease his anxiety about his mother's illness."
4. When receiving positive feedback, simply say "thank you." This response demonstrates to the compliment giver that the evaluation was acknowledged.
5. Allow the richness of the compliment to penetrate. Positive feedback is a means of generating energy. It is a gift. Enjoy it.
6. Encourage further compliments by adding: "I appreciate that you shared that with me."

The selection of encouraging words, however, is not enough. Nonverbal communication must be congruent with the spoken communication. Positive words are perceived as positive when the body language conveys the same message. Inconsistency between verbal and nonverbal communication results in the receiver responding more to the facial and vocal expressions than to the words (Mehrabian, 1971). To convey a willingness to listen, use direct eye contact and "open" body gestures (eg, arms to the sides, not folded across the chest).

A positive tone in work settings is contagious. Concerted energy toward establishing rapport can influence an entire work group. Just one nurse's efforts can encourage others to look at work as a meaningful challenge in which strengths are identified and shared and there is clarity in and congruence between words, expressions, and gestures.

Total quality leaders draw out their workers. They encourage the contribution of ideas, creativity, and attention to detail and processes, so that employees work at their greatest capacity (Covey, 1991). Such positive environments build foundations for the development of collegial relationships.

DEVELOPING COLLEGIAL RELATIONSHIPS

Collegiality occurs when one nurse reaches out to another to establish a relationship in which both exert equal influence or power. It is only when a "power balance" exists among two parties (ie, a willingness to collaborate or share power resources) that a collegial relationship can occur (Figure 9-1).

For example, suppose an experienced nurse chooses not to help a newly assigned nurse because no one helped when that nurse was new. You can be sure that if this "power imbalance" continues, it will not take long before an adversarial relationship develops between these two nurses. The experienced nurse has a great deal of power in the form of information and expertise, whereas the new nurse has very little. Only when the experienced nurse shares information and expertise freely will the power between the two be balanced and a collegial relationship established.

This power-balancing process incorporates the interactional components of setting a positive tone. Nurses must be motivated to work together, to appreciate differences, and to communicate directly and freely. Nurses must develop clear communication patterns and skills and set personal goals for building teams and being team players.

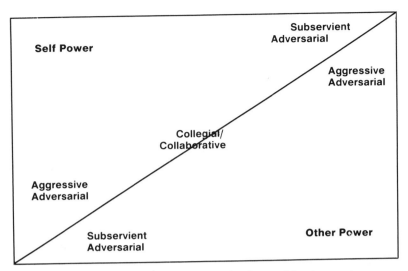

FIG 9-1. Model for developing collegial relationships in nursing.

BUILDING TEAMS

Building teams and encouraging teamwork does not occur just because a group of individuals happens to work together. Because work groups are composed of human beings they can be considered "organic." Therefore, to function fully, teams must be carefully planned and must mature. A Team Effectiveness Model (Plunkett & Fournier, 1991) provides a simplified approach to building a team. Nurses who want to build a team must concentrate on team goals, member roles, processes, and relationships.

Well-functioning teams include the following five R's (Jackman & Waggoner, 1991):

RESULTS	The team envisions the goals.
RULES	Guidelines govern the team members' behavior.
RITUALS	There is team action to meet goals.
ROLES	Members fill a variety of roles, and timelines are established.
RECOGNITION	Strengths of team and team members are identified.

With the many changes now taking place in nursing care delivery, it has never been as important for the nurse to incorporate "team thinking" into a repertoire of skills. According to Bragg (1992), members of effective teams:

- Share leadership responsibilities
- Cooperate
- Share ideas freely
- Listen attentively and accommodate the concerns of others
- Seek creative solutions when viewpoints differ
- Forego personal recognition for the sake of the team
- Recognize and support the contributions of other members

Team players are the most important ingredients for a successful team. Teamwork is not always easy. There are many different individuals to deal with on a daily basis, and challenges often occur (eg, when members block any one of the above guidelines). As a result, it is crucial to understand conflict and to know how to deal effectively with differences among people.

MANAGING CONFLICT

Whenever two persons come together, there is a potential for conflict because individuals have unique ways of perceiving or "seeing" situations and understanding information. Consequently, when perceptions and understandings of situations or information differ, conflict occurs. Therefore, conflict may be defined simply as "differences" between and among individuals or groups. Interpersonal conflict occurs between individuals or groups, whereas intrapersonal conflict takes place within an individual (eg, a nurse having difficulty choosing one job over another).

Conflict within the work setting is a natural phenomenon. If no conflict ever occurred and there was always complete agreement, everyone would think alike, much like robots. Not only would the work environment be dull and boring, but no progress would be made. Creativity would not exist. Although conflict occurs as a normal part of work, it quickly grows in intensity if ignored. Thus, the goal in conflict management is to intervene quickly and positively.

Confrontation can be an exciting challenge, and the results well worth the investment. When conflict is handled well, a great deal of learning and an understanding of different interactions can occur. Communication between persons increases as relationships grow. However, liking a person better is not the intended outcome. Being able to work together more effectively is the goal. Other positive outcomes of conflict include the generation of new ideas and new solutions to difficult problems.

Conflict abounds in our health environment. There are conflicts between health care organizations and society as persons ask for health services in quantities and at levels of quality that cannot be delivered. Changing demographics and limited finances have stimulated professional groups to vie for the client's attention. Conflicts occur between the private and public sectors as federal and state governments attempt to determine their appropriate roles in the financing and delivery of care. As resources become scarce, health care organizations encounter increased internal conflicts, in which personnel or work units compete for their "fair share." With a health care environment facing shrinking resources and increasing demands, it has never been more important for nurses to become comfortable with conflict management.

Managing conflict is much like assessing and intervening when there is a client problem. Often, causal factors must be identified by determining the differences that created the conflict. For instance, there may be conflict because a nurse did not provide enough or accurate information to make the most effective decision. The causal factor may be conflicting facts, emotions, perceptions, or values. Knowing the cause of the conflict helps determine the ease with which it can be resolved. It is much easier to deal with difference in information than to come to terms with differing values, such as the ethics related to the "right to die."

Successful conflict management must account for personal emotional barriers, including differences in individuals' perceptions of conflict. One's perception of conflict arises from messages sent over time by parents and significant others. Suppose a nurse learns as a child that conflict is negative and should be avoided. When this nurse encounters conflict, he or she may avoid the issue rather than confront it. Likewise, nurses who perceive that conflict is harmful or threatening may take an aggressive stance.

Perceptions of conflict have been linked to traditional gender roles. Many women were socialized into believing that they were not suited to the vagaries of conflict. Being angry was not considered an acceptable response, and women were expected to avoid conflict or to accommodate others when differences occurred. This message can cause women to feel fearful and powerless when confronted with conflict. Today, gender socialization and parental messages about conflict are changing. Children are being taught that conflict can be positive. Nonetheless, the remnants of the past still influence a great segment of our population.

The frustration and anger associated with conflict are major barriers to conflict management. Anger occurs as a result of a perceived threat, for example when one nurse "puts down" another by criticizing client care skills. The criticized nurse then makes assumptions about the intensity of the threat and determines how much power is needed to ward it off. If the threat is not perceived as dangerous or if the nurse feels powerful enough to confront it positively, the nurse will not become angry. If, however, the threat is perceived as dangerous or if a feeling of powerlessness emerges, anger erupts for protection (Kelley, 1979). This process is circular and can intensify as conflicts repeat themselves (Figure 9-2).

Although anger is a common response to conflict, it can become a barrier to conflict management because it is difficult to problem solve rationally while feeling intense emotions. Dealing with these emotional barriers is one of the most difficult aspects of conflict management. To help control such emotion and manage conflict effectively, a problem assessment and intervention process using positive confrontation should be employed. This rational approach includes six steps:

Assess

1. Analyze the situation. Identify the type of conflict to determine the time investment. Review the facts and validate any assumptions through further investigation. Examine who is involved and the role played. Determine if the situation can be changed. Become aware of personal messages that are blocking the ability to act. Realize that the other individuals involved may be dealing with similar blockage.

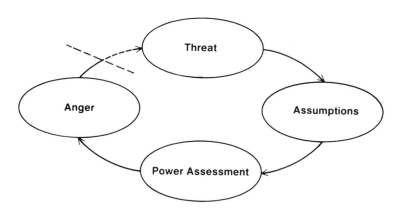

FIG 9-2. The anger cycle. (Illustration by John E. Jones and Anthony G. Banet, Jr. Reprinted from Pfeiffer JW. Jones JE [eds]: The 1976 Annual Handbook for Group Facilitators. San Diego. University Associates, Inc., 1976 Used with permission)

2. Identify and confine the issue. Describe the problem and prioritize the issues. Often, there are many issues, some of which are more critical than others. Determine which issue is crucial to solving the problem and start with that one. Attempting to resolve more than one issue at a time can lead to confusion and frustration.
3. Set the objective. Visualize and describe the outcome of positive confrontation.

Identify

4. Manage the feelings. Anger is a personal choice that can be avoided by identifying what triggers it. Each person has a unique response to certain words, actions, and expressions. Whatever the situation, should that word, action, or expression be used by another individual, anger will quickly emerge. It could, for example, result from a particular tone of voice that may sound condescending. If a person is aware of the trigger, then becoming angry is truly a choice.
Check the reality of assumptions that are made. Assumptions are the stimulus for assessing power. The more factual the assumptions, the stronger the feeling of power. The intent is to feel as powerful as possible. The equation is simple. As the feeling of power increases, the probability of becoming angry decreases.

Intervene

5. Enter the conflict believing that it will be resolved. Identify what the positive outcome will be.
6. Select the appropriate method for resolving the conflict. Conflicts require different methods of resolution. Selection of a method depends on desired outcomes. Each method requires a different set of skills (Table 9-1).

Two methods often selected for conflict resolution are compromise and collaboration. The major difference between them lies in the intended outcome and the time needed to reach it.

Of the two methods, collaboration is considered more growth producing even though it takes a considerable amount of time. The goal of collaboration is to have both parties win: No one is asked to give up anything. The problem-solving process continues until each individual is satisfied with the resolution. Both time and skills in prob-

TABLE 9–1 METHODS FOR RESOLVING CONFLICT

METHOD	RESULTS	APPROPRIATE	INAPPROPRIATE	SKILLS REQUIRED
Denial or withdrawal	Person tries to solve problem by denying its existence; results in win–lose	When issues are relatively unimportant; when issue is raised at inopportune time	When issue is important, when it will not disappear, but will build to greater complexity	Judgment of what is needed in the situation
Suppression or smoothing over	Differences are played down; results in win–lose	Same as above; also when preservation of relationship is more important than issue	When evasion of issue will disrupt relationship; when others are ready and willing to deal with issue	Empathy
Power or dominance	Authority, position, majority rule, or a persuasive minority settles the conflict; results in win–lose	When authority is granted by one's position; also when group has agreed on method of decision making	When those without power have no means to express their needs and ideas, especially if this lack of opportunity has the potential for future disruption	Decision making; running effective meetings
Compromise or negotiation	Each party gives up something to meet midway; results in some loss of each side's position	When both sides have enough leeway to give; when resources are limited; when win–lose stance is undesirable.	When original position is inflated or unrealistic; when solution must be watered down to be acceptable; when commitment by both parties is doubtful	Attentive listening and paraphrasing; problem solving
Collaboration	Individual abilities and expertise are recognized; each person's position is clear, but emphasis is on group solution; results in win–win. When time is available to complete process; when parties are committed to and trained in use of process	When time is limited; when parties lack training in or commitment to collaborative efforts	Attentive listening and paraphrasing; problem solving	Attentive listening and paraphrasing; problem solving

(Hart, L.B.: Moving up! Women and leadership. New York: AMACOM [1980]. Leadership Dynamics. P.O.Box 20. Reprinted with permission) lem assessment, identification, and intervention are essential. Compromise, on the other hand, takes less time and skill, but requires that both parties be willing to give something up (Hart, 1980; Bolton, 1979).

Collaboration is an important intervention when nurses or departments must work together over a long period and when performance is measured by the accomplishment of the same objectives (eg, the laboratory and a particular work unit). However, if the period of working together is very short or limited, compromise may be a better intervention. It is much easier to give up something if there is little investment. Although the outcomes of compromise and collaboration differ, the approaches are similar. The cornerstone of both is mutual respect. Listening skills are critical. All facts, assumptions, and feelings must be "heard."

Positive confrontation is integral to effective conflict management. It is a technique that can be used to verbalize facts, assumptions, and feelings. Positive confrontation offers a nondefensive, rational approach. Nurses can effectively communicate their perceptions of another person's behavior, their feelings about that behavior, and the effects the behavior has on them. This three-part script is planned ahead of time and is both verbally and nonverbally expressed as clearly and succinctly as possible. Communicating the script effectively requires that all three parts are shared in the following way (Bolton, 1979):

"When you . . ."
—State the behavior in descriptive terms.

"I feel . . ."
—Disclose feelings.

"Because . . ."
—Talk about the consequences of the other person's behavior.

When the script is shared, listen and then deal with the response. For example, two nurses were in conflict because one continually asked the other to do "little favors" on a consistent basis. These "little favors," such as checking IVs, were clearly part of the requesting nurse's client assignment. The "little favors" were never very "little"; they took more time than calculated and interfered with the other nurse's performance. The times when the nurse needed "little favors" herself and asked for help, the other nurse "did not have time." At first the nurse being asked to do the favors did not mind because she was a team player. But when the requests did not cease, anger became a normal reaction and the relationship between the two deteriorated. Intervention was necessary.

After problem assessment and identification, the intervention chosen was positive confrontation. The goal was to collaborate. The script used was as follows:

> "When you continually ask me to do your 'little favors' and then don't offer to help me when I get behind . . ."
> "I feel angry . . ."
> "Because the "little favors" take time away from the care I need to give my assigned clients, I fall behind. . ."

The next step is to listen and then respond to the response. Negotiation is used to reach a mutual decision.

NEGOTIATION

Negotiation is a communication process in which a mutual decision is made (Fisher & Ury, 1981). If the decision is to move toward a win–win strategy, collaboration should be used. If concessions are appropriate, a compromise should be reached. In any case, Nierenberg (1981) asserts that a basic ingredient in negotiation is preparation. Nurses must be clear about desired outcomes and be sensitive to what is happening during the entire resolution process. In the example above, negotiating a resolution could be accomplished by both nurses listening to each other and focusing on an acceptable outcome. It is important that no assumptions be made regarding motives, intent, or reasons why the nurse keeps asking for favors. If it is assumed that the nurse is lazy, incompetent, or doing this "on purpose," resolution will be difficult or impossible. In this situation a change in behavior might be appropriate. One request might be:

> "I am willing to help you as long as I am also able to finish my assignments. I am requesting that, if I am willing to help you, you will reciprocate when I ask you for help. If you are willing to do this, the positive outcome for both of us is that our assignments will be completed."

The above is a process that requires negotiation. Should it not occur, then consequences for noncompliance must be shared. Unfortunately, the consequences might be that requests for help in the future will be refused or carefully scrutinized.

Negotiation is critical for managing conflict and obtaining the necessary resources or materials for departmental or personal objectives. Negotiation is a method for reaching agreement using both cooperative and competitive elements—getting a mutually acceptable agreement and the best results for both parties involved. Three conditions must be present for appropriate negotiations: conflict of interest, ambiguity about the right solution, and an opportunity for satisfaction by both parties (Schoonaker, 1989). Preparation is essential.

The method used for negotiation separates people from the problem, focuses on interests not positions, invents options for mutual gain, and uses objective criteria (Fisher & Ury, 1981). Nurses should plan the desired objectives and "bottom lines." For example, if a nurse were negotiating for a different schedule, the "bottom line" would be a clear idea of what would *not* be acceptable, such as working every weekend. The other person's position should be analyzed and possible "bottom lines" projected.

If possible, when negotiating, pick a "neutral" area for a discussion. Clearly communicate the position (eg, "I can work every third weekend") using congruent body language. Learn the other person's position as quickly as possible. Strategies such as getting all of the issues on the table, allowing bargaining room, sending consistent signals, and ensuring that agreements are made clear at the end of the negotiation are crucial (Schoonaker, 1989).

Nurses now find themselves in a variety of situations that require negotiation. Clarity in thinking and communication and effective listening skills are critical, as are rational problem solving and an ability to focus on positive outcomes. It is important for nurses to remember that negotiation requires planning and sensitivity to others. Being a skilled negotiator will not happen overnight. In this case, practice does have a direct impact on success.

SUMMARY

Working in today's health care organizations can be an exciting challenge for nurses. Establishing rapport by developing a positive work philosophy and focusing on the strengths of colleagues sets a tone for the sharing of power resources. This "power balancing" is critical to the development of collegial relationships.

A benefit of developing a positive climate is the enhancement of relationships with others. When those relationships are challenged or when there are differences, conflict management is imperative. Positively confronting a situation to bring conflict to resolution requires the ability to overcome personal emotional barriers using a logical process to assess problems and select the appropriate method for conflict intervention. Methods such as compromise and collaboration suggest that conflict resolution should be based on respect and mutual problem solving. Negotiation is a crucial skill for nurses in the current health care environment. The ability to secure needed resources and solve conflicts of interest will promote positive working relationships and provide opportunities to achieve organizational and departmental goals.

DISCUSSION QUESTIONS

1. What specific challenges or barriers might prevent nurses from establishing positive work climates in hospital, clinic, and community health settings? What strategies could be used to overcome these challenges or barriers?
2. Think about the last conflict you had with someone. What were your feelings? Did they get in the way of resolving the conflict? In what way? If you had to deal with the conflict now, what would you do to have a positive outcome?
3. Discuss a negotiation you had with a supervisor, peer, family member, or merchant. What happened with the negotiation that made it successful or unsuccessful?

REFERENCES

Bolton, R. (1979). *People skills*. Englewood Cliffs, NJ: Prentice-Hall.

Bragg, D. D. (1992). Team basics: How to develop teamwork in training organizations, *Performance and Instruction, 31*(9), 10–14.

Covey, S. R. (1991). *Principle-centered leadership*. New York: Summit Books.

Fisher, R., & Ury, W. (1981). *Getting to yes: Negotiating agreement without giving in*. Boston: Houghton-Mifflin.

Hart, L. B. (1980). *Moving up! Women and leadership*. New York: AMACOM.

Jackman, M., & Waggoner, S. (1991). *Star teams. Star players*. New York: Henry Holt.

Kelley, C. (1979). *Assertion training: A facilitator's guide*. La Jolla: University Associates.

Mehrabian, A. (1971). *Silent messages*. Belmont: Wadsworth Publishing.

Naisbitt, J., & Aburdene, P. (1990). *Megatrends 2000* (p. 300). New York: William Morrow and Company.

Nierenberg, G. I. (1981). *The art of negotiating*. New York: Simon and Schuster.

Plunkett, L. C., & Fournier, R. (1991). *Participative management. Implementing empowerment*. New York: John Wiley and Sons.

Richardson, J., & Margulis, J. (1981). *The magic of rapport*. San Francisco: Habor Publishing.

Schoonaker, A. N. (1989). *Negotiate to win. Gaining the psychological edge*. Englewood Cliffs, NJ: Prentice-Hall.

SUGGESTED READING

Blanchard, K., Carew, D., & Parisi-Carew, E. (1990). *One minute manager builds high performing teams*. New York: William Morrow.

Block, P. (1987). *The empowered manager. Positive political skills at work*. San Francisco: Jossey-Bass.

Dawson, R. (1992). *The secrets of power persuasion*. Englewood Cliffs, NJ: Prentice-Hall.

Francis, D., & Young, D. (1992). *Improving work groups*. San Diego: Pfeiffer.

Jandt, F. E. (1985). *Win–win negotiating: Turning conflict into agreement*. New York: John Wiley & Sons.

Nanus, B. (1992). *Visionary leadership*. San Francisco: Jossey-Bass.

Yates, D. (1985). *The politics of management*. San Francisco: Jossey-Bass.

Priority Management

Nancy R. Kruger

LEARNING OBJECTIVES

This chapter will enable you to:

1. Understand principles of time management.
2. Understand variables that affect priority setting.
3. Learn to set priorities.
4. Identify barriers to successful patient care management.

Vestal, K.W. Nursing Management:
Concepts and Issues, 2 ed.
© 1995 J.B. Lippincott Company

PRIORITY MANAGEMENT

Today's health care climate demands that all care givers make the maximum use of their resources. To take advantage of resources, it is important to use time wisely by establishing priorities for patient care responsibilities and then integrating service to patients with professional development and personal time. Developing skills in time management and priority setting will help you function more effectively and will help prevent burnout (Salmond, 1986).

Learning to care for patients in an organized fashion is often overwhelming for a new graduate. It is common for the new nurse—or not-so-new nurse for that matter—to feel intimidated by the workload in caring for patients. Yet there are several things you can do to diminish your anxiety and your workload. Start by developing sound time management. Time management is self-management. By investing time in how you manage your activities, you prevent other people and circumstances from managing them for you.

WHAT IS TIME MANAGEMENT AND HOW DO I DO IT?

Time management is the planned, organized evaluation of when and for how long you do something. Effective time management requires diligence, discipline, and flexibility (Brown & Wilson, 1987). To begin the process of managing your time, some basic assumptions about your work area need to be questioned:

- What are the expectations of your job? How do you spend your time in relation to formal job expectations and informal ones?
- Does peer pressure influence how you spend your time?
- How do the institution's philosophy and policies affect your time?
- What is the institutional norm for managing your time?

Then ask yourself:

- What do I do with my time?
- How appropriate is the time I spend completing a task?
- Am I doing tasks appropriate to my job responsibilities?

You may, for example, be expected to spend time instructing patients about their post-hospital medication regimen and exercise and diet plan. How much time do you spend performing this activity? Peer norms include such things as going to lunch or to break at the same time with the same people whether or not it has an impact on patient treatments. Does everyone always spend the first half-hour of the shift talking about the latest movie, the most recent sales in clothes, or who is dating whom? Is the institutional philosophy one in which only the physicians are permitted to give patients instructions about aftercare? How long do others within your unit typically spend doing certain tasks, such as giving the report at the change of shift? Does everyone typically leave the unit by a certain time every day, regardless of the work to be done? Answers to such questions about your work time and your time outside work should help you determine how you spend your time and help you begin managing it more effectively.

To develop a picture of how you spend your time, keep a record of your activities for about 1 week. On a log, indicate how you spent your time with a brief notation (Fig. 10-1). Whenever you are interrupted, write the reason for the interruption in the "comments" sec-

TIME	ACTIVITY	COMMENTS	PRIORITY
7 AM			1 2 3 4
7:30			1 2 3 4
8 AM			1 2 3 4
8:30			1 2 3 4
9 AM			1 2 3 4

1 = Must complete the task right now

2 = Necessary to complete the task sometime today

3 = Nice to complete the task today

4 = Unnecessary to do

FIG 10-1. Log book.

tion. Circle the number that indicates the relative importance of the activity. Later, you can compare the relative importance of each activity with the goals you have set for your patient that day.

Rank each item immediately after completing the activity. Although this may seem tedious, it is important that you reflect your work accurately. If you overstate or understate the amount of time spent or its importance, you will not be able to accurately identify areas where you can make significant improvement. Remember, the purpose of keeping the log is to help you evaluate how efficiently you use time. To be effective is to do the right job. To be efficient is to do the right job in the right way (Winston, 1983).

ANALYZING YOUR WORK

After you have filled in your log for about 1 week, analyze the results. Compare your data with your job description and expectations. First, review the specific elements of your job description (Fig. 10-2).

POSITION DESCRIPTION

TITLE: Clinical Nurse	DEPARTMENT: Nursing Service		F.L.S.A STATUS:
REPORTS TO: Head Nurse	GRADE 14	POSITION CODE 1406	X Non-Exempt
POSITIONS SUPERVISED: Staff Registered Nurses' Ward Clerks and Nursing Assistants			Exempt _____ Administrative _____ Executive _____ Professional

PRIMARY FUNCTION:
Responsible for Clinical management of patient care on the unit.

PRINCIPAL DUTIES AND RESPONSIBILITIES:

1. Assist the staff nurses' with nursing process by making daily clinical rounds and reviewing the patient care and patient documentation with the staff nurse.

2. Review patient care plans and update daily with the staff nurses.

3. Holding patient care conferences at least monthly with the staff nurses to establish clinical care practices and review of these practices. Encourage staff to participate in the area.

4. Review, revise and develop written care plans protocols through nursing Standards Committee.

FIG 10-2. Job description.

5. Participate in the evaluation of these protocols and the staffs ability to implement these protocols. Implement all policies and procedures with staff.

6. Participate and coordinate with the Head Nurse and Assistant Director for Education al Programs in the orientation of new staff.

7. Provide assistance to the staff for the Discharge Planning Process—utilizing the patient, family, Utilization Coordinator and Social Service Department.

8. Coordinate with the Nursing Quality Care Committee and follow-up recommendations from the committee.

QUALIFICATIONS:

Education: Registered Nurse—Pennsylvania—BSN

Experience: One year-Med/Surg. 6 months ophthalmic—demonstrated ability in all steps of Nursing Process.

Certification/Licensure: Current licensure in Pennsylvania

WORKING CONDITIONS: Lifts weights over 25 pounds, repeated bending, squatting, stooping, Pushing and pulling movements. Prolonged walking and standing. Exposed to infections occasionally, cuts when handing instruments and hazardous gases in anesthetized areas. Exposed to electrical and radiant energy hazards.

DESCRIBED BY:	DATE:	APPROVED BY:	DATE:

Position Title	Department	Subdivision	Work Area
Clinical Nurse	Nursing Service		Patient Care Floor Operating Room

9. Self continuing education. Attend a minimum of two "outside," and eight inhouse conferences/year.

10. Monthly rotations on evenings nights as needed.

11. Provides staffing relief as needed.

12. Additional functions as assigned by the Assistant Director for Patient Services.

FIG 10-2. Position description. (Continued)

Important elements of this document include your title, your supervisor, personnel you are expected to supervise, the primary function of the job, and a list of duties. Other important details that should be listed on the job description are qualifications and working conditions, including equipment you may be expected to use and possibilities for hazardous exposure. Such information can be helpful when you plan your day. For example, if you are expected to work with patients who are being treated with chemotherapy or radioactive material, plan carefully to limit the amount of time you are exposed to these patients.

Second, clarify the job expectations with your nurse manager. Although the job description indicates your formal job duties, there are likely to be some unwritten rules that informally define certain expectations. Every institution has those jobs that "must be done," those that "should be done," and those that are "nice to do" (Feldman, Municken, & Crowley, 1983).

As part of this review, look at the job descriptions of your coworkers. It can be helpful to review the job descriptions for secretaries, therapists, assistants, licensed practical nurses, and nurse aides. Knowing the duties and responsibilities of others will help you know whom you can ask for consultative advice (eg, a clinical nurse specialist) or to whom you can delegate certain jobs (eg, ask the secretary to fill out lab slips).

Next, develop a list of activities that you think are the most important. This should be done independently of how you spend your time, as reflected in your log. In a study done by Hendrickson and Doddato (1989), nurses were asked to indicate those activities that they believed were professional nursing functions. They were then asked to indicate those tasks that they believed they would be unable to perform if the day became busy. The results indicated that tasks such as medication administration and IV therapy were usually completed, even when time became limited. But tasks such as teaching, discharge planning, and attending team conferences were left undone, despite the fact that teaching activities were ranked higher on the list of necessary functions of a professional nurse. Avoiding such activities often leads to inadequate preparation for discharge. Patients consequently are unable to comply with post-discharge treatment plans.

Returning to your log, compare what you did with your time with what you believe to be important. Now you will begin to learn how to set priorities. If you believe you are not spending enough time on professional nursing functions, identify what you now do that can be done by others. By delegating these tasks to others, such as secretaries, therapists, and environmental health workers, you will free up time for the higher priority nursing activities.

VARIABLES THAT AFFECT PRIORITY SETTING

Each institution has rules that guide the nurse in setting priorities. For example, patients may get to their various therapy treatments on time because the nurse manager places a high priority on making sure the pa-

---

DISPLAY 10-1. LIST OF PROFESSIONAL NURSE ACTIVITIES

Planning Activities (Professional nurse required)
- Developing a care plan
- Participating in nursing conferences
- Participating in nursing and medical rounds
- Conferring with patient's families
- Counseling and teaching patients
- Assessing patient condition and diagnosing problems
- Evaluating patient changes and responses to treatments

Functional Activities (Professional nurse or associate worker such as an LPN or nursing assistant)
- Documentation of care
- Preparing medications, giving medications
- Administering treatments
- Assisting with routine activities of daily living

Other Activities (Non-nursing personnel)
- Tidying up the patient's room
- Filling out lab slips, answering unit phone, giving directions to visitors
- Transporting patients
- Personal time such as break

(Modified after Hendrickson, G. & Doddato, T. [1989]. Setting priorities during the shortage. *Nursing Outlook, 37* [6], 280–284.)

---

tients get to physical therapy. If your patients are taken to physical therapy, however, they may not receive medications on time or may miss an important conference that you have arranged with the social worker.

Institutional variables that may affect priority setting include policies and procedures. Take, for example, the schedule for collecting laboratory specimens. If the lab has a routine time to pick up 24-hour urine specimens, you need to be certain the patient's specimens are available at the designated time and place. This may mean delaying another patient's care, a dressing change for instance, to meet the deadline imposed by the lab.

Another institutional variable is the model of practice used to deliver patient care. Today, much emphasis is placed on collaborative practice and patient management by interdisciplinary teams. For the nurse to set priorities and manage time successfully, an understanding of the model of practice and a willingness to work within its boundaries are essential.

Many collaborative practice models or interdisciplinary teams are using critical pathways or "care maps" to provide a structure for meeting patient care goals. Typically, each day is mapped out in terms of the treatment plans prescribed by the physician and the nurse. These plans are preprinted, and the expected duration and course of care is indicated on the pathway. The nurse and other members of the care team are then able to measure the patient's progress against the map. Using the care maps, team members set goals for each day's care. A problem can arise when critical pathways for several patients must be followed by one nurse. Competing priorities can emerge within a specific patient pathway and among several patient pathways, so new priorities must be set for these competing goals before work can begin for the day.

For many years, multidisciplinary teams have been established to develop protocols of care for specific patient populations. More recently, they are being developed to better manage larger delivery systems within an institution. An example of how such a team collaborates can be seen at the large university teaching hospital where I work. Concern about the way children were being managed through painful diagnostic procedures led to the creation of a conscious sedation program by a multidisciplinary team. When this plan was implemented, the time that the nurses performed certain activities had to be changed, shifting their daily priorities. Physicians and child-life personnel altered some of their activities to afford a higher priority to the administration of conscious sedation, and clinic schedules, nursing assignments, and child therapeutic play activities were changed.

DISPLAY 10-2. VARIABLES AFFECTING PRIORITIES	
Institutional	Model of practice; nursing department policies and procedures; fiscal considerations; level of automation of the medical record; accreditation; type of facility (eg, teaching, non-teaching, acute care, rehabilitation, long-term care)
Patient	Level of patient according to Maslow's hierarchy of needs (physiologic, safety, love, self-esteem, self-actualization)
Professional	State licensure, code of ethics, certification, professional standards of practice
Individual	Skill level, years of experience, educational background, level of comfort according to Maslow

Professional variables affect the priorities you set. The kinds of technical skills that individual employees are permitted to practice is one variable. For example, administering anesthesia is limited to certified registered nurse anesthetists (CRNAs). In many instances, licensure dictates what can be done. In other situations, a priority may be set by professional standards or a code of ethics. Spending time with a dying patient will supersede the patient who is asking for a backrub.

Finally, the skills that an individual nurse possesses can act as variables for determining care priorities. The nurse directly responsible for a patient's care, for example, may not be able to insert an IV catheter. If the patient requires an IV, it may have to wait until the nurse who can perform the task is available.

LEARNING TO SET PRIORITIES

Priority setting for specific patients can be structured around Maslow's hierarchy of needs (Fig. 5-2). The nurse first considers the patient's physiologic integrity, followed by his or her need for safety, love, self-esteem, and self-actualization. In practice, you must first be certain your patients are physiologically stable before you can reassure them they are. When the patients feel secure enough to absorb information, you begin teaching. If your patients appear unable to comprehend instructions, it is essential that their families understand the therapeutic plan. Nurses, too, function within Maslow's hierarchy of needs. Until nurses feel safe in what they are doing, they will be unable to reach self-actualization in the performance of patient care. Sophisticated judgments about care priorities, then, come after much practice and validation by managers.

The key to learning to set priorities is taking time to **plan** when, where, what, how, and why you are going to do something, then **organizing** the personnel and equipment that are needed, and finally, **directing** the care.

There are several handy ways to plan your time and activities. "To Do" lists are particularly helpful. You can select a preprinted calendar like the one shown in Figure 10-3. Develop a "To Do" list for a month by inserting your work schedule and your activities outside work. Remember, one facet of your life influences the other.

Next, develop a more detailed list for the week, which includes your work schedule and any meetings or classes you must attend during your work time. Finally, develop a "To Do" list for the day's activities, including the work you will be doing with your patients. Your list for setting patient priorities may actually be your assign-

Sunday	Monday	Tuesday	Wednesday	Thursday	Friday	Saturday
OFF	7-3	7-3 Class 6-9	OFF	7-3 Computer Inservice 10-11	7-3	7-3
7-3	3-11	OFF Class 6-9	3-11	3-11	3-11	OFF 8 pm concert tickets
OFF	3-11	OFF Class 6-9	3-11	3-11	3-11	3-11
3-11	3-11	OFF Class 6-9	3-11	3-11	3-11	OFF
OFF	7-3	7-3 Class 6-9 Term paper due	7-3 Dentist appt. 430 pm	7-3 Drug Inservice 130-2	OFF	7-3

FIG 10-3. Calendar for one month.

ment list, which is an excellent tool for directing you toward a practical goal.

New graduates often set idealistic goals such as "giving the best nursing care I can" (Predd, 1989). Although admirable, such goals provide little help in setting priorities of care. More practical goals, such as keeping the patient safe and comfortable or providing the patient and family with medication education, allow you to complete the job even if you cannot check off every item on your day's list. You can then go home feeling good about having attained the day's goals. The following case study will help you use goals to plan, organize, and direct care as you set your priorities.

CASE STUDY

You have just come on-shift and received the following report:

Mark Hill, 66, exploratory laparotomy 6 days ago, chronic renal disease with 3-year history of hemodialysis for renal disease. Central line with hyperalimentation, NPO, OOB with assistance, incontinent of stool today.

Bertha Bilger, 59, admitted from the ER last night with acute abdominal pain, postop laparoscopic cholecystectomy 1 week ago. Awaiting surgery.

Susan Clinton, 44, postop cholecystectomy 1 week ago. Now has a retained stone in the common bile duct. Today she had an ERCP, and a piece of the endoscope broke off in her common duct and was left behind after the procedure. She continues to have pain, is NPO, and has a peripheral IV infusing.

Nancy Thompson, 21, with Crohn's disease. She is postop a temporary colostomy 1 month ago and was readmitted to the hospital yesterday with dehydration. Last night she developed leg tenderness in the right calf and was diagnosed as having a DVT. She had a heparin drip infusing. In addition, she has purulent drainage coming from the bottom of her midline incision. She had a barium enema through the afferent loop of the colostomy during the night and returned from radiology covered with barium and feces. She has been reported by the off-going nurse as crying softly in her room.

Jake Hammer, 75, readmitted 3 days ago for peripheral vascular disease, diabetes, and a groin infection. He has a right heel ulcer that needs wet-to-dry dressing changes. He is alert and oriented.

Harry Ortiz, 66, 6 days postop CABG. Yesterday he developed atrial fibrillation with a rate of 140. His procainamide was adjusted to 1000 mg b.i.d., and he is now NSR with occasional PACs. Pending drug levels, he is scheduled for discharge tomorrow.

You have been called by the MICU and told that you will be getting a transfer patient, a man who took an overdose of clonidine and is wanted by the police for armed robbery. There is some question of ETOH abuse.

STEP 1: PLAN

After listening to the report, take a few minutes to think about your patients and their priorities. Ask yourself:

- Which patients are physically or mentally unstable and need frequent checks?
- Which patients are in pain and need regular medication and position change?
- Which patients have complicated treatments or dressing changes that require a significant amount of time to complete?
- Which patients require counseling and teaching reinforcement?
- Which patients will be discharged within the next day or two?

These questions will help you set priorities as you complete the following assignment. You know that Thompson will require frequent checks because of the DVT and the possibility of a pulmonary embolus. Bilger will be going to the operating room and is on-call for her preoperative medications. When she returns to the unit, probably on your shift, you will need to monitor her at least every half hour. Hammer, because of his

Date: 10-25-92
Charge RN: JONES

Narcotics
Code Cart ✓

MD/RN work rounds: 10³⁰-11¹⁵
Inservice 11³⁰-12

Room	Patient	Adm Date	Problems	Priority
34	Hill 66 ♂	10-18	Exp. lap. 10-18 Chron. Ren. Fail. Hemo, Dia / HAL. NPO, 008 Depressed	✓
36	Bilger 59 ♀	10-24	Abd. pain to OR for Exp. lap. on CALL – NPO	✓
37	Clinton 44 ♀	10-15	Postop chole (10-15) Readmitt for retained stone. ERCP pain NPO, IV	
43	Hammer 75 ♂	10-23	PVD, Diabetes, Postop fem-pop RT. Heel ulcer wet-dry dressing readmitted for infected groin	✓
47	Ortiz 66 ♂	10-19	CABG x2 A.F. @ 140 ↑ Procan to 1000mg BID→NSR Disch AM	
60	Thompson 21 ♀	10-24	Crohn's Dis. Temp. colost. DVT c̄ Hep Drip Dehydrated Pain, IVBs	✓

TIME Transfer from MICU 354.0. ♂ c̄ ETOH abuse.

7	
8	
9	
10	
11	
12	
1	
2	
3	

Comments:

FIG 10-4A. Assignment sheets.

age, bed rest, and disease, will also require frequent monitoring. Hill is on hyperalimentation and will need to go to hemodialysis for his routine treatment. He will leave the unit by 9:00 AM and be away until after lunch. Place a check mark by these four names: Thompson, Bilger, Hammer, and Hill (Fig. 10-4*A*).

Review the list again. This time look for patients who will require pain medication or IV fluid administration. Both Clinton and Thompson have IV infusions, and Clinton has abdominal pain and Thompson has a DVT. Bilger will require attention when she returns from surgery. Place a check by each of their names (Fig. 10-4*B*).

Now look at your assignment list again. Who needs treatments or procedures that are time consuming? Hammer and Thompson have complex dressings; each will take about a half hour. Place another check next to their names (Fig. 10-4*C*). Teaching, counseling, and discharge planning will be needed more immediately for Thompson, Ortiz, Bilger, and Hammer than for your other patients. Add a check next to these four names. Of course, you will be able to obtain more information from the patient, patient care plan, and the medication record when you make your initial patient care rounds.

STEP 2: ORGANIZE

The next part of the process involves organizing your workload. Consider what personnel and supply resources you will need. Analyze each patient's condition by answering the following four questions as you prepare to set your priorities:

- What needs to be done immediately?
- What is the major problem?
- What systems are involved?
- What complications are possible?

Take Nancy Thompson as an example. You already know you will need to check her vital signs and inquire about any new chest pain or difficulty breathing because of her potential for a pulmonary embolus. You will need to assure yourself of intravenous access in case you need to administer medications quickly, so you will have to check her IV site. Next, check the supplies needed to change her dressings and her colostomy. You will need a block of time, and you may need assistance. These procedures will have to be done within the first hour because she has a lot of drainage on her dressings and her abdomen. Finally, you will need to visit frequently to monitor for possible signs of infection, provide emotional support, and teach colostomy care.

Date: 10-25-92

Charge RN: Jones

Narcotics

Code Cart ✓

MD/RN work rounds: 10³⁰ - 11¹⁵

Inservice 11³⁰-12

Room	Patient	Adm Date	Problems	Priority
34	Hill 66 ♂	10-18	Exp. lap 10-18 Chron. Ren. Fail, Hemo Dialysis - Glu., HAL, NPO, OOB Depressed	✓
36	Bilger 59 ♀	10-24	Abd. pain to OR for Exp. lap. ON CALL - NPO	✓✓
37	Clinton 44 ♀	10-15	Post op. Chole. (10-15) Readmit for retained stone, ERCP, pain, NPO, IV	✓
43	Hammer 75 ♂	10-23	PVD, Diabetes, postop fem-pop readmitted for infected groin Rt. heel ulcer IV → wet to dry drsg.	✓
47	Ortiz 66 ♂	10-19	CABG x 2 A.F. Q 140↑ procan to 1000mg BID → NSR Disch. in AM	✓
50	Thompson 21 ♀	10-24	Crohn's Dis. Temp Colost., DVT c̄ Hep. Drip Dehydrated, pain, IV, B.E	✓✓

TIME	Transfer from MICU 35 y.o. ♂ c̄ ETOH Abuse
7	
8	
9	
10	
11	
12	
1	
2	
3	

Comments:

FIG 10-4B. (Continued)

Date: 10-25-92

Charge RN: Jones

Narcotics

Code Cart ✓

MD/RN work rounds: 10³⁰ - 11¹⁵

Inservice 11³⁰ - 12

Room	Patient	Adm Date	Problems	Priority
34	Hill 66 ♂	10-18	Exp lap (10-18) (Chronic Ren Fail., Hemo Dial ↓ Glucose HAL, NPO, OOB, Depressed	✓
36	Bilger 59 ♀	10-24	Abd. pain to OR for Exp. lap. ON CALL - NPO	✓✓✓
37	Clinton 44 ♀	10-15	Post op Choley (10-15) Readmitt for retained stone ERCP, pain, NPO, IV	✓✓
43	Hammer 75 ♂	10-23	PVD, Diabetes, post op. fem-pop readmitted for infected groin	✓✓✓
47	Ortiz 66 ♂	10-19	CABG x2 A.F. Q 140 ↑ Procan to 1000 mg BID → NSR Rt. heel ulcer wet → dry drsg. IV Disch. in AM	✓
50	Thompson 21 ♀	10-24	Crohn's Disease Temp. Colostomy, DVT c̄ Hep. Drip Dehydrated, pain, IV, BE ↓ ↓ ↓	✓✓✓

TIME Transfer from MICU 35 y.o. ♂ ETOH Abuse

Comments:

FIG 10-4C. (Continued)

Refer to your assignment sheet (Fig. 10-4C). You have planned to complete your evaluation of your patients on rounds between 7:20 AM and 7:40 AM. You have planned to change Ms. Thompson's dressing between 7:45 AM and 8:30 AM. She has four check marks next to her name and is your first priority after rounds.

Review your patient assignment list again and indicate what time during the shift you plan to complete your other patients' care. Don't forget to include your lunch and break time. You will need to include any educational programs or multidisciplinary rounds you plan to attend. As you complete each task, draw a line through it. This shows that you are achieving your goals and will give you a sense of satisfaction.

Now determine the lower priority activities you want to accomplish during your shift. Consider such things as a review of the medication and activity plans for Mr. Ortiz because he is expected to go home tomorrow. You will need to confirm a regular heart rate and the absence of chest pain. The exact time you do these things is not necessarily important, but you need to complete these activities during this shift.

What supportive tasks would you like to do, if you have time? You might want to follow up with Ms. Clinton about the piece of material that was inadvertently left behind during the ERCP. You know the doctor has spoken to her about it, but she will need reassurance.

In case of a crisis, such as when Nancy Thompson suddenly stops breathing and the patient who has just been transferred from the medical intensive care unit suddenly starts vomiting blood, you can drop everything to take care of these emergencies. Give your list to a colleague who can help to cover your other patients. The other nurses will know what you have done because your "To Do" list indicates what has been accomplished by the items lined out. They will know what needs to be done because your list is already in order of priority. Your colleagues need only continue down the list and mark items off as they go.

STEP 3: DIRECT THE CARE

Remember that you are part of a team. Other members are available to help. Use them. A licensed practical nurse can help pass medications (assuming this policy is sanctioned in your institution), whereas a transport aid may take a patient to radiology. The secretary is available to transcribe physician orders on the new patient transferred from the intensive care unit.

In many care settings, much of the work associated with charting and care planning is done on a computer. If this is the practice where you work, you may need to plan at what point you will need to "get on the computer." This activity is essential so that you can share your data with others and retrieve important information such as laboratory results or a list of medications.

Access to computers may be required to order supplies for patient treatments and dressing changes. Although the nurse may not be required to perform such activities, you may need to check whether the secretary has placed the appropriate order. Again, this takes planning so that you don't find yourself in the middle of a procedure and lack an important supply to complete it.

The final step in directing the care is recording a patient's progress so that further planning and execution of the treatment plan is possible. Record information as you complete an activity. Record vital signs when you obtain them, for example, instead of carrying them around in your pocket on a piece of paper. Many institutions keep flow sheets on clipboards that hang at the end of the bed to make this convenient for the nurse. Similarly, if you have bedside computers, enter the data as soon as you obtain it. You may need to save some time at the end of the shift to record final observations about each of your patients. Or you may wish to comment on each of your patients' problems. This will be one of the variables that is set by your institution, so you will need to become acquainted with the expectations for charting and recording information.

TIPS TO SAVE TIME

Display 10-3 is a list of tips that you may find helpful when planning your day. These tips will help you gain confidence and help relieve the anxiety and stress that can interfere with your ability to function to your greatest ability. Try using them.

BARRIERS

To be successful in learning to set priorities and reaching your goals, it is important to know some of the internal and external barriers you may encounter, so that you can avoid getting caught up in time-wasting activities. Internal barriers are those activities over which you have direct control, whereas external barriers are those produced elsewhere but which infringe upon your ability to complete your job. Among the most important internal barriers for the new nurse to concentrate on controlling are ineffective communication, failure to delegate,

---

DISPLAY 10-3. TOOLS TO STRUCTURE YOUR TIME

1. Memorize the routine protocols that you use daily. This saves time and instills confidence.
2. Find a comfortable way to assess patients uniformly, and then do it the same way every time (eg, systems assessment, etc.).
3. Learn where information is written on your chart forms. This facilitates retrieval when information is needed in a hurry.
4. Anticipate patient needs.
5. Learn the location of all equipment you may need.
6. Block out chunks of time for writing, planning, and thinking.
7. Group similar tasks together, like phone calls. Cluster information so you make one call instead of several calls to the same person.
8. Review the critical pathways patient plans, and schedule patient care accordingly.
9. Try to balance different types of activities such as meetings, classes, and patient care.
10. Control patient care interruptions. Tell team members when you are going to be engaged in a lengthy task, and then shut the door to the patient's room to ensure privacy as well as decrease interruptions.

---

failure to evaluate your own time effectiveness, procrastination, indecision, lack of self-discipline, poor listening habits, and excessive socialization.

Each time waster prevents the nurse from achieving patient care goals. Fortunately, there are remedies. Ineffective communication may be remedied by clearly stating what you want. Ask for feedback to be sure your request is understood. When looking at your "To Do" list, note which tasks coincide with your job description. Note which tasks can be performed by the secretary or housekeeper. Delegate those tasks to the appropriate people.

Procrastination may be tackled by identifying aspects of care that you find difficult to perform. Break the task into smaller parts. Promise yourself a reward (eg, a coffee break) after you have completed an unpleasant chore. Schedule unpleasant jobs early in your shift so you get them out of the way.

Excessive socialization can be a real time waster. Although you certainly want to enjoy your colleagues and to work as a team member, your goal is to provide nursing care to your patients. Save socializing for coffee and lunch breaks or for outside the workplace. Avoid gossiping, which wastes time and often is destructive to colleagues and patients.

External barriers are more difficult to control. Telephone calls, for example, may present a problem. A physician calling to check on a patient's lab results so that additional orders may be given should be

---

DISPLAY 10-4. TIME WASTERS

Internal Barriers
Ineffective communication
Procrastination
Failure to delegate
Indecision
Failure to evaluate your own time effectiveness
Poor listening habits
Excessive socialization
Lack of self-discipline
Tendency to act without thinking
Not focusing on your job
Emotional and personal stress
Inability to limit time with patients

External Barriers
Telephone
Lack of protocols for common problems
Insufficient supplies
Crises or unexpected situations
Unclear lines of authority
Responsibilities of resource personnel unclear

---

responded to immediately. When a family member calls about your patient's condition, however, you might ask the secretary to get the number. Then arrange a specific time to return the call so you can give it your full attention.

Protocols are excellent tools for helping you handle common problems. If you work on a unit where telemetry is common, specific drug protocols for the treatment of rhythm disturbances are particularly useful. These allow the nurse to initiate treatment without wasting precious time waiting for a physician to return a phone call.

Finally, know your limits. Other resources are available to you. For example, if you are unsure of how to complete a dressing change, find the procedure manual and read how to do it. Then, collect all of the supplies that are necessary and assemble them at the bedside. If necessary, write down the steps of the dressing change on a piece of paper and take it with you so that you can refer to it as you complete the procedure. You can ask a nurse who has had experience with this type of dressing change to come with you for supervision while you change the dressing. This way, your colleague can give you some helpful tips as you proceed while providing you with support and assuring you that you are accurately and safely performing the procedure.

There are other areas of limitation, including the limits of your knowledge of and experience with drugs and their expected effects and side effects. You may have limited knowledge about the practice patterns of some of the physicians with whom you come into contact. Limitations may exist in how the particular institution handles system problems such as the delivery of supplies or transport of patients to diagnostic tests or procedures. In each instance, refer to written procedure guides and to your colleagues. Your supervisory personnel and coworkers will be able to assist you. Ask for their help.

SUMMARY

Setting priorities for patient care is essential if you are to use your time effectively to achieve patient care goals. Managing your time through priority setting will help you diminish job stress and avoid burnout. Not only will you enjoy your work more, but by applying these principles to your personal and professional life, you will enjoy all aspects of your life more fully.

DISCUSSION QUESTIONS

1. How would you reset your priorities when Mr. Ortiz develops chest pain at 11:00 AM? What would you do first, and why? What additional things would you need to consider when changing his plan of care?
2. How would you handle your assignment if one of your colleagues' patients needed assistance and you were requested to administer medication to four additional patients at 2:00 PM?
3. How would you manage to distribute your patients' lunch trays at the same time you received a call from the postanesthesia recovery unit to come and pick up Ms. Bilger for return to her room?

REFERENCES

Brown, M., & Wilson, C. (1987). Time management and the clinical nurse specialist. *Clinical Nurse Specialist, 1*(1), 32–38.

Feldman, E., Monicken, D., & Crowley, M. (1983). A systems approach to prioritizing. *Nursing Administration Quarterly, 7*(2), 57–62.

Hendrickson, G., & Doddato, T. (1989). Setting priorities during the shortage. *Nursing Outlook, 37*(6), 280–284.

Predd, C. S. (1989). Great tips for setting priorities. *Nursing, 19*(10), 120–126.

Salmond, S. (1986). Time management: The time is now. *Orthopedic Nursing, 5*(3), 25–32.

Winston, S. (1983). *The organized executive.* New York: Norton.

SUGGESTED READING

Brown, S. (1985). Time management: The foundation of a smoothly operating NICU. *Neonatal Network, 4*(2), 44–48.

DeBaca, V. (1987). So many patients, so little time. *RN, 50*(4), 32–33.

Frings, C. S. (1988). Effective time management. *Medical Laboratory Quarterly, 20*(7), 43–45.

Gruber, M. (1988). Practical time management for GI nursing staff. *SGA Journal, 10*(3), 150–152.

Hartley, B., & Spiegel, S. (1986). Time management: Teaching strategies to prevent the white rabbit syndrome. *Canadian Nurse, 82*(11), 14–17.

Ledford, J. (1988). First things first: Setting priorities. *Professional Medical Assistant, 21*(6), 18–19.

Lynch, M. (1991). P-A-C-E yourself: Tips on time management. *Nursing, 21*(3), 104, 106, 108.

Marriner, A. (1983). Time management through planning. *Journal of Continuing Education in Nursing, 14*(1), 21–26.

Marriner, A. (1984). Time management for career development. *Nursing Success Today, 1*(2), 4–7.

McAlvanah, M. F. (1988). Time management: A key to fulfilling job expectations. *Pediatric Nursing, 14*(6), 536.

McConnell, E. A. (1983). Ten tactics to help beat the clock. *RN, 46*(9), 47–50.

McFarlane, M. (1991). It's time to manage your time. *Dermatology Nursing, 3*(3), 172–182.

Morano, V. (1984). Time management: From victim to victor. *Health Care Supervisor, 3*(1), 1–12.

Poteet, G. W. (1985). Teaching time management for ward clerks. *Journal of Nursing Staff Development, 1*, 128–130.

Rutkowski, B. (1984). The nursing approach to better time management. *NursingLife, 4*(5), 52–57.

Rutkowski, B. (1985). The perennial problem of problem solving. *Nursing, 15*(2), 89–92.

Salome, P. B. (1986). Tips and techniques for balancing work, home, and personal responsibilities. *Perioperative Nursing Quarterly, 2*(3), 36–42.

Scott, P. P. (1986). Coping with the time trap. *Canadian Critical Care Nursing Journal, 3*(2), 10–12.

Short, B., Woodburne, C., & Sumner, S. (1990). Making the most of your time . . . by involving others. *Nursing, 20*(1), 99–100, 102, 104.

Solie, C. J. (1989). How to make time when you need it. *RN, 52*(10), 19–20.

Ulrich, B. (1985). Time management for the nurse executive. *Nursing Economics, 3*(6), 318–323.

11

Managing Change

Katherine W. Vestal

LEARNING OBJECTIVES

This chapter will enable you to:

1. Understand the practical approaches to managing change.
2. Describe the role of a change agent.
3. Develop various change scenarios expected in health care in the 1990s.

Vestal, K.W. Nursing Management:
Concepts and Issues, 2 ed.
© 1995 J.B. Lippincott Company

Managing change has become the password for the 1990s. There is hardly any facet of your personal and professional life that has escaped the onslaught of changes in health care, the economy, and the social structure in which you live. Although you probably would describe yourself as a champion of new things and resilient to the chaos in the environment, it is likely that managing the many changes has not been easy.

When you decided to pursue professional nursing as a career, you elected to add new knowledge, new skills, and new job opportunities to your life. The process of becoming a nurse undoubtedly produced many changes in your life. Now, in your role as a new nurse, you will manage and promote changes that will affect many lives—those of patients, families, and coworkers. Many people will look to you for guidance and leadership as a professional member of a health care organization that will itself undergo transformation in the 1990s.

THEORY VERSUS PRACTICE

Management gurus have proposed many theories about change. These theories offer approaches for understanding and managing the process of organizational change. They provide a framework for thinking through the steps of a change process and are useful in providing a disciplined approach to the change cycle.

One of the most useful frameworks describes *unfreezing, moving,* and *refreezing* as three distinct phases of change. In the unfreezing stage, a problem is identified that requires change. This need for change must be accepted by others, who will provide the impetus to move forward. The process of unfreezing occurs differently for individuals; some see the need immediately, whereas others resist acknowledging it.

Once the need to change is acknowledged, the next phase is the exploratory moving phase. People move toward change by exploring options, formulating plans, and implementing the change. Although this second phase may sound easy, the positioning of alternatives for implementation can be a difficult process.

The final phase requires refreezing the new changes and reestablishing a stability around the changes. Refreezing keeps others from going back to the "old" and provides an infrastructure on which to build. In reality, people in a group tend to vacillate, moving at different speeds in different directions. Ultimately, they must converge to have the change be permanent. Thus, the theory of change is heavily influenced by the practicality of change when individuals are involved.

In practice, people find change to be more personal than theoretical. No matter what the issue is, you must personally make a decision to act, think, or feel differently to have a different outcome. To some, changing the way things happen is a comfortable situation; in fact, they relish change. To others it is an affront that they fight in hope of maintaining the status quo.

At this time in history, maintaining the status quo in health care is unthinkable. A static organization would surely be doomed to failure as more nimble competitors left it in the dust. Therefore, the challenge of getting you and your colleagues to support organizational change is more than an isolated event. It is the constant need for continuous change and improvement that will ensure future organizational success. This need and goal must be shared by all. Getting people to embrace change as an organizational constant requires consistent messages, superb communication throughout the organization, and frequent renewal of information so that you can make educated and reasonable decisions as they are needed.

Duck (1993) cautions that managing change requires balancing many change initiatives simultaneously as a part of a whole. She cautions that fragmenting change projects or processes into isolated pieces will not produce the effect needed for the whole organization. For example, if you elect to make one isolated change in your nursing practice without considering its impact on other providers, departments, or practices, it is likely that the overall system of care will be compromised further. Likewise, if your nursing team conducts a total quality management initiative to change a work process without including other involved providers, the effect on the organization may not be positive.

It is easy to see that the multiple change initiatives ongoing in your workplace require that you understand the big picture of the patient care process and organizational goals, in addition to your local unit issues. Having a big picture of the organization will make it easier for you to understand and support ongoing changes. The more you know about your organization, workplace, and environment, the more effective you will be as a professional.

CHANGES IN PATIENT CARE DELIVERY

There are a multitude of changes taking place in patient care delivery that will have an impact on your role as a professional nurse.

HEALTH CARE REFORM

The 1990s will be chaotic for health and social policy as the nation grapples with quality, cost, and access issues. These changes are being played out in the public forum and promise to produce a new commitment to guaranteeing health care to all citizens. At this time, no one knows what the outcomes will be in terms of providers, delivery systems, or patient care. However, you must know that these new systems will have a significant impact on your role as a nurse—an impact that can only be speculated about in seminars, classes, and personal conversations.

INTEGRATED HEALTH CARE SYSTEMS

In response to the pending changes in health care reform, health care providers with services along the care continuum are rapidly repositioning their organizations to be successful in the future. Providers are linking together to form integrated systems that can provide health and illness services to large populations of people at an affordable cost. These systems are being formed by acquiring, partnering, and collaborating to provide comprehensive services for their health care enrollees.

Inherent in these changes is a renewed interest in health and wellness, a more efficient and effective system for treating illness, and a microscopic focus on costs. As a professional nurse, these changes will impact your practice immensely. Your knowledge needs will change, your career options will expand, and your professional competencies will be expected to support the increasing complexities of care.

NEW PATIENT CARE DELIVERY SYSTEMS

As integrated care networks expand, the care of a patient will be managed across the continuum from cradle to grave. The historic fragmentation of care will be better managed by more knowledgeable providers, improved information technology, and, in managed care plans, increased focus on costs per month per enrollee. These changes will necessitate new jobs, new care processes, new work environments, and new methods of outcome measurement. These changes will in turn require different ways of thinking about patient care, new approaches to quality management, and more knowledge about cost management.

As a professional nurse, you will be expected to lead, manage, and ensure changes that will reinvent health care delivery. Professional nurses have the opportunity to influence positively an enormous amount of change and to help others understand the new order. As a nurse, you are expected to lead, not just follow; to embrace creative solutions, not just make incremental change; and to support organizational initiatives with a positive attitude, not veiled resistance.

From the macroscopic health care scene to the microscopic unit-based activities, the professional nurse plays a major role in managing change. Knowing that a part of your role is to be a proactive member of a health care team sets the stage for you to make important contributions for the ultimate good of the patient and your profession.

OVERCOMING RESISTANCE TO CHANGE

Some people cling desperately to the present and to the past. These people seek to hang on to the familiar, to protect old habits, and to dig in their heels to resist new initiatives. It is not hard to understand why some people approach change in this manner. After all, they risk losing stability, control, and predictability as they face new challenges. Some fear they do not have the skills or knowledge to succeed in a different environment. Others don't understand the big picture and fear that the change will produce bad results.

Regardless of their motives, people who resist change in organizations slow down the wheels of progress. In the fast-paced health care environment, this resistance can be fatal to the organization or, at the least, to the individual's ability to succeed at work.

Dealing with resistance to change requires that you understand the events that led to the need for change. Determine for yourself why the organization is initiating changes. What are the compelling reasons for what's going on? Study the situation both outside and inside the organization. Then, in your role as a professional, help educate those around you about the overall picture and the need for new approaches. Guide your coworkers along the path of change by demonstrating successes and measuring results. Maybe then you will convert the resisters—actions often speak louder than words.

Resistance to change is real and can affect the whole milieu in which your team works. One of the greatest skill sets you can possess is the set of tools to support change. It will help you for a lifetime.

GUIDELINES FOR SUPPORTING CHANGE

In their handbook for organizational change, Pritchett and Pound (1992) set forth some myths and realities of organizational change. They believe that you have the opportunity to frame a situation and then to reach conclusions that will cause you to resist or embrace and support change. By weighing the situation against a broad, informed, and objective view of reality, you can interpret change accurately and deal with it effectively.

CHANGE IS HERE TO STAY

Despite the often held view that "this too shall pass," organizations undergo constant change. Those who wish for the "good old days" are focusing their energy on the impossible. The health care administration will better serve you and your patients if it constantly looks for ways to adapt, to adjust as fast as possible, and to protect the future of your organization.

YOU CONTROL YOUR REACTIONS

Yes, you have complete control over your reactions to change. As one wise person said, "You can go to Pity City, but just don't stay there." Getting upset with a change contributes little to progress, so acknowledge your feelings and then move forward. Nobody else is in charge of your attitude, so be upbeat and get the credit.

PROGRESS SOMETIMES FEELS LIKE TROUBLE

It is easy to feel like a victim in organizational change. Your job, your team, and your activities may change, making you feel like your entire career is up for grabs. But don't jump to conclusions too soon. Take a broad look at the issues, give the change time to work, and find the opportunities inherent in the change. If you don't see them immediately, keep on looking, or make your own opportunities!

CHANGE REQUIRES CHANGE

If your organization is undergoing major change or even minor adaptations, it is inconceivable that your role can stay the same. If you don't change, you will quickly be out of step with the new beat in the organization. When you see changes in the corporate culture, work priorities, or management style, take that as a new set of directives for you. Get ahead of the change by adopting behaviors that will ensure your success.

PROBLEMS ARE A PART OF CHANGE

It is impossible to institute new ways of doing things without creating some problems in the transition. If change were perfect, no one would resist it! Sure, there will be problems as progress takes place and sometimes the new instability increases job stress. The alternative would be much worse—no change, no stress, no future organization. So remember, handling problems is your job; some do it better than others.

MANAGEMENT MAKES TOUGH DECISIONS

The process of guiding change requires giving out information, managing the process, and attending to the sensitivities of information. Because change is so personal, the manager often must assist each worker individually with the process of change. In some organizations, the magnitude of change is so great that this becomes difficult. So before you add to a manager's stress, recognize that he or she isn't perfect but is trying to do the best job possible. Perhaps you can help work with your team to support the manager and the changes as they occur.

MAKING CHANGES WORK

In today's turbulent health care settings, there is hardly time to recover from one change before you are on to the next. The time available to restabilize the organization is short, creating an environment that feels constantly in motion. Rather than spending time second-guessing the managerial strategies, why not defend the organization that issues your paycheck and determine how you can help make the future a success. That doesn't mean you don't question decisions—it only means that once the discussion is completed, you move into the future as a team player.

BECOMING AN EFFECTIVE CHANGE AGENT

Throughout your professional career, you will be called on to be an agent of change. Assuming that you are committed to your employer and the values of the organization, becoming a change agent can be an exciting and fun part of your professional role. This does not require that you react to all change with glee and delight but, rather, that you approach changes with thoughtful sensitivity to others around you.

One thing is certain. First you have control over your attitude and the way you manage changes. You can choose to be a pioneer, an explorer, and a positive, enthusiastic player. You can focus on removing obstacles and moving forward. It is not hard to see that nurses with a "can-do" attitude will be in high demand and will be sought out to become leaders in the organizations future.

Second, to be an effective change agent, you will need to take ownership of the changes. It is not enough to "not be resistant." Nothing less than taking personal responsibility for moving forward will be enough. It is your future that is being formed, so help form it in a way that you will want to spend your career.

Third, protect your political capital by carefully choosing the issues you will challenge. To be sure, some issues are worth a challenge. Others, in the bigger scheme of things, are not. Ask yourself, "Is this a hill to die on?" as you debate whether or not to take on a battle. More often than not, altering your approach will gain you most of the benefits in a less confrontational way. There are always trade-offs. Select yours carefully.

Fourth, it may seem simple, but try to keep your sense of humor. Sure, organizational change is difficult, so being a change agent is more difficult. But things are bound to occur that deserve a chuckle. Taking yourself or the change so seriously that you are mired in stress is not healthy for you or the organization.

Finally, stay focused on inventing a new future rather than trying to fix the past. Think of new ways to do things and new opportunities for growth. Focus on what's coming and anticipate how you can acquire the knowledge and skills to succeed in the new environment. It's possible that what you do so well now may not even be needed in he future. Therefore, ensure your success by anticipating the future organizational success. Align your future with that of the organization.

SUMMARY

Managing change will be a big part of your future both personally and professionally. It would be interesting to know if people who look optimistically to the years ahead have learned to master change in a productive way, constantly moving forward with a positive outlook. It is a sure bet that all health care organizations, professions, and jobs will undergo substantial change in the years to come. Your role as a professional nurse will be to lead, guide, and manage change. Many of the resources for this role come from within yourself—your mind, your attitudes, and your resilience to change. Other resources come from around you—your peers, your managers, your organization. The combination of all these supports is staggering. There's not much you can't do if you want to. Isn't that a powerful thought?

DISCUSSION QUESTIONS

1. Describe a change taking place in a clinical area and develop a plan for your role as a change agent.
2. Analyze a change process that did not go well and determine how it might have been handled better.
3. Profile a person who is resistant to change and develop approaches for managing his or her transition into a positive supporter.

REFERENCES

Duck, T. (1993). Managing change: The art of balancing. *Harvard Business Review, 72*(1), 71–76.

Pritchett, P., et al. (1992). *The employee handbook for organizational change.* Dallas: Pritchett Press.

SUGGESTED READING

Kanter, R., Stein, B. & Jick, T. (1992). The challenge of organizational change. *New York Free Press.*

Mariner-Tomey, A. (1992). *A guide to nursing management.* St. Louis: Mosby.

Mohrman, A., Mohrman, S., Lidford, G., Cummings, T. & Lawler, E. (1988). *Large scale organizational change.* San Francisco: Jossey-Bass.

Morgan, G. (1988). *Riding the waves of change.* San Francisco: Jossey-Bass.

Quality Management

Ruth Miller

LEARNING OBJECTIVES

This chapter will enable you to:

1. Understand the basic history of health care programs for quality assurance, quality assessment and improvement, and risk management.
2. Discuss the impact of regulatory and accreditation agencies on these programs.
3. Describe how quality improvement and risk management activities intersect with and complement each other while performing separate organizational functions.

Vestal, K.W. Nursing Management:
Concepts and Issues, 2 ed.
© 1995 J.B. Lippincott Company

THE HISTORY OF QUALITY MANAGEMENT

To understand what is now called *quality assessment and improvement* (or *total quality management*) and *health care risk management*, the professional nurse must have a basic knowledge of the people and organizations that have contributed to the development, growth, and refinement of health care standards, practice, and risk management. The purpose of this chapter is to provide this basic knowledge and to encourage further study of the subject.

The monitoring and evaluation of the quality of patient care and outcomes began as early as the 1880s with the work of Florence Nightingale. In her work is found the inception and evolution of systems for quality assurance, quality assessment and improvement, continuous quality improvement (CQI), total quality management (TQM), and patient outcomes, with the accompanying action phase of monitoring and evaluating care.

In the middle to late 1800s, Florence Nightingale, after her experiences as a field nurse during the Crimean War, developed techniques for patient care, originated the concept of the patient care ward, and conceived the modern profession of nursing. Nightingale's concepts included the separation of intensive care patients from acute care patients, fresh air and good ventilation, and manageable nurse-to-patient ratios. Her attempts to standardize and analyze hospital statistics formed the beginning of health care quality assessment programs (Saunders, 1988).

In *Notes on Nursing* (1859), Nightingale defined nursing as the care of sick and well persons in homes or hospitals by nurses, both professional and nonprofessional. She wrote that nursing is either good or poor and that symptoms and suffering can result from poor nursing or lack of nursing. There are laws, canons, or basic rules of nursing, and the laws of health and the laws of nursing are said to be the same laws. These laws hold for both the well and the sick.

As early as 1913, a few physicians persistently called for defining hospital quality on behalf of the patient and in terms of the actual outcomes of patient care. One of these was Dr. E. A. Codman of Boston, who remarked that "A factory which sells its products takes pains to ensure that the product is a good one, but a hospital, which gives away its product, seems to regard the quality of its product as not worthy of investigation." He also stated that the only firm ground for evaluating a hospital was by actual results (Stevens, 1989). These statements are frequently quoted today in publications

196

and presentations dedicated to quality assessment and improvement and to TQM.

In the following years, the medical and nursing professions began to organize on the national level because of concerns about quality of care, fee splitting, lack of practice standards and regulation, and inadequate medical education (Stevens, 1989). Hospital administrators, most of whom were medical superintendents, organized to articulate their interests at the national level. The Association of Hospital Superintendents of the United States, established in 1912, became the American Hospital Association (AHA) in 1913 (Stevens, 1989). Although the AHA agreed in principle that there was a need to inspect, classify, and standardize hospital care to improve patient care and outcomes, they did not have the funds or the power to launch a major hospital inspection program (American College of Surgeons, 1946).

It was the American College of Surgeons that set up a committee on the standardization of hospitals. This committee initially met in 1913 and, after nearly 5 years of work, finalized the informal content of Minimum Standards to be used in surveying hospitals (American College of Surgeons, 1946). The Minimum Standards were published in the March 1918 issue of the *American College of Surgeons Bulletin* and in the April 1918 issue of *Surgery, Gynecology and Obstetrics*. Inspection of hospitals with 100 beds or more began on April 1, 1918. Although the initial three standards requiring case (medical) records, clinical laboratories, and prohibition of division of fees applied to physicians only, the authority for enforcing the standards was given to the hospital trustees or the governing authority. With these voluntary inspections, the prerequisite of which was conformance to standards, the health care industry was changed completely and forever.

Financial constraints prohibited the American College of Surgeons from continuing the hospital accreditation and standardization program, and in 1951 the Joint Commission on Accreditation of Hospitals, which included the Canadian Medical Association, was formed. The standards evolved by the American College of Surgeons over a period of some 35 years were adopted by the Joint Commission. The Joint Commission officially began to survey hospitals on January 1, 1952, using 11 standards that addressed the following: a modern physical plant free from hazards and properly equipped; a competent, well-trained chief executive officer or administrator with requisite authority and responsibility granted by the governing board; an adequate number of efficient personnel, properly organized and under competent supervision; group conferences of the administrative and medical staff to review their respective activities regularly and thoroughly; and a humanitarian attitude in which the best care of the patient is always the primary consideration (American College of Surgeons, 1946).

During the following years, the number and scope of the standards grew. The contributors to these standards were medical, nursing, and other health care professionals who, along with the paid Joint Commission staff, proposed and composed new standards and reviewed existing standards to determine the need for revision or elimination. Draft copies of proposed standards and recommendations on revision or elimination of standards were sent to accredited hospitals for review and comments.

In 1935, the Social Security Act was passed. This act was the direct result of the continuing efforts to establish public health legislation by organizations such as the American Association for Labor Legislation and by some members of Congress. The prototypes used in these efforts were Bismark's 1883 Sickness and Insurance Act, which was passed in Germany to help stem the growth of socialism, and the 1911 National Health Insurance Act enacted under the Liberal Party in England (Sidel & Sidel, 1984).

Three decades later, Public Law 89-87 created the Medicare and Medicaid programs. The law was signed by Lyndon Baines Johnson on July 30, 1965, and became effective January 1, 1966. Written into the Medicare Act was the provision that hospitals participating in that program were to maintain the level of patient care that had come to be recognized as the norm. The standards of the Joint Commission on Accreditation of Hospitals and the American Osteopathic Hospital Association's accreditation program are specifically referred to in the law. The original Conditions of Participation for Hospitals as published by the Social Security Administration reflected the 1965 standards of these organizations.

Under this law, hospitals continuing to meet the voluntary accreditation status of either of these organizations have "deemed status." In 1972, as the result of problems with the voluntary accreditation survey process in relation to the "deemed status," the Social Security Act was amended under Public Law 92–603, which provided for validation surveys (ie, a surveying of the surveyors; Johnson & Johnson, 1988).

HEALTH CARE RISK MANAGEMENT

Health care risk managers recognize the actions taken by Nightingale and others to prevent and reduce losses resulting from adverse patient care and credit them with changing the image of the hospital from that of a place to die to a place to recover health (Saunders, 1988).

Health care risk management, however, is relatively new. Before 1965, losses as the result of casualty, workers' compensation, and professional liability were fairly low. The case of *Darling v. Charleston Community Memorial Hospital* (1965) set a precedent. It effectively made the medical personnel who use the hospital part of the enterprise whether staff employees or independent practitioners, thereby holding the hospital directly liable for the failure of administrators and staff to properly monitor and supervise health care delivery within the hospital. As a result, health care organizations began to experience larger losses from untoward events. To make matters worse, many states began to liberalize their workers' compensation laws into no-fault programs, leading to an increase in claim settlements. As a result of these risk burdens, hospitals were forced to search out and create viable alternatives to commercial malpractice insurance. This led to the development of self-insurance programs and the need for an individual to administer this program and all activities of a health care organization attendant to financing risk.

Under self-insurance programs, activities that had been the responsibility of commercial carriers, such as claims management, investigation of incidents, and loss control, became the hospital's responsibility (Goldman, 1991). Self-insured hospitals were required as a condition of participation in Medicare to have a risk management program (ECRI, May 1992). As a result, by the mid-1970s, the discipline of risk management emerged with a unique focus on reducing the risk of patient injury and minimizing medical malpractice claims (Goldman, 1991). It was not until 1989, nearly a decade after quality assurance standards appeared, that the Joint Commission standards required hospitals to have risk management programs.

Several states require the reporting of any event that results in risk or harm to the life or safety of a patient or employee. For example, the Division of Health Facilities Evaluation and Licensing in New Jersey includes as reportable events any unscheduled interruption for 3 or more hours of the physical plant or clinical services essential to the health and safety of patients and employees and any alleged or suspected crime that endangers the life or safety of patients or employees, including crimes reportable to the police department or those resulting in an immediate on-site investigation by the police (ECRI, December 1991). Events must be reported by telephone, with a written follow-up report within 7 calendar days of the event, unless determined unnecessary by the department. As of May 1992, 10 states have passed legislation requiring the establishment of internal risk management programs (ECRI, May 1992).

THE DEVELOPERS OF TQM AND CQI IN INDUSTRY

Three of the most recognized leaders in the TQM process are W. Edwards Deming, Philip B. Crosby, and J. M Juran. Their methods have been found to be effective in the health care industry, and the decision to use (or not to use) the methods of one or the other is strictly up to the organization.

The W. Edwards Deming Management Method

There are 14 steps to the Deming method, with the goal being continuous improvement of the quality of the product or service. Deming's "chain reaction" concept is perhaps easier to address than the 14 steps. With better use of time and materials, productivity improves, enhancing the ability to capture the market with better quality and lower price. This in turn improves the potential for staying in business and the continued ability to provide jobs (Walton, 1986). The Deming chain reaction improves quality, thereby decreasing costs because of less rework and fewer mistakes, delays, and snags.

The Philip B. Crosby Method

Crosby also has a 14-step quality management process. He is best known for his statement (and book by the same title), "Quality is free" (Crosby, 1980):

> Quality is free. It's not a gift, but it is free. What costs money are the un-quality things, all the actions that involve not doing jobs right the first time. Quality is not only free, it is an honest-to everything profit maker. Every penny you don't spend on doing things wrong, over, or instead, becomes half a penny right on the bottom line.

Crosby's maturity grid, which uses measurement categories and states of development of quality management in the work setting, has been described and tested as a diagnostic tool to measure the maturity of organizational quality management in the health care setting (Masters & Schmele, 1991).

The J. M. Juran Method

J. M. Juran's method is known as the *Juran Trilogy* because there are three inter-related processes: quality planning, quality control, and quality improvement.

Quality Planning.   Determine who the customers are and what their needs are. Develop product features responding to the customers' needs and develop processes that are able to produce those product features. Transfer the resulting plans to the operating forces.

Quality Control.   Evaluate actual quality performance, compare actual performance to quality goals, and act on the differences.

Quality Improvement.   Establish the infrastructure needed to secure annual quality improvement. Identify the specific needs for improvement (ie, improvement projects). For each project, establish a project team with clear responsibility for bringing the project to a successful conclusion. Provide the resources, motivation, and training needed by the teams to diagnose causes, stimulate establishment of a remedy, and establish controls to hold the gains (Juran, 1989).

QUALITY MANAGEMENT AND HEALTH CARE RISK MANAGEMENT TODAY

CURRENT STANDARDS

Quality

The first quality assurance standards appeared in the 1980 *Accreditation Manual for Hospitals.* These standards required the governing body to establish, maintain, and support, through the hospital's administration and medical staff, an ongoing quality assurance program that included the objective assessment of important aspects of patient care and the correction of identified problems (Joint Commission on Accreditation of Healthcare Organizations [JCAHO], 1993).

In the 1993 *Accreditation Manual,* the chapter titled "Quality Assessment and Improvement" describes hospital activities designed to assess and improve the quality of patient care. There are 27 listings under the heading of "Quality Assessment and Improvement" in the index of the manual, some of which refer to the quality assessment and improvement chapter and others to specific areas of the manual for further detail.

Risk Management

Reference to risk management in the 1993 *Accreditation Manual* is found under the following areas: Management responsibility (MA.1.6.1), medical staff role in (MS.5.1.7), quality assessment and improvement, coordination with (QA.4.2.2, QA 4.2.3), and in safety management program (PL.1.2.2, PL.1.3.1.4).

CURRENT REGULATIONS

Quality Regulations

482.21 Medicare Conditions of Participation: Quality Assurance (QA): The governing body must ensure that there is an effective hospital-wide quality assurance program to evaluate the provision of patient care. The interpretive guidelines, under survey procedures for 482.21, state that a hospital that continually evaluates the quality of care generally provides high-quality patient care.

Risk Management Regulations

Risk management regulations remain the same for hospitals participating in the Medicare program. If a facility is self-insured, it must have a designated risk manager. Hospitals are also subject to individual state regulations.

Other Regulations: Federal, State, and Local

At the federal level, the Occupational Safety and Health Administration (OSHA) is responsible for safety in the workplace. OSHA regulations cover basic safety and the complex issues of disposal of hazardous wastes and handling of chemical spills. The Bloodborne Pathogen Standard (March 1992) addresses the safety of employees with a potential for exposure to bloodborne diseases such as human immunodeficiency virus and hepatitis B virus. Also at the federal level is the Food and Drug Administration (FDA), which may inspect any facility in which drugs or medical devices are used for investigation of a specific device-related problem or to conduct an on-site audit for compliance.

At the state level are the licensing agencies for health professionals and the Hospital Licensing Standards, with which all hospitals must be in continued compliance. The state agency responsible for enforcing the licensing standards also approves the renewal of the hospital's license to operate.

At the local level, there are county or city regulations. For example, local fire marshals are responsible for the annual fire-safety survey before license renewal. They monitor hospitals on a random basis for continued compliance with applicable city, state, and National Fire Protection Agency (NFPA) requirements. Another example is the city's Department of Health, which is responsible for routine inspections and issuance of the sanitary license in food preparation and storage areas.

The preceding information may seem overwhelming, but in your role as a professional nurse, it is essential that you have at least this basic understanding of the various regulatory and accrediting agencies and of the impact they have on the hospital. In addition, it must be understood that individual professionals, by their actions or inactions, have a significant impact on the hospital's ability to be in continued compliance with Medicare Conditions of Compliance for Hospitals, licensing laws, voluntary accreditation standards, and other applicable regulations. Health professionals must be aware that attorneys for the plaintiff understand and keep current with this information.

QUALITY ASSURANCE VERSUS QUALITY IMPROVEMENT

The term *quality assurance* frequently indicates a focus on clinical aspects of care rather than on the full series of interrelated governance, managerial support, and clinical processes that affect patient outcomes. Activities often are compartmentalized by hospital structure. The focus is on the performance of individuals and especially on problem performance. Frequently, action is initiated in response to an identified problem rather than in an attempt to develop better processes. The appropriateness of care (was the right thing done?) and effectiveness of care (was it done right?) are separated from the efficiency of care. Efforts to improve patient outcome frequently are not integrated with efforts to improve efficiency or value (JCAHO, 1993).

Quality assessment and *quality improvement* are the terms found most frequently in literature, probably because the Joint Commission's terminology tends to become the current terminology. The 1993 *Accreditation Manual* defines quality assessment as "the measurement of the technical and interpersonal aspects of health care and services and the outcomes of that care and service" (JCAHO, 1993).

Quality improvement is defined as the ongoing study and improvement of the processes of providing health care services to meet the needs of patients and others. Quality assessment and improvement denotes the ongoing activities designed to evaluate objectively and systematically the quality of patient care and services, to pursue opportunities to improve patient care and services, and to resolve identified problems. Standards are applied to evaluate the quality of a hospital's performance in conducting quality assessment and improvement activities (JCAHO, 1993).

TQM and CQI are essentially the same concept as quality assessment and improvement. Through continual examination of and focus on patient outcomes, the goal is to deliver the highest quality product or service by continuous learning and improvement of processes, products, and services (ECRI, May 1992). There is a paradigm shift in TQM and CQI from emphasis on provider to customer, job to process, functional to cross-functional, vertical to horizontal, inspection to prevention, reactive to deliberate or provocative, and problem people to problem processes (Moore, 1992). The introduction to the 1992 *Accreditation Manual* refers to "drawing upon the insights of the originators and major developers of continuous quality improvement such as W. Edwards Deming, Joseph Juran, and Philip Crosby" (JCAHO, 1992). The introduction to the 1993 manual is silent on the subject.

Regardless of the word coined for the program or which program is used, the goal is essentially the same—to bring the results of patient care and services into a more desirable condition (ie, to improve them). The following statement appears under the heading of "Quality Assessment and Improvement" in the 1992 *Accreditation Manual*: "Even if performance is meeting some objective standard, quality can still be improved" (JCAHO, 1992). To modify an old adage, "If it ain't broke, it can be improved."

Any and all of the preceding goals can be achieved by establishing expected patient outcomes and outlining critical pathways or other monitoring and evaluation tools. The outcomes and critical pathways must be multidisciplinary. Regardless of the tools used, outcomes, not processes, must be measured and evaluated. In other words, do not measure whether something was documented, but measure the patient's outcome as reflected in the documentation. For example, ask "Did the patient receive adequate pain relief postoperatively?" instead of "Did the nurse document the response to the pain medication within the required period of time?" The process is valuable as a mechanism to identify and resolve problems on chosen aspects of patient care and the processes related to care.

To keep CQI meaningful and relevant, the tools in place for this process should be simple and the indicators relevant. Direct patient care staff should participate in the development of indicators so that the focus is not on something that has to be done for the Joint Commission but on something that has to be done for the patient. Additionally, try not to restrict data-collecting activities and sharing of information to a select few. The sharing may be done in innovative ways (eg, dedicated bulletin boards, posters, and "games") and in the traditional meeting format. All tools should contribute to answering the frequently asked question, "How will this really impact my practice and what difference will this make in the patient's outcome?"

These quality assessment and improvement activities do not deal with financial concerns, except in direct relation to patient care issues such as unnecessary surgery, unjustified admissions, excessive use of ancillary services, or other inappropriate or unnecessary care (ECRI, May 1992).

RISK MANAGEMENT: CLINICAL VERSUS FINANCIAL

The goal of clinical risk management is to prevent and reduce potential losses resulting from adverse patient care events. Trends and isolated occurrences are examined to improve quality, limit liability, and reduce the financial impact on the institution of even a single compensable event.

Financial risk management involves minimizing the probability of events that have adverse physical or psychological effects on patients, visitors, and staff or result in physical losses to plant and equipment; overseeing expenditures by the hospital to insure against the occurrence of such events; and monitoring compensation paid and associated legal and administrative costs when such events result in injury, death, or damage (ECRI, 1984).

RISK MANAGEMENT AND QUALITY ASSURANCE: INDIVIDUAL FUNCTIONS AND OVERLAP

Risk management functions include claims and insurance management, workers' compensation, contract and policy review, safety, medical/legal problems, and general liability issues. Quality improvement functions include department or physician actions taken to improve practice, care, and outcomes; disciplinary measures; ongoing patient monitoring; and review of use and practice problems.

There is some overlap between the risk management and quality improvement functions. Both identify problems leading to adverse events (eg, generic screening); intervene to reduce likelihood of recurrence (eg, policy/procedure change or corrective action); share a database; focus on patients; use continuous monitoring systems to prevent recurrence of identified problems; analyze information; require clinical and managerial expertise and staff education; and report to a governing board (ECRI, May 1992).

THE IMPORTANCE OF TQM, CQI, AND RISK MANAGEMENT

The importance of TQM, CQI, and risk management activities in daily nursing practice cannot be overemphasized. These activities include continuous compliance with the following: approved hospital, departmental, and unit-specific policies and procedures; federal, state, and local laws and regulations, including Medicare, OSHA, and fire prevention standards; regulations of agencies such as the state Department of Health, which is responsible for licensing hospitals, and the state boards regulating professional practice; and, in an accredited hospital, the voluntary accreditation standards of either the Joint Commission or the American Osteopathic Hospital Association. Another important consideration in CQI and risk management activities is professional practice accountability, as related to knowledge and use in daily practice of the standards of professional practice established and defined by the American Nurses Association and specialty nursing organizations.

Risk management is the prevention and reduction of potential losses resulting from adverse patient outcomes. Its focus is not only on improving quality but also on reducing the financial impact of adverse occurrences to the institution. It is in this area that risk management and CQI programs can best improve efficiency and effectiveness by sharing information and avoiding duplication of effort (ECRI, May 1992). Risk management and CQI activities must be coordinated to manage risks effectively and efficiently while maintaining control over the quality of care.

Adverse occurrences to patients, especially those in the preventable category, pose the greatest risk of severe financial loss to health care institutions. Financial loss means not only payouts to individuals for claims and lawsuits, but also long-term damage to the reputation of the institution. The focus of CQI is to provide the highest quality patient care and services and, through ongoing monitoring and evaluation, to identify trends and patterns to improve patient care and outcomes (JCAHO, 1993). Although the prevention of financial loss is one of the benefits, it is not the goal of an organized and effective quality improvement program.

The following fictitious case review, created for purposes of this chapter, should help explain the different yet complementary roles of risk management and continuous quality assessment and improvement.

CASE REVIEW: LUMBAR LAMINECTOMY WITH SPINAL FUSION

The orthopedic unit of a large metropolitan hospital, with the cooperation and agreement of physicians and the multiple disciplines involved in the care of their patients, has established multidisciplinary critical pathways specific to the various diagnoses of the patient population.

The pathways are used in planning the care of all patients, and the patient teaching protocols used on admission are an extension of the pathways. The staff has found that the patients not only like the process used, they benefit from it. Pertinent to this case review are the established activity and teaching goals as described in the "Lumbar Laminectomy with Spinal Fusion" pathway.

> On the third postoperative day, a patient who had a repeat lumbar laminectomy with spinal fusion was without evidence of postoperative complications. However, the patient resisted efforts to assist him in attaining the established ambulation goals, preferring to do it his way. His way did not include adhering to instructions to use the lumbar sacral support or the immediately accessible call bell to summon assistance.
>
> Sitting on the edge of the bed, the patient attempted to slide his feet into his slippers, which were not easily accessible. As he positioned himself to reach the slippers, the bed began to roll away from him because the wheels had not been locked. As the bed rolled further away, the patient quickly attempted to stand, but his legs gave way, and he slid and sat down "hard" on the floor.
>
> Staff members hurrying to his room in response to his cry of pain and call for help attempted to stand him up. But he apparently had no feeling in his legs and could not stand. He was lifted into bed, the side rails were put in place, the call bell was placed within reach, and, belatedly, the bed wheels were locked. In accordance with policy, the physician, nurse manager, and the risk manager were notified.
>
> After obtaining the necessary information, the risk manager immediately opened up a file on the case as a potentially compensable event and began making plans for a review of the occurrence with the nurse manager and for scheduling interviews with the staff members involved. The RN responsible for the care of the patient assumed charge of the immediate issues of patient comfort, physician notification, and carrying out of any orders. The nurse manager, using the person assigned responsibility for unit quality assessment and improvement functions, began clinical investigation of the case for the possibility of a breach in standards of care and in anticipation of questions from the physician and risk manager.

In this case study, the nurse manager's investigation would include a review of documentation to determine if preoperative teaching was done and if the preoperative interview or the patient's response to teaching about the importance of ambulation postoperatively revealed the possibility of problems related to ambulation. If problems were anticipated, the review would determine whether physical therapy consultation was called for earlier than usual and whether established protocols were followed when the patient resisted ambulation goals.

One of these persons would immediately contact the appropriate persons to examine the wheel-locking mechanisms on the bed to ensure that there was no mechanical failure. On the basis of the findings, an investigation into the apparent breach of prudent safety policies related to the locking of bed wheels would begin.

Because the record may not be silent about the incident, they would have to ensure that the event was recorded in an objective fashion to include assessment of injury, timely notification of physician, initiation of appropriate treatment, continued observation of the patient and injury, and safety precautions. This documentation is significant because, in case of claims made, silence in the record could possibly suggest to a lawyer that the practitioners thought they did something wrong and, therefore, omitted this significant event. Finally, the usual protocol for filling out and submitting incident or adverse occurrence reports would be followed.

On completion of the preceding activities, the nurse manager, quality representative, and the risk manager would work together to look for trends or similar events on that unit or with the particular staff involved. Based on the findings, a conclusion would be reached regarding actions to be taken.

Discussion

The review of the medical record found documented evidence that the established critical pathway and approved preoperative teaching protocols had been explained to the patient. There was also evidence that the patient verbalized understanding and did not anticipate any problems with compliance.

Also, in accordance with protocols, there was evidence that this teaching was reviewed on the first postoperative day and that the patient verbalized understanding and was prepared to comply with plans for ambulation and sitting in the chair with lumbar support. Documentation after that was silent about compliance or noncompliance.

Patient Outcome

Although the diagnostic studies after the fall were negative, with the patient's neurologic status documented as intact, the patient's length of stay was extended by 5 days. During this time, the patient reported that feeling had returned to his legs and he was able to attain maximal functional mobility.

Conclusion

In this patient's case, the preventable adverse occurrence was most likely due to two factors: lack of compliance with established patient care and lack of compliance with safety protocols. The fact that the patient apparently suffered no permanent damage was not because of, but in spite of, the actions of the multidisciplinary care givers.

A planned, multidisciplinary, and mandatory inservice program was given for all personnel on all shifts. Each session reinforced the established unit goals of all disciplines working cooperatively to enhance the efficiency, safety, and effectiveness of the established patient outcomes program. These sessions contributed to the development and reinforcement of preventive behaviors. Preventive behaviors should help prevent adverse occurrences such as those described in the case review by identifying and reducing sources of error in care, documentation, and safety.

The continued use of preventive behaviors should reduce the need for reactive behaviors such as incident investigation, bill adjustment decisions, and insurance reserve manipulation. Reactive behaviors are not desirable because they are designed to respond to errors and claims after they occur.

LEST WE FORGET

Health care professionals must be careful about becoming immune to the negative evaluations patients can give on what we perceive as routine. A 2:00 AM awakening for vital signs or medications, for example, may be accompanied by bright lights, loud voices, and what the patient perceives as less than gentle handling. Other examples are cold meals or no meals because of tests; walks in corridors with a urine-filled catheter bag clutched in hand; transportation by wheel chair with johnny gown open; no posterior or frontal covering of patient; and forgetting that routine invasive techniques such as IVs might be found extremely anxiety-producing to the average adult. A feeling of discontinuity can be created by shift changes, so that the patient and family feel that there is no one in charge or responsible for their care (Press, 1992).

Expecting patients to surrender autonomy and conform to clinical schedules, treatment modes, and behavioral requirements puts us on a crash course with them. These expectations often are reinforced by our actions, which can imply that we are too busy to consider patients' feelings about their lost identity and dignity as individuals (Press, 1992).

Another "lest we forget" is the danger of not understanding or of underestimating the significance of family members on patients' perceptions of care. Transforming a patient's impressions of care and services that could lead to litigation can begin with either the patient or the family. Patients rarely initiate lawsuits without consulting significant family members. If the family and the patient have had negative interactions with the hospital, the predisposition to claim is greater. For this reason, measures must be taken to assist family members who overtly or covertly demonstrate anxiety or have emotional outbursts (Press, 1992).

OTHER CONCERNS IN PATIENT OUTCOMES AND RISK MANAGEMENT

Patient Confidentiality

It is important to respect the confidentiality of patients and family by not engaging in "loose talk." Beware of hall conversations or conferences on patients. Patients or their families who accidentally overhear staff members talking inappropriately about the patient or the patient's condition, whether on the unit, in the cafeteria, or in the elevators, may feel that their rights have been violated and seek legal assistance.

Medication Administration

To help prevent medication errors, adhere to the five "rights" of medication administration: right patient, right dose, right order, right route, and right time. Don't forget the importance of verifying and documenting allergies or untoward reactions to medications.

Documentation

Documentation is an important area of risk management for all health care professionals. Documentation has been identified as the most important nonmedical issue leading to liability for the hospital. Cases often have to be settled out of court because of charting and documentation errors, even when the care provided was acceptable. Everything done for a patient should be documented on the chart in a clearly legible manner. A chart that is complete and accurate can prevent a claim from being filed or can serve to bring the case to a successful conclusion (Odom, 1990).

A frequent documentation problem is omission. Legally, if a service was not charted, it is very difficult to prove that it was done. Deliberately falsifying, altering, or tampering with a chart can increase malpractice awards by millions of dollars. Such acts are unethical and constitute fraud. Correction fluid should never be used. Any late entry should be labeled as such and any correction should be made properly (Odom, 1990). Do not criticize other health care professionals in the chart or use words that reveal a negative attitude toward your patient. Do document any information that you report to the physician (Iyer, 1991).

If an unreadable page must be recopied, the following applies: At the top of the page, identify that the page was rewritten with the statement, "Notes copied from original of (date)." Do not destroy the original; place it in the chart with the copied page (Iyer, 1991).

Controlling Patient Nosocomial Infections

Nosocomial infections may prolong hospital stays for weeks or even months and may cause death or permanent harm. Adherence to the health care organization's comprehensive infection control program designed to prevent or reduce nosocomial infections should be mandatory. Comprehensive programs include strategies for preventing cross-infections between patients, universal precautions for preventing transmission of disease between patients and staff, control of visitor traffic, procedures for instrument and equipment sterilization and for sterile technique during surgical and invasive procedures, and revision and implementation of policies, procedures, and educational programs in response to new legislation and regulations (ECRI, September 1992).

Safety

"Safety practice is the identification, evaluation and control of hazards to prevent or mitigate harm or damage to people, property or the environment." (ECRI, November 1992) Safety, security, and loss prevention are essential components of risk management and CQI programs. Monitoring hospitals for prevention of patient falls, violent crimes, infant abductions, and disaster planning are all part of safety management.

SUMMARY

It is the responsibility of all professionals to know standards and regulations, to know the programs in place in their facilities, to keep current with health care news, and to "know the future," so they can continue to grow in and with the profession of nursing.

DISCUSSION QUESTIONS

1. Discuss the differences and interrelations among quality assurance, risk management, and TQM initiatives.
2. Review several patient records and evaluate the quality and completeness of the documentation.
3. Describe the professional nurse's role in TQM within a health care setting.

REFERENCES

American College of Surgeons Bulletin. (1946). *21*(4).

Crosby, P. B. (1980). *Quality is free.* New York: Penguin.

Goldman, T. A. (1991). Risk management concepts and strategies. *Journal of Intravenous Nursing, 14*(3).

ECRI and Pennsylvania Insurance Management Company. (1984). *Hospital Risk Control: Perspectives.*

ECRI and Pennsylvania Insurance Management Company. (1991). *Hospital Risk Control: Perspectives.*

ECRI and Pennsylvania Insurance Management Company. (1992). *Hospital Risk Control: Perspectives.*

Darling v Charleston Community Memorial Hospital (1965). 33 Ill. 2d 326, 211 N.E. 2d, 253 (Supreme Court of Illinois), Certiorari denied, 383 U.S. 496, 86 S. CT., 1204, 16 L.Ed. 2d 209 (1966).

Federal Register. (December 6, 1991). *56*(235)

Iyer, P. W. (1991). Six more charting rules to keep you sane. *Nursing 91 21(7), 36.*

Johnson, E. A., & Johnson, R. L. (1988). *Hospitals under fire* (pp. 128–132). Rockville, MD: Aspen.

Joint Commission on Accreditation of Healthcare Organizations. (1992). *Accreditation Manual for Hospitals.* Oakbrook, IL: Author.

Joint Commission on Accreditation of Healthcare Organizations. (1993). *Accreditation Manual for Hospitals.* Oakbrook, IL: Author.

Juran, J. M. (1989). *Juran on leadership for quality: An executive handbook.* New York: The Free Press.

Masters, F., & Schmele, J. A. (1991). Total quality management: An idea whose time has come. *Journal of Nursing Quality Assurance 5*(4),13.

Medicare Conditions of Participation, Interpretive Guidelines and Survey Procedures for Hospitals. (1986).

Moore, K., et al. (1992, September). *Principles and values of continuous quality improvement in healthcare.* Paper presented at Management Conference, St. Luke's Episcopal Hospital, Houston, TX.

Nightingale, F. (1859). *Notes on nursing: What it is and what it is not.* London: Harrison & Sons.

Odom, J. L. (1990). The emerging role of risk management. *Journal of Post Anesthesia Nursing, 5*(2), 122–123.

Press, I. (1992). *Hospital risk control: Perspectives—6: "The predisposition to file claims, the patient's perspective."* Plymouth Meeting, PA: ECRI (published for Pennsylvania Management Company), 3.

Saunders, L. M. (1988, July). *Designing for productivity.* American Hospital Association.

Sidel, V. W., & Sidel, R. (1984). *Reforming medicine: Lessons of the last quarter century* (p. 66). New York: Pantheon.

Stevens, R. (1989). *In sickness and in wealth.* New York: Basic Books.

Walton, M. (1986). *The Deming management method.* New York: Putnam.

Nursing Informatics

Roy L. Simpson

LEARNING OBJECTIVES

This chapter will enable you to:

1. Understand the historical role nursing has played in shaping patient care technology and how and why that role is changing.
2. Understand the basic definitions of nursing informatics and nursing information systems as seen both by the American Nurses Association and by most system suppliers.
3. Understand the impediments to the advancement of nursing information systems.
4. Understand the basic concepts of technology evaluation.
5. Understand how systems are selected and what role nursing managers and clinical nurse specialists play in the process.

Vestal, K.W. Nursing Management:
Concepts and Issues, 2 ed.
© 1995 J.B. Lippincott Company

The field of nursing informatics is relatively new, having been designated a true nursing specialty by the American Nurses Association in 1992. Historically, most information systems in health care have centered on financial and administrative systems. Only recently has emphasis been placed on the role of high technology in assisting clinicians and primary care givers.

That technology is changing, growing, and adapting at breakneck speed. Today's solution may be tomorrow's old news. Although this chapter does not focus on the actual systems available today (except in the most general terms), it will help readers understand the dynamics behind patient care technology. More importantly, it will provide guidelines for how nursing leaders, managers, and staff can protect their interests in the selection and management of information systems.

HISTORICAL OVERVIEW OF NURSING INFORMATION SYSTEMS

In the late 1970s and early 1980s, many hospitals and health care institutions began using technology to help manage the seemingly limitless amount of data related to patient information and financial accounting. The first hospital information systems were actually administrative and financial systems. The reason was simple: financial information and patient data are relatively stable. Financial information also has its own set of universally accepted data standards. As a result, financial and administrative systems were more easily built and were used by just about every kind of organization within 10 years of their introduction.

By the middle to late 1980s, it became clear that information technology had to move to the clinical arena to provide greater value. Yet because most clinical systems started out as financial and administrative systems, administrative and financial managers continued to make purchasing decisions—even for systems used in patient care settings. This caused many problems for the nursing profession, whose needs for clinically sensitive technology often were ignored, despite the fact that information technology can be a viable solution to the relentless nursing shortage and that nurses are the primary users of patient care systems.

Because nursing was often "outside the loop" when it came to selecting patient care systems, the Joint Commission on Accreditation of Healthcare Organizations (JCAHO) mandated nurse participation in the selection process in 1991. In the *Accreditation Manual for Hospitals,*

216

the Commission specified that nurses be involved in evaluating, selecting, and integrating all systems that affect patient care. There were other movements demanding nursing's involvement, including the Institute of Medicine's (IOM) vision for a computerized patient record. Because entering observations and managing patient care information is primarily the domain of nursing, nursing leaders began to see the importance of having a say in how computerization of the patient record affects patient care and nursing care delivery.

These new pressures increased the need for nurses to be properly educated about technology to make appropriate decisions. It is for this reason that in1992 the ANA designated nursing informatics as a specialty. More and more nursing schools are offering graduate programs in the specialty.

WHAT IS A NURSING INFORMATION SYSTEM?

The ANA defines nursing informatics in the following way:

Nursing Informatics is concerned with the legitimate access to and use of data, information and knowledge to standardize documentation, improve communication, support the decision-making process, develop and disseminate new knowledge, enhance the quality, effectiveness and efficiency of health care, empower clients to make health care choices and advance the science of nursing.

Basically, nursing informatics involves all aspects of technology related to nursing care delivery, which could include financial and patient care applications. For example, nursing managers typically receive regular reports from the organization's financial or cost-accounting system about staff productivity and quality of delivered care. Even though the information is generated from a "financial system," it is used to evaluate nursing care and thus falls within the realm of nursing informatics.

Information systems are typically identified as a hospital information system (HIS) or a nursing information system (NIS). The HIS encompasses the information processing needs of the entire health care organization—from administrative to clinical functions. It typically includes the automation of ancillary departments such as radiology, pharmacy, and laboratory. Nevertheless, there is no single universally accepted definition of an HIS. Each vendor or supplier may have a slightly different understanding or definition. That's why nursing managers should always be vigilant about establishing the minimum requirements of an HIS and clarifying the vendor's operating definition.

The NIS is commonly understood to be a subset of the larger HIS, although linked or integrated with it. The Center for Healthcare Information Management (CHIM), defines the NIS as:

> . . . a software system that automates the nursing process from assessment to evaluation, including patient care documentation. It also includes a means to manage the data necessary for the delivery of patient care, e.g., patient classification, staffing, scheduling and costs. It is not separate, but an integral part of the healthcare organization's overall information system.

As such, the NIS typically includes the following functions or subsystems:

- Patient acuity or patient classification for assistance with staffing and scheduling
- Care planning and documentation to reduce the inordinate amount of time (up to 40%) nurses spend managing, communicating, and documenting patient information
- Quality assurance for evaluating the quality of nursing services based on a number of factors, including patient records, nursing care plans, and patient care criteria based on predetermined standards
- Order management/results reporting, to significantly enhance and streamline communications between nursing and other departments, including radiology, clinical laboratory, nutrition, and pharmacy
- Inventory, for streamlining communications between the nursing department and materials management for supplies
- Discharge planning, for standardized discharge plans
- Evaluation of nursing services by reports or "query" capabilities (ie, you can "ask" the system to report on nonstandard requests)

In the future, NISs may include bedside or point of care systems that involve sophisticated technology small enough to be portable and easily hand-held and used at the bedside. Although such technology already exists, few health care organizations can afford it. Many predict that it won't be until the late 1990s that this technology "trickles down" to most major health care settings.

KEY BARRIERS TO NURSING-RELATED TECHNOLOGY

One of the IOM's criteria for a computerized patient record is that "it supports structured data collection in a manner that adequately supports practitioners' direct entry and stores that information according to a defined vocabulary." (Simpson, 1991)

The key phrases here are "structured data collection" and "according to a defined vocabulary." Unfortunately, nursing does not have a universally accepted "defined vocabulary," taxonomy, lexicon, or minimum data set. Nearly every other health care constituency already has its own minimum data set—hospitals have UHDDS, physicians have ICD-9-CM, finance has standard billing codes (UB-82), and so forth. Nursing is the only major health care player without its own minimum data set.

The problem is that technology must operate from a universally accepted minimum data set. For example, bank teller machines all have a universal minimum data set. In other words, at almost every automatic teller you can expect the same kinds of codes or questions. You expect the system to be universal. Otherwise it would be chaotic. The purpose of a minimum data set is to help nurses compare data across clinical populations, geographic areas, and time. To do so, data categories, variables, and elements must be identified and accepted.

For example, the term *patient immobility* should mean the same thing in Miami as it does in Alaska. But it is possible that each nursing service organization could have a slightly different definition for what constitutes immobility. The problem then arises of which definition vendors should use to create their NIS. By not having a universal minimum data set and taxonomy, we place the burden on the vendor, supplier, or developer to define nursing terms and, in a sense, nursing practice.

Currently, the American Nurses Association has backed the adoption of the data elements approved for classification by the North American Nursing Diagnosis Association (NANDA). The NANDA data elements puts the control of nursing information back in the nurses' hands. Once there is consensus within the entire nursing profession (which, at press time, there is not), system developers will be able to incorporate nursing data and nursing definitions into patient care systems more successfully.

EIGHT STEPS TO TECHNOLOGY EVALUATION

Publicly supporting a system that is clinically and organizationally inappropriate can be a professional and personal nightmare for a nursing manager. Not only does a "mistake" cost thousands (usually millions) of dollars, it seriously erodes nursing staff confidence in its leadership. To avoid mistakes, it is helpful to understand basic concepts of technology evaluation. These concepts include architecture, data evolution, communication, data access, information security, hardware, resources, and support.

1. **Architecture.** Architecture refers to a system's data-handling capabilities. There are two types of architectures—"open" and "closed." Open architecture refers to the system's ability to accept information from other internal and external systems, regardless of format. Closed systems don't accept data outside their system limits without the use of complicated interface programs. Many vendors today are moving toward open systems because they protect the existing technology investments.

2. **Data Evolution.** Data evolution refers to the ability to manipulate or alter data according to your specific needs at any specific moment. This is usually a function of a "report writer" or "query system." With the latter, you can ask the system to contrast and compare data not typically contrasted and compared. Data manipulation can be quite complex. Generally, the more complex the system, the more complex it is to use. Therefore, sophistication should always be balanced against usability. After all, what good is a really "smart" system if nobody uses it because it is so difficult?

3. **Communication.** Does the system allow for easy communications between users and systems? Ideally, your system should let you communicate easily with systems in other departments, with other users, and even with systems in satellite centers.

4. **Data Access.** How easily is data accessed from multiple sources? When there are multiple systems in one hospital, it usually means that there are different "languages" and operating systems in use. In these cases, an interface that "translates" the languages is required. Although an interface can be very effective, there is always the risk that the true meaning (in this case, the integrity of the data) will be communicated ineffectively. The problem of data access is universal in a business environment in which there is a wide variety of technological choices, platforms, languages, and operating systems.

5. **Information Security.** In the clinical setting, data security is critical. With stringent security measures, data such as confidential patient information can and will be protected from data mismanagement, hackers, and system breakdown. It is imperative that nursing leaders examine all solutions and options available for protecting patient data.

6. **Hardware.** Hardware is the actual "box" the system runs on (whereas "software" is the application that runs on it). Hardware can be anything from a small personal computer to a huge, multi-million dollar mainframe. The hardware you choose will have a lot to do with the protection of and the speed with which you access it. Many health care organizations, however, are committed to specific hardware platforms, which may or may not dictate future technological decisions.

7. **Resources.** What resources will be needed to meet technological requirements and user demands? No system should be selected without a thorough understanding of how every user and system in the organization will be affected.

8. **Support.** The level of support you expect to receive is extremely important. An HIS or NIS typically requires a great deal of support or "hand holding" from the vendor or developer during the implementation and initial stages of use. Nursing managers must articulate the kind of support they want, in what amount, who will provide that support, and how that support will be accountable.

SELECTING AND MANAGING AN INFORMATION SYSTEM

Selecting an HIS or NIS can take as long as 2 years. The process is quite complex, particularly when clinical information is involved. Nursing leaders must balance the needs of their nurses with the sometimes competing needs of physicians, other clinicians, and administrators. Most software contracts last a minimum of 7 years.

For effective systems selection, nursing managers must be ready to oversee the following steps:

1. Perform a systems inventory. Before you can choose what you want, you have to know what you have in your organization. For example, if your organization has committed itself to a specific platform, your options are limited. You need to know that up front.

2. Understand the organization's budgetary limits. This is a basic point, but it bears reviewing because of the constantly changing nature of technology. Bedside terminals, for example, promise great things for the efficiency of nursing services and for the improvement of quality care. However, their cost is astronomical (all new technology is very expensive at first; prices fall after the

technology is proven and becomes more available). Nursing leaders must understand financial constraints before pursuing technology options.

3. Understand the organization's strategic plan. It is imperative to understand the organization's position, not just technologically, but its future direction and how that direction will impact nursing. Without that understanding, all decisions will be made in a vacuum. More and more nursing leaders are creating Nursing Strategic Plans, which fold into the vision of the larger organization's plan but also articulate the goals and strategies for nursing service.

4. Create a business plan for an NIS. The idea of creating a business plan for a system may seem foreign to nurses, but it is actually standard practice in most industries and professions. A business plan helps you identify the kind of system you want. It also helps you prioritize your needs and articulate your vision to the board of directors of the organization.

5. Understand the RFP (Request for Proposal). The RFP is the standard way in which organizations specify what they want in a system. It is distributed to key suppliers, who are then asked to "answer" how their system would meet those requirements. The supplier who fulfills the most requirements usually wins. When it comes to nursing requirements, be specific to a fault (even if it means stating the obvious). In other words, never assume that suppliers have the same understanding of nursing terms that you have. Spell it out for them to avoid confusion or disappointment later. (For example, patient classification may mean one thing to you, but something entirely different to the vendor.) Define what you mean by common phrases as best as you can.

6. Assign a clinical nurse specialist to serve with you on the selection committee. Nursing must have representation on the selection committee, as mandated by the JCAHO. However, it is not enough to have management's perspective. Because the system will be used by clinical nurses, it is imperative that a clinical nurse specialist be assigned to serve with you on the committee. This way, you can effectively cover both clinical and management issues.

7. Accept the fact that selecting a system requires a great deal of education. The nurses on the selection committee must understand that systems selection can be a long process that requires a great deal of knowledge. Many nurses in these situations either enroll in postgraduate courses to understand the basics of nursing technology or do a lot of "weekend reading." One excellent source for self-education is networking through the many national, regional, and local nursing associations. Many have nursing infor-

matics subgroups that provide the opportunity to learn from those who have selected and implemented systems or are in the process of doing so.

8. Create an advisory committee of key clinical nurses and other clinicians (including physicians). By creating a clinical advisory committee, you can ensure that patient care issues will always remain at the forefront of the selection process. There is strength in numbers, and by including key clinical players, you will likely obtain early "buy-in" from key players within and outside your department.

9. Demand veto power. You and your clinical nurse should have both affirmative and veto voting powers. Having veto power is particularly important—after all, if the system doesn't meet your standards, you should have the right to vote against it. Retain the right to say "no" if the system doesn't meet nursing's needs.

10. Participate in contract negotiations. Once a system is selected, many nurses think the job is over. Rest assured, it is not. Negotiating the contract is a crucial part of the process through which you can protect nursing's interests by clarifying such issues as warranties, intellectual property, maintenance agreements, maintenance fees, maintenance obligations, and upgrade management. This process can be quite complex, and many nurses often seek outside consulting assistance.

Once a system is selected, nursing managers must be ready to handle the cultural changes that occur as a result of implementing a new system. For the most part, people are resistant to change—even if it is for the better. To prevent problems, nursing managers must understand why people resist change and how to assuage concerns about quality, productivity, and job preservation. In addition, nursing leaders should solicit "buy-ins" from key individuals and constituencies early on in the process to avoid surprises later.

Finally, nursing leaders should be prepared to be "change sponsors" and assign "change agents." A change sponsor is a high-level executive who champions the system and is able to motivate lower levels of managers and staff. Change agents are typically staff-level people who can "speak the language" and act as liaisons between technical and clinical departments.

SUMMARY

It is important to understand that nursing has only recently entered the world of information systems management. Participation in the selection process was officially mandated in 1991, whereas Nursing

Informatics was not named as a specialty until 1992. Despite the fact that it is a fairly young field, there is much that nursing can do to advance the interests of nursing information technology.

Nursing must support a uniform, universally accepted minimum data set. Without these data elements, nursing technology is virtually at an impasse. In the meantime, nurses should understand the basic concepts of technology evaluation, which include architecture, data evolution, communication, data access, information security, hardware, resources, and support. Finally, nurses must be ready to manage the selection process by emphasizing self-education, representation on the selection committee, veto power, and change management.

DISCUSSION QUESTIONS

1. Why is the lack of a minimum data set an impediment to the advancement of nursing technology?
2. Why is it important for nursing to have veto power on the selection committee?
3. Why is the concept of "change management" important to nursing managers in the process of selecting a new information system?

REFERENCE

Simpson, R. (1991). Computer-based patient records, Part I. The Institute of Medicine's Vision. *Nursing Management*, 22(10), 21.

SUGGESTED READING

Austin, C. J. (1988). Evaluating and selecting a computer system. In *Information systems for health services administration* (3rd ed.). Ann Arbor, MI: Health Administration Press.

Johnson, J. (1988). *The nurse executive's business plan manual.* Rockville, MD: Aspen.

Saba, V., Johnson, J., Halloran, E., & Simpson, R. (1992). *Computers in nursing management.* Kansas City, MO: American Nurses Association.

Saba, V. K., & McCormick, K. A. (1986). *Essentials of computers for nursing.* Philadelphia: JB Lippincott.

Simpson, R. (1990). Technology: Nursing the system, a series of articles on nursing informatics. *Nursing Management*, July 1990 to the present.

Simpson, R. (1993). *The nurse executive's guide to directing and managing nursing information systems.* Ann Arbor: Center for Healthcare Information Management.

Simpson, R., & Somers, A. B. D. (1991). The role of the clinical nurse specialist in information systems selection. *Clinical Nurse Specialist*, 5(3), 1–163.

Simpson, R., & Waite, R. (1989). NCNIP's system of the future: A call for accountability, revenue control and national data sets. *Nursing Administration Quarterly*, 14, 72–77.

SECTION

II

FOCUS ON PROFESSIONAL SUCCESS

Becoming a Successful Employee

Donna Richards Sheridan

LEARNING OBJECTIVES

This chapter will enable you to:

1. Explain the relationship between a good student and a good employee.
2. List 10 characteristics of good employees.
3. Describe the written sources of job expectations in a health care setting.
4. Explain how to assess cultural and informal expectations in a health care setting.
5. Describe the interrelation of motivation, goal setting, and performance appraisal.
6. Explain ways you can take responsibility for your professional development.

Vestal, K.W. Nursing Management:
Concepts and Issues, 2 ed.
© 1995 J.B. Lippincott Company

Your responsibilities as a nursing employee begin on your first day reporting to work for your first paid nursing position. No doubt this moment will be filled with excitement, enthusiasm, a willingness to do well, and perhaps a touch of apprehension. You are ready to be a good nurse providing quality patient care. It's not new; you did it as a student, you tell yourself.

On your way to becoming a good nurse, you learned to be a good student (or you would never have made it to this point). As a student, your nursing goal was to learn. Your focus had to be on yourself—obtaining the necessary knowledge and skills to become a professional nurse. Now your focus needs to shift so that you can use that knowledge and skill within the framework of an organization. Although your primary focus will shift, much of what you learned about succeeding as a student will help you succeed as a nurse.

According to Newmann (1986), good employees:

- Are able to follow and to lead
- Learn about and contribute to their professions
- Seek out challenges
- Respect fellow students and workers regardless of grade or job level
- Are patient
- Have a probing mind and ask questions
- Have the courage to challenge injustices
- Care equally for people regardless of religion, race, or sex
- Contribute to the school or hospital
- Are dedicated
- Have a sense of humor and are cheerful

Looking over this list, it becomes apparent that learning to be a good employee is a lifelong task. What makes a good student also makes a good nurse and a good employee. They are the amorphous characteristics that make a good person. You have been working on this all your life and hopefully will continue to grow in this way throughout adulthood and your nursing career. These characteristics will help you now to be a good employee.

Pol (1986) highlights the key points: "I think a good employee is one who has goals (long-term and short-term) both personal and professional. This employee must also be loyal, flexible, and kind. This person should be able to accept the client (patient) at client level

228

of education and background. The employee should be a person interested in people and their dignity."

In *The Seven Habits of Highly Effective People* (1990), Stephen Covey explains how effective individuals move from a state of dependence by becoming proactive, beginning with the end in mind, and putting first things first. Using these three habits, you can move to a state of independence. Three more habits will then move you to the higher state of interdependence. These include win–win thinking, seeking first to understand then to be understood, and using synergy. Covey warns that the successful person must also continue to "sharpen the saw." This habit includes regular balanced renewal with a commitment to continuous improvement. The good employee moves toward interdependence and continually strives for self-improvement.

EXPECTATIONS OF THE EMPLOYER

Besides the amorphous "good" characteristics defined above, what does your employer expect? An employer, any employer, has a responsibility to get a quality product "out the door" in a way that keeps employees happy or satisfied enough to make them want to continue "churning out the product." In health care, the product is service. In nursing, the product is bringing people to the highest level of health and self-care or helping them to die with dignity, within the constraints of the economy, the law, and other imposed limitations. No organization can exist unless it operates within these limitations. So the job of your hospital employer, no matter what level, is to produce quality patient care. This is accomplished indirectly by using employees. Therefore, the employer is responsible for producing satisfied employees—nurses—who produce quality patient care.

Your direct employer probably is a nurse administrator. This person defines what quality patient care "looks like" for your unit. The organization adds what quality patient care looks like for your institution. The expectations your employer has of you come from a variety of levels and are found in a variety of places.

A job description offers you the fastest clues to your employer's expectations. Your job description will tell you your job classification (title), a brief description of the job, the specific qualifications for the job, to whom you report, and your functions and responsibilities in the job. It clarifies what your role is in contributing to the overall purpose of the organization. Weber (1978), "the father of modern bureaucracy," recognized the need for rules to guide bureaucracies and the need to break down an organizational purpose into tasks. Weber then proposed hiring only persons qualified to serve the organizational purpose for jobs described by those delineated tasks. Thus, your job description contains tasks essential to the organization's goals.

Your organization's job descriptions may list expectations very specifically, such as "obtains and documents a nursing history upon admission of each assigned patient through a planned interview." In this case, your learning needs are clear—you may begin by finding out what form and what format are used for the nursing history and for the documentation? Your organization may not have job descriptions that delineate your tasks so clearly and may state your job expectations broadly, such as "uses the steps of nursing process to deliver quality patient care." If this is the case, other procedural documents may be available to clarify your job, for example, the "standards of care" that define "quality patient care" for your unit or organization.

The performance standards of your position may be found in skills checklists. These checklists often are used during orientation to assess your beginning skills. More delineated skills measurement may be found in a competency program. Used especially for new graduates, Competency-Based Orientation (CBO) is a program that explains each skill in measurable and behavioral terms and suggests resources for learning. Competency programs extend beyond CBO and exist for cross-training, learning to use new products or equipment, and correcting problems for improved quality.

Although hospitals provide opportunities to improve competence, it is your professional responsibility to maintain competence as a registered nurse. Code Five of the *Code for Nurses*, adopted by the American Nurses Association in 1950 and revised in 1985, states that "the nurse maintains competence in nursing." Although much of your job expectation is explained to you in orientation, it is a good idea to know if and where expectations are written to serve as a resource to you as needed.

Reviewing policies and procedures may be helpful in understanding your job if you have broadly written job descriptions. Read through the policies and procedures related to the specific functions of your job. For example, if you want to know if it is your job to administer a certain type of chemotherapy drug, a policy will state "who" can administer the drug. Further, you can find "how" to administer the drug in a procedure. Policy and procedure manuals are located on each nursing unit.

Job descriptions in your organization may be in the form of a clinical ladder. Clinical ladders address the fallacy of the old concept "a nurse is a nurse" or "all nurses have the same skills." A clinical ladder differentiates and defines the clinical expectations of each nursing level. Of three or four levels, each one increases in responsibility and authority.

Usually a Staff Nurse One is a new graduate. This person is still learning how to be a nurse in a particular organization. A Staff Nurse Two is a fully functioning staff nurse who performs the expected daily operations and whose lower level needs of physiology, safety, and security are met. Herzberg (1966) claims that employees are dissatisfied if lower level needs are not met (eg, if health care benefits are inadequate). However, meeting lower level needs does not motivate or satisfy an employee. It merely removes dissatisfactions. If health care benefits are inadequate, adding benefits will remove this dissatisfaction. However, adding more and more health care benefits after removing the dissatisfaction will not increase job satisfaction. Job satisfaction can only be increased by meeting upper level needs.

Removing dissatisfactions is essential to job satisfaction but will not, in itself, motivate employees. Satisfiers, according to Herzberg, will motivate employees after the dissatisfiers have been removed. Some job satisfiers you may want to seek out include greater autonomy, responsibility, and accountability. Remember that these satisfiers and motivators are different from one nurse to the next.

There are some consistencies mandated that address lower level motivators. On a basic level, employees expect to be treated fairly. Over the years, fairness abuses by industry have led to unions and legal actions that now ensure basic employee expectations as legal rights. Personnel departments and union representatives (where there is a nursing union) can inform you of your rights should you have a grievance against your employer. In these situations, it is important for you to seek assistance because both employee and employer must follow the policies, procedures, and labor laws.

Beyond basic fairness, Fitzgerald (1984) describes another consistent factor in motivation that addresses higher level needs: "Workers will be motivated if they have a job that makes them feel good about themselves. Individuals need to feel they have a future in the organization and their work load must be perceived as reasonable." Successful organizations increase motivation by building a shared vision. Senge (1990) proposes that this shared vision binds people around a common identity and sense of destiny. He claims that where a genuine vision exists, people excel and learn because they want to, not because the they are told to. Being a part of the creation and unfolding of the vision of your organization will increase your enthusiasm for your job, enhance your motivation to contribute, and improve your opportunities to grow.

Besides spending time thinking about what motivates you, think about the future in your organization. Look for "fits" between what the organization needs, what your employer expects, and what motivates you.

PERFORMANCE APPRAISAL

Any deficits between the job expectations of your employer and your current abilities constitute your growth needs. You and your employer need to assess your strengths to do the job and how you "fit" with the unit and the organization. When you do not yet have the ability to do the job or to do it within your new setting, you and your employer need to plan together how you will gain this needed knowledge or skill. Identifying and planning how to meet the needs you have in this new job should be done with your employer. This establishes a baseline for your performance and for your future performance appraisals.

Considering the organizational unit and patient needs along with your motivations should be part of a goal setting process with your supervisor. Setting goals, priorities, and realistic time frames are important to your success in growing and moving ahead. Your goals should include subgoals and feedback sessions with your employer so you can be sure you both have the same understanding of where you are going and how soon you will get there. Both of you should be clear about your goals and how you will accomplish them. Goals need to be stated in measurable, behavioral terms and should have realistic time frames, with subgoals rewarded and celebrated along the way.

A more sophisticated way to grow as a professional is by seeking peer input. If your organization does not provide this system, you can do it informally. In a private setting, ask a colleague whom you respect and trust, "What do you see as my strengths?" "What is one suggestion you have that would improve my performance?" Consider including a peer suggestion in your goals.

Performance appraisal sessions are your opportunity to share with your employer your perceptions about your progress. Together you can look at how you have grown and look for new goals or areas in which you need to grow. A performance appraisal session offers the opportunity to receive individualized feedback, a pat on the back, some shared concerns, and some chances to grow. Performance appraisals should not be a shock to either party. There should not even be surprises. If you have a problem or see a problem developing, go to your employer and discuss it in a timely manner. Ask your employer to do the same with you.

SUMMARY

One of the most important aspects of being a good employee is taking responsibility for yourself. Use your initiative to understand and "fit" into your organization—to grow, to learn, and to look for your own goals. Be proud of your profession and your organization and seek out ways to contribute—that's what makes a good employee.

DISCUSSION QUESTIONS

1. What are the major expectations your new employer will have when you come to work?
2. How will you know what to do in your new job to be successful?
3. What is the purpose and process of performance appraisals?

REFERENCES

American Nurses Association. (1985). *Code for nurses with interpretive statements.* Kansas City, MO: American Nurses Association.

Covey, S. R. (1990). *The seven habits of highly effective people.* New York: Fireside, Simon & Schuster.

Fitzgerald, P. (1984). Workers perceptions: The key to motivation. *Health Care Supervisor, 3*(1), 13–18.

Herzberg, F. (1966). *Work and the nature of man.* New York: World.

Pol, M. (1986). What makes a good employee? *Stanford Nurse, 8*(1), 12.

Senge, P. M. (1990). *The fifth discipline: The art and practice of the learning organization.* New York: Bantam Doubleday Dell.

Weber, M. (1978). Bureaucracy. In J. M. Shafritz, & P. M. Shitbeck (Eds.), *Classics of organizational theory.* Oak Park, IL: Moore.

SUGGESTED READING

Deal, T. E., & Kennedy A. A. (1982). *Corporate cultures.* Menlo Park, CA: Addison-Wesley.

Drucker, P. F. (1974). *Management tasks, responsibilities, practices.* New York: Harper & Row.

Maslow, A. H. (1959). *Motivation and personality.* New York: Harper & Row.

Newmann, E. (1986). *Survey of what makes a good student and what makes a good employee.* Unpublished manuscript, City College School of Nursing, New York.

Sheridan, D. R., Bronstein, J. E., & Walker, D. D. (1984). *The new nurse manager: A guide to management development.* Gaithersburg, MD: Aspen.

Short, E., & Farratt, T. W. (1984). Working unit culture: Strategic starting point in building organizational change. *Management Review, 73*(8), 15–19.

Stoner, J. A. (1982). *Management* (2nd ed.). Englewood Cliffs, NJ: Prentice-Hall.

Successful mergers require a mesh of corporate cultures. (1983, March). *Savings and Loan News, 104*(3), 94.

Creating Career Success

Katherine W. Vestal

LEARNING OBJECTIVES

This chapter will enable you to:

1. Describe the difference between a job and a career.
2. Construct a career map to serve as a development guide.
3. Recognize and use the tools, both written and verbal, necessary for career success.
4. Define the methods for career evaluation.

Vestal, K.W. Nursing Management:
Concepts and Issues, 2 ed.
© 1995 J.B. Lippincott Company

In entering the nursing profession, you have made a decision. You have chosen a career in a field that offers numerous opportunities. The nursing field is growing, diversifying, and changing in such a way that nurses have almost limitless career options. The key to career success is deciding which direction to go and then strategizing to reach your goals.

Although career planning may sound easy, the diversity of opportunity in nursing has, in fact, made it more difficult. Many nurses begin their professional lives simply by looking for a job. They soon find that there are many jobs, and the decision is which one to accept. Despite an over or under supply of nurses in small geographic pockets, the general job situation for nurses remains good. There are jobs, although the hours or locale may not be ideal. Nevertheless, a nurse *can* get a *job*.

Then there are those nurses who want a *career*. A career is a means of finding professional growth, satisfaction, and self-fulfillment. More clearly stated, it is a progression of jobs that leads to additional skills, rewards, and recognition. Having a career implies a commitment that entails constant effort and progress toward achieving success. To know if you are successful, you must clearly understand what success means to you. Success is subjective; it is a set of achievements that you define for yourself. People often define success in terms of what others want, such as, "my mother wants me to teach nursing," or "my friend says the only way to make it is to be a manager." In the final analysis, the person who must define success is you. What are the achievements to which you aspire, and what measures will you use to know if you have arrived?

Success is dynamic. Your criteria for success will probably change many times in your career. As you achieve one milestone, you will re-examine your personal expectations and move forward. Or you may reach the point you strive for and discover that you no longer find it an indicator of success. So you rethink your goals.

Career planning and strategizing is an ongoing process that is a part of your overall professional activities. It should be viewed as fun and as an opportunity to be creative, to let others advise you, and to determine directions that you want to take. One thing is clear: to make no decision is in reality to make a decision. Rather than actively participating in your career planning, you are allowing others to do it for you. And you may not like the results.

Career development is not easy. A sense of cautious optimism is probably reasonable. It is a conscious and deliberate process that attempts to match the trends of the profession to the personal and life stages of the nurse and to mesh these often divergent patterns into a planning model. Out of this analysis may come a contract with yourself about the pace you wish to maintain, the people on whom you will have an impact, and the price you are willing to pay for your success. Many nurses find that the costs in time, energy, and trade-offs are higher than they are willing to pay and revise their career goals accordingly.

In a 1985 survey conducted by *RN* (Lewis, 1985), nurses were asked why they entered the nursing profession. Job security and opportunity for professional advancement were both ranked high. Other reasons for choosing nursing included the desire to follow a strong drive toward a goal and the desire to do work perceived as personally rewarding. From this standpoint, work can be the ultimate seduction in life. It can become a passion, which is not necessarily bad. If you find work rewarding and are able to do it successfully, how can it be bad? There is a tendency to overwork that nurses must confront when embarking on a career. Some nurses are comfortable with becoming work directed; for others, it is uncomfortable. Each person adjusts and finds a way to balance a personal and a professional life.

Another important factor in considering a career in nursing is the rapidly changing health care system. Models of delivery, organizational structures, and forms of nursing care are evolving at a rapid rate and will give rise to unprecedented opportunities. The economic situation has placed increasing emphasis on cost containment, innovation, and the creation of new delivery models. As always, nursing will be the framework for these systems. Nurses will increasingly venture into nurse-controlled, nurse-owned, nurse-compensated, and special-function roles.

Career strategizing requires a commitment to a future in nursing. The dilemmas of career professionals are inherent in a nursing career but present many manageable challenges. Career moves are rewarding, fun, and always a part of a bigger picture. At the start of your career in nursing, begin to plan your strategies for success. All nurses want to do well, to progress, and to feel that they are making a difference. These aspects of career accomplishment are important and can best be accomplished with clear goal setting and career strategizing for success. A job may "just happen," but a successful career is made. The new graduate must determine how this can be done.

CAREER DEVELOPMENT

Inaccurate perceptions of specific careers often keep people from fully exploring options. In the long run, they may be cheating themselves of rewarding experiences. Once a person does choose a career, he or she may find that even the good choices have many rough edges. Nurses may spend 6 to 8 years "getting into a role." Once they feel truly competent, they often become apprehensive. Suddenly they find themselves asking, "Is this all there is?" They feel they should be running the second lap, yet they don't know where to go.

Career anxieties are common. These anxieties can play havoc with a person's sense of control over his or her life. Those who have high career expectations may feel pressured to move ahead very quickly. Because an employee's future depends in part on helping the employer to succeed, employees tend to contribute a good deal to help ensure that the organization will succeed.

A study of the work force in the United States reveals interesting demographics. One half is now under 35 years of age, up from just over one third at the end of the 1950s. The work force is increasingly better educated. It is composed of flexible, mobile, and highly skilled workers who are intensely aware of the changes taking place in the labor markets (Brody, 1985). Traditional wage structures have broken down, and new structures have replaced them. Partly in response to this restructuring, young workers have become more interested in acquiring new skills and more willing to change jobs, including locations, to seize opportunities. In addition, they tend to speak highly of their current employers. They may have their gripes, but their post-Depression work ethic has produced new attitudes toward employers. A new generation of young workers has grown up seeing kaleidoscopic changes, and they are in the middle of these changes, learning whatever new skills they have to learn, moving a hundred or a thousand miles to find a job, and keeping the wheels of the economy turning.

These trends are important in considering career development because the nursing profession as a whole, the trends in health care, and the national state of the economy are inextricably intertwined. The new nurse entering the work force must be competent and competitive with others vying for the same career advancement. Developing careers becomes a matter of strategy and good decisions, not a matter of luck. The nursing license is not a ticket to nirvana but rather a way of life that can be as difficult as it is rewarding. It is a career that comes with demands as well as privileges.

A CYCLICAL PROCESS

Career development is a cyclical process. After developing career options, the process of continual reassessment and redevelopment begins. The frequency of the reassessment and redevelopment will depend on your level of ambition, the pace at which your career is moving, and the changes around you that may prompt you to reconsider your needs. Although you may occasionally assess your career position daily, it is more likely that you will formally assess it yearly.

The process of career strategizing is best compared to the nursing process. There are four basic components: assessment, definition of goals, implementation, and evaluation. These components provide structure for the process, which is necessary to avoid a cursory or shallow analysis of career issues. Being methodical in your analysis will yield higher quality results in the long run.

As a new nurse, career planning provides you with a sound direction for the initial steps in your profession. In time, you may feel that your career is stalled, and you may need to make considerable efforts to advance it.

Throughout the career development process, keep in mind three basic competencies necessary for success. The first is *analytic competence.* This is the ability to identify, analyze, and solve problems without complete information. The second is *interpersonal competence,* which is the ability to influence, supervise, and control behaviors. The third is *emotional competence*, or the capacity to be stimulated by emotional and interpersonal crises rather than debilitated by them. These attributes become the framework for career success, and the strategies become the catalysts.

CAREER MAPPING

Career mapping is a method of creating a master plan. Like a strategic plan developed by a business, a career plan can serve as a map for career advancement. People rarely take adequate time to plan careers and, consequently, react haphazardly to opportunities that arise. Just because an opportunity becomes available does not mean that it fits into your plan for your career.

A career master plan should serve as a methodical future-mapping system. It can identify whether you need more education, what types of experience are necessary to meet your goals, and a target income. These plans pinpoint opportunities in your field, project potential opportunities in other fields, and define career movement patterns. They can provide direction concerning the type of networking you will need, the professional associations to which you should belong, and the requirements for your continuing education.

In addition, the plan introduces the element of time, describing certain career stages that should be achieved within set time limits. The element of time is important because it can easily elude you until you suddenly realize that too many years have passed with no real advancement. Then you become frustrated at an outcome you could very well have controlled.

CAREER FOCUS: NARROW OR BROAD

A frequent dilemma of the new nurse is how to choose a clinical area in which to work. Your educational experience has provided many diverse clinical experiences, most of which you probably enjoyed. So how can you pick just one area in which to work?

First of all, recognize that your first job is just that—*a first job.* You will hold many others in your career, each of which will enrich your total nursing knowledge. So look at the initial job as the first opportunity in a series of many.

Second, new nurses often face pressure to specialize in a narrowly focused area. This too can be dealt with by assuming that the decision to develop a narrow or broad focus will evolve through your dynamic career planning. The ultimate need for a broad background may be evident, but a current practice that is narrow may well suit your situation. For example, if your goal is to be director of maternal and child health services, you know this requires a broad base of experience in all maternal and pediatric services. It is understandable, however, that your first job will be in labor and delivery because you must start somewhere. Later, the planning for broad experience will be crucial to career development.

PRODUCING A MAP

Producing a career map involves four steps:

1. Assess your skills and interests.
2. Determine your goals.
3. Create a map.
4. Develop strategies to support the map.

These processes are simple and, in the end, produce a written plan that you can reflect on and share with others for their advice.

Assessing Your Skills and Interests

As a new nurse, it is particularly important that you realistically determine your present set of skills. Initially, you may feel that they are few. On closer examination, you should find that you have a long list. This list may look like a basic inventory of strengths and interests. Write down these items, and make the lists as detailed as possible (Table 15-1). You will use this information for the map and for interviews.

Determining Your Goals

Next, give thought to what you want to accomplish. This may be done in the form of a 1-year, 5-year, or 10-year plan. Some new nurses are absolutely certain of their ultimate career goals when they enter the profession, whereas others are quite confused. Knowing that this plan is dynamic and can be changed any time you want permits you to establish goals and develop a plan without feeling committed forever.

Creating a Map

The map should begin with where you are now and end with your goal. The steps outlined in between will be those steps you will need to take, in terms of experience and education, to meet your goals.

TABLE 15-1. LIST OF SKILLS AND INTERESTS

SKILLS	INTERESTS
Interest in people, epecially children	Pediatrics
Ability to establish rapport	Families in crisis
Good knowledge of nursing process	All MCH areas
Skill at writing nursing care plans	Management of people
Good communication skills	Learning new things
ICU nursing skills good	
Even-headed in crisis	
Good organizational skills	
Ability to manage time well	

TABLE 15-2. A TEN-YEAR CAREER MAP

Experience/ Years	2	2	1	2	3	Year 10
New Graduate B.S.N.	Labor and Delivery	Postpartum Staff Nurse	Pediatric Staff Nurse	Pediatric Head Nurse	Pediatric ICU Head Nurse	Director MCH
Education	MCH Continuing Education	Masters in MCH		Management Continuing Education		

A typical career map is shown in Table 15-2. In this plan, the new nurse starts in a staff nurse position and aspires to be a director of maternal and child nursing services in 10 years. This seems to be a reasonable goal that could be met if all of the preparatory elements were accomplished. The nurse will need varied clinical experiences, additional education, and hard work to meet the goal. The map shows that she worked and went to school for her master's degree at the same time to reach her 10-year goal. If she had elected to stop working to go to school, her experience factor would be different, or the time factor would need to be lengthened to compensate.

If the map were designed to prepare a teacher, clinical specialist, or home health care nurse, the process would be the same. Determining the goals and then putting a map on paper is essential in converting dreams to realities.

Developing Strategies to Meet the Goals

Once the goals and map are in a form that can be shared, talk to others about it. Ask nurses who have accomplished goals similar to yours how they did it and what advice they could give you. Explore educational programs, both formal degree and continuing education, to determine your options. Will you have to move to another area to get the experience or the education?

Next, develop an active list of activities to be accomplished, including skills to be learned, leadership roles to fill, ways to achieve visibility in the organization, and ways to market yourself in a positive manner. These plans can be incorporated into an overall strategy for developing your career.

Sounds like a lot of work? It may be, but compare it to the amount of work you will do that may not contribute to your career goals if you don't have a plan. This time will be well spent and may save you years of random progress.

LATERAL OR DOWNWARD MOVEMENT

In today's changing organizations, lateral and downward movement is becoming a more openly employed and less stigmatized method of managing people. In fact, under certain circumstances, lateral and downward movement can be good for you and for the organization.

With the movement of the baby boom generation into the ranks of middle management in organizations, a phenomenon of slow upward movement has developed. The youth of the work force and the economic recession have resulted in fewer available jobs for young people and tight upward mobility. Recognizing these factors is important in career planning because if a specific experience requirement exists and constant upward involvement is not possible, both lateral and downward moves may be the answer.

In your parents' careers, lateral or downward movement indicated that career growth was virtually over and advancement unlikely. In your career, this stigma should not prevail because the job market and organizational designs are drastically different. Instead of dwelling on whether a move is up, down, or sideways, focus on whether or not the experience is essential to your career plan. If that experience is essential for your future plans, then there is no question that you should pursue it.

A temporary lateral move to put you in a better position for future growth is a small price to pay now for a much larger reward later. For example, if the nurse striving for the maternal and child health role had not had labor and delivery experience, which is essential for the role, she may have had to return to a role as labor and delivery staff nurse after her tenure as a pediatric head nurse. A 1-year "downward" move to the position of labor and delivery staff nurse would prepare this nurse for the role of director. One year is not a high price to pay. By keeping the long-range goal in mind, the stops along the way make sense. Thinking of the long-term goal shows that you are willing to delay gratification and take risks. You will take a job that is not easy because you understand that you need the experience.

IS MANAGEMENT THE ONLY WAY UP?

Nurses often believe that the only road to advancement is through managerial jobs. This is a misconception, but it is one easily formed when looking at many hospitals and clinical settings. It would be nice if all health care institutions had developed routes upward through clinical work, education, and research, but such career paths are found at only a few enlightened organizations.

This is why it is important to map your career. If you can clearly state your goals in education, research, or clinical work, then you can plan your moves accordingly. Becoming a manager only because you want a promotion generally results in disaster. You must enjoy work to do it well.

To progress in areas other than management, you may have to select an organization that has those tracks for advancement. Or you may need to find alternative career options such as consulting, specialty companies, or self-employment. Don't buy into the idea that management is the only way up until you do some research to validate or invalidate your assumptions.

TOOLS FOR CAREER BUILDING

Career building is a composite of theory, practice, and evaluation. Designing a career entails an enormous amount of time and energy, and even more to implement one. There are several critical tools that are essential in career progress. These include developing a professional presence, presenting yourself in writing, and promoting yourself in person. These factors are often crucial in determining whether you progress.

DEVELOPING A PROFESSIONAL PRESENCE

It is probably not possible to define the term "presence." It is a subjective feeling that one either has or does not have. A nurse with "presence" can enter a room, and everyone will know he or she is there before any words are spoken. A nurse with presence always projects a professional image through attire, language, and conduct. Nurses with this nebulous quality of presence can work at the staff level or the executive level; they may be in positions of little or great power. Presence is not a function of role, but rather a function of demeanor.

A useful way to look at presence is to identify persons who you think possess this quality. Then analyze the behaviors they exhibit that promote this aura, and decide which of those behaviors might be useful for you. Individualize them to fit *your* personality. The aura of presence can be learned, and in fact, *must* be learned for career success.

Research has shown that attractive people are generally viewed positively and that this attitude follows over into the job market. That does not mean that you must look like a fashion model, but your grooming, from hairstyle to clothing, will affect how you are perceived by an interviewer. You should dress for the role you want to play on the job. Research has shown that recently graduated students who dressed more formally for job interviews were noticeably more assertive. They believed that they made a favorable impression on the interviewers.

Career confidence requires that you no longer act like a student when you are looking for a job. Career confidence means you are ready to step forward without stepping on the wrong toes. Positive attitudes rather than aggressive methods work best. Think through the encounters you are about to have, plan as many details as possible, and be mentally prepared to deal with the mini-crisis that may occur. Above all, be as calm, cool, and collected as possible. It helps promote your image as a true professional, at ease with your new role.

PRESENTING YOURSELF IN WRITING

A great portion of your professional life will involve writing. The writing may be clinical (eg, nurses' notes or nursing care plans), managerial (eg, memos or requests), or educational (eg, teaching plans and tools, or research-oriented materials). In addition, you will be required to perfect your personal writing in the form of letters and thank-you notes. An often overlooked business tactic, the thank-you note, should be carefully examined from the standpoint of both etiquette and business.

The habit of writing a note to network with persons you meet at a conference, to thank colleagues who help you with a problem, or to acknowledge someone's recent accomplishment is a powerful tool in business. Thank-you notes are appropriate after interviews to reiterate your interest in the job and to thank the interviewer for her attention. This is an important way to keep your name up front.

Another important written presentation is the resume. An essential tool in applying for a job, the resume is useful for many other professional activities. Spending the time to develop a concise resume is essential.

The Resume

The *resume* is a summary of your qualifications and accomplishments and contains a concise account of your work history, interests, and goals. The *curriculum vitae (CV)* is a form of resume used mostly in academic circles to summarize educational, professional, and scholarly accomplishments. Although the two terms generally are used interchangeably, this text will use the term "resume."

A resume will be presented to prospective employers or others who want a concise history of *you*. It summarizes years of pertinent experience in a few pages. Although many persons advocate a one-page resume, as your accomplishments accumulate it may be impossible to condense the information onto one page and still do yourself justice. Be as concise as possible, but at the same time mention all important aspects of your career.

The format of a resume may vary, but it must look professional and be accurately typed on a top-quality paper; these are essentials. There are many books that show different formats for resumes. Select the format that appeals to you; after all, it is your personal career tool. More importantly, make sure that all the information is completely honest, correct, and complete. Misrepresentation of information is easy to spot and can lead to immediate dismissal.

Information Files. It is important to begin immediately to keep accurate files of your accomplishments so that you can easily retrieve information when it is needed. Although you may update your resume only once a year, it is necessary to keep the information needed for updating in a safe and convenient place. A simple means of doing this is to use a manila folder labeled "Personal File 1994." Place all pertinent pieces of information into this file, such as brochures of programs you attended during that year, copies of projects you developed, important letters, and so forth. On the file cover, list the committees of which you are a member, professional organization involvement, and speeches you may have made. At the end of 1994, file the folder in a safe place, and start a new one for 1995.

In this way, you will always be able to reconstruct important activities of each year. You may rewrite your resume many times to refocus it, and accurate information is essential. There is always a tendency to forget details, and, without solid data, it will be impossible to reconstruct your career activities over time.

Resume Information. The resume is your personal marketing tool, so you must make important decisions about what you want to include in it. There are no rules that dictate content. For example, if you want to include your age and feel that it will be helpful to you, do so. If you feel it would be detrimental, do not.

The basic components of a resume are your name, address, phone number, education, experience, continuing education, honors, professional work, and personal interests. These components can be arranged in any order, but keep in mind that the reader will go from top to bottom and left to right on the page. So strategically arrange the information that is most important to you.

Display 15-1 gives an example of a resume for a new nurse. Note that Mary Smith, RN is applying for her first job in nursing, and her resume is designed to reflect that goal. After more experience, Mary will rewrite the resume, adding new material. In future years, her resume goal will read "to become director of maternal child nursing in a large teaching hospital."

At the present time, Mary's job experience in retailing and as a student nurse are included because they reflect her ambition and accomplishments as a valuable employee. Again, as years of nursing experience grow, she may elect to start her chronicle of work experience with her first professional nursing job and to add committee work and other professional activities.

In summary, resumes are important tools for career success. Be sure that they are free of typographical errors or misspelled words and that they are absolutely accurate in content. Top-quality originals and copies are essential and are easy to make using a word processor.

Cover Letters. A cover letter to a prospective employer should accompany your resume. This cover letter serves to introduce you, express your interest in the organization, and explain briefly what you can offer it. Like the resume, it should be flawlessly typed, professionally constructed, and *addressed to the proper person.*

Asking for information to be sent to you ensures a reply and will be an indication to you that your letter has received some attention. You should follow up with a phone call.

PRESENTATION IN PERSON

Presenting yourself in person to an employer typically happens in the form of a job interview. This is a structured discussion, usually taking place in the work setting, in which you assess the organization and

Text continues on page 250

DISPLAY 15-1. A RESUME

MARY A. SMITH, R.N.
1206 Edison
Houston, Texas 77000

PERSONAL DATA:
Birthdate: 6/27/71
Place of Birth: North Carolina
Marital Status: Single
Health: Excellent

PROFESSIONAL GOAL:
To practice as a staff nurse in Labor and Delivery.

EDUCATION:

Place	Degree	Year
University of Texas	B.A. English	1992
University of Kansas	B.S.N	1994

OCCUPATIONAL EXPERIENCE:

Sales Associate, Neiman Marcus, Dallas	1989–1991
Student Nurse, Kansas General Hospital	1992–1994
(Worked as staff on weekends)	

PROFESSIONAL MEMBERSHIPS:

American Nurses Association	1994–present
Sigma Theta Tau	1993–present

CONTINUING EDUCATION:

Nurses Role in High Risk Delivery	University of Kansas	1994
NAACOG Convention	Atlanta, GA	1992
Grand Rounds in OB	University of Kansas	Monthly

INTERESTS:
Writing articles for publication
Painting
Marathon running

References Upon Request

DISPLAY 15-2. A COVER LETTER

1206 Edison
Houston, Texas 77000
January 1, 1994

Dr. Karen Myers, R.N.
Vice-President for Nursing
General Hospital
Salem, California 44000

Dear Dr. Myers:

I am interested in joining a progressive nursing organization that has a need for my skills and can provide opportunities for my professional growth. I understand that the Maternal Child Services at General Hospital offer opportunities that meet my interests.

I have a B.S.N. from the University of Kansas. The attached resume further outlines my qualifications. As you will note, I am seeking an entry level position as a labor and delivery nurse, but would be willing to discuss other MCH openings you may have. I would eventually like to progress to a nursing management role in the MCH field.

If you would like to discuss my experience in detail, I would be glad to come for a personal interview. I would appreciate receiving information about your hospital, and in particular its nursing organization.

I look forward to hearing from you.

Sincerely,

Mary A. Smith, RN., B.S.N.

Enclosure

it assesses you. What each of you is probing are strengths, weaknesses, and the potential "fit" within the organization. Depending on the job, interviews have different formats, including individual interviews, multiple interviews, group interviews, stress interviews, and reinterviews. It is important to be prepared for the interview. Knowing in advance the form it may take will help you prepare.

Individual Interviews

A one-on-one interview usually takes place between a nurse recruiter or nurse manager and you. During a specified amount of time, each of you will have the opportunity to ask and answer questions. Because you may be nervous, it is helpful to write out your questions in advance and to take notes during the interview. It is easy to say "I'm a little nervous and I want to be sure I remember the things we discuss. Would you mind if I make notes as we go along?" Then take only the notes necessary to trigger your memory. Do not take notes as if you were attending a lecture. Eye contact and interaction with the interviewer is imperative.

This interview should include a brief tour of the area in which you may work and an overall discussion of work benefits. It may not include salary negotiations, especially if there are other interviews to follow.

Enter the interview with confidence and with professional presence. At the end, if you feel that certain aspects of the interview did not go well, review and rehearse these points before your next interview. There should be few surprises in the interview because the questions are almost standard:

Why do you want to work *here?*
What are your strengths and weaknesses?
What are your nursing goals?
What will you bring us as a professional nurse?

In turn, your questions should focus on the organization and what it can offer you. Ask about its promotional policies, career philosophies, orientation practices, and commitment to professional growth.

The important thing is to relax and let the interviewer structure the meeting. However, be sure you have met your informational needs before you leave. In addition, determine when you can next expect to hear from the organization and when it can expect to hear from you.

Multiple Interviews

These interviews are designed to reduce the risk of hiring the wrong person. In this situation, all the major individuals you will work with interview you. This may include persons from personnel, recruitment, nursing management, and the patient care team on the unit. Although multiple interviews are becoming more common for staff nurse positions, they are frequently used as you move up in the organization. The interviewers generally ask questions that have a specific job relationship within their area of responsibility. They want to be sure you have the knowledge and, more importantly, that you will "fit in."

Multiple interviews can sometimes get out of hand, with as many as 15 to 25 persons interviewing the candidate before a job offer is made. For multiple interviews, be sure you are consistent throughout the many sessions and that you treat each interviewer as if he or she were the key person in the decision-making process.

Group Interviews

These interviews are frequently used in the health care profession and involve meeting with 5 to 20 persons at one time. Each person may have been assigned an area of questioning, or the interview may simply be an open session. A group interview can be a useful test for a job that requires sophisticated communication skills or people skills. Your strategies should include frequent eye contact with each person and projection of a professional but relaxed manner.

Stress Interviews

A few years ago, stress interviews were popular. The theory was that by subjecting candidates to a stressful situation their ability to react properly under stress was tested. For example, although the candidate was filling out an application, persons would interrupt or create distractions, then watch to see the applicant's reaction. The problem with stress interviews was that top candidates were often turned off and could not imagine why an organization would subject prospective employees to such treatment. If you are subjected to a stress interview, project self assurance and remain poised. Recognize it as a test, not a personal affront.

Reinterviews

It is common for organizations to request a reinterview after some initial screening has taken place. Once all applicants have been seen, the top three of four are called back for interviews that are more precisely focused. Treat all the interviews as essential. They are a valid means of selecting qualified employees. The time lapse between the initial interview and the actual hiring may be much longer than you anticipate. Check back often with the organization to determine if you are still under consideration. Never assume you are not until you receive confirmation that you are no longer a candidate.

Presenting yourself professionally in writing and in person are essential tools for success. Prepare your written materials carefully before mailing them. Practice your interview skills, arrive on time, and participate enthusiastically. The organization will make every effort to select the applicant with the most interest and potential. You want to be that person!

THE NEXT STEP: PROMOTION

Every nurse who strategizes for career advancement looks forward to the day when he or she is promoted. A promotion involves the same process of submitting your resume, interviewing, and competing for a job. This job, however, provides upward mobility rather than entry level possibilities. The stakes may be higher in that you might be an internal candidate vying for promotion over your peers or competing directly with a colleague for the job.

It is important to recognize that the organization will want to select the best candidate for the job. Although being an internal candidate may offer an initial advantage, it will not ensure promotion. You must be competitive and meet the new job requirements, just as all candidates must. So the same factors of education, experience, maturity, and other requisite skills will come into play. In addition, there will be the inevitable and ever-present office politics.

If you are seeking promotion, you must take an active part in your career planning. You must have a clear idea of your immediate supervisor's views. Assuming added responsibility, establishing and pursuing goals, and acquiring the education needed at the next job level will contribute toward your chances of advancement. If chosen for the job, you will experience excitement, challenge, and, ultimately, opportunities to advance even further. You can increase possibilities of promotion by being visible and promoting yourself in strategic ways. The more persons who know who you are, what you do, what you know, and what you can offer, the more opportunities will come to you. These new opportunities are crucial to your success, so become comfortable talking about yourself; regard self-promotion as a benefit to others.

An important aspect of self-promotion is to market yourself, rather than merely bragging. Prepare by writing down every possible detail about yourself and become adept at retrieving such information when it is needed. Describe in detail who you are, what you do, what you know, and what you want. Probe deeply to find the heart of the information—your values, attitudes, enthusiasm, and confidence.

Evaluating Job Offers

If you are offered a job, you will need a way to determine whether it is to your advantage to accept the position. Ginsburg recommends the seven C's for systematically assessing realistic job opportunities (Ginsburg, 1983).

1. *Content of the position:* Will this job train and position me for advancement?
2. *Challenge of the position:* Is the challenge too much, too little, or just right?
3. *Climate of the position itself and within the organization:* The work environment is critical to success.
4. *Chemistry:* What is your feeling about how well you will get along with your immediate supervisor?
5. *Concern for results and people:* What importance does the organization place on those who work for it?
6. *Compensation:* Is the total monetary package with benefits satisfactory for you?
7. *Community:* Is the job in a community where you would want to live?

In making a critical decision about a new job, be sure you possess as many facts as possible. Just because the job is offered to you does not mean you should accept it. Weigh the factors carefully before making a decision.

If You Are Passed Over

Being passed over for promotion can be a big disappointment. You felt you were the perfect choice, and you now feel rejected and slated for obscurity in the organization. How can you recover and go on to be highly productive, a candidate for future promotions?

It is helpful to have open communication with your manager during the entire selection process. She is in a position to diffuse some of your distress and to reassess your current role in the organization. Assuming she wants you to continue to work in that capacity, it is useful to seek the counseling or assistance needed to deal with your feelings.

Then work with your manager to evaluate options for increased involvement in your work setting. Assume more responsibility or find new opportunities so that you feel you are progressing. Talk with the persons who did *not* hire you in a candid, nonthreatening manner to determine the areas in which you were not competitive. Using this information, shore up your deficiencies. Then you will be ready the next time! The employee who is passed over is by no means passed by, and opportunities will arise in the future.

CHANGING JOBS

All nurses will change jobs at some point in their careers, and probably at many points. Changing jobs may not necessarily mean changing organizations, because it is possible, over time, to have many roles in the same organization. However, some job changes may involve going to a new setting, a different part of the country, or entering a new facet of the health care field. These changes can be positive experiences if handled well, or negative if handled poorly.

In the past, persons who changed jobs frequently (ie, more than 3 times in 5 years) were regarded as job-hoppers. This stigma often made employers reluctant to hire the individual for fear they would invest significant resources in training and orientation without reaping long-term productivity. However, in the past few years, the economy and business world have dictated a new set of circumstances. It is common now to see mergers, acquisitions, closures, and consolidations, all of which lead to a reduction in staff. Persons lose jobs more frequently, and the search in the job market is more fluid.

Thus, the nurse who changes jobs must have a clear statement about why the change occurred. Was the job change due to an organizational restructuring that eliminated your position, or to career development needs, or to a relocation? As long as the explanation is factual and plausible, there is little problem. However, if you have changed jobs 3 times because you didn't like your supervisor, the prospective employer will look more critically at you.

Job Dissatisfaction

Job dissatisfaction may one day become a reality for you. It may be that you will lose interest in your job or that the demands are too high for the rewards. Or it may be that you envision yourself in a different role or setting. Whatever the reason for your dissatisfaction, the result will be that you begin to search for another job. Statistically, persons change jobs at least 3 times in their work life.

Be sure you distinguish *job* dissatisfaction from *career* dissatisfaction. In the former, you change jobs and put your current knowledge and skill to work in a different milieu. In the latter, the nature of the work, the tasks to be performed, and the purpose to be served have become so distasteful that you begin to think about a different career. Often nurses mistakenly believe they are dissatisfied with nursing as a career, when a problem exists simply with their current job. For each person, the answer to the dilemma will be vastly different.

In the case of job dissatisfaction, you must take time to analyze the cause of the dissatisfaction. Otherwise, it is highly probable that you may change jobs and find the same set of circumstances in another setting. What are the causes of your problems? Goal blockage? Uncertain expectations? Contradictory demands? Poor relationships with co-workers? Organizational restrictions? Policies of the institution? Recognition gaps? A sense of being overworked or undervalued? The answers to these questions will help you determine whether the problem is simply job dissatisfaction or a more serious discontent—career dissatisfaction.

RISK MANAGEMENT IN CAREER PLANNING

The concept of risk management that you are familiar with in health care delivery can be applied to the management of your career. There are five steps involved in the process (McEwan, 1984):

1. *Risk Identification:* What is important in your life and how can you position yourself for success rather than increased risk? By identifying where you want to be at certain stages of your career, you can then identify those issues that might prevent you from reaching each plateau.

2. *Risk Evaluation:* After you identify the risks, you can estimate the probability of an adverse outcome due to the risk.
3. *Opportunity Identification:* Besides identifying potential risk situations, you can identify and evaluate potential opportunities.
4. *Implementation:* Once action steps are identified, you can be in control of your career progress. Timing is an important factor and one that should be given due consideration.
5. *Monitoring:* Because situations can change, and a decision made on today's facts may not hold up tomorrow, you must try to keep on top of events as far as career risks and opportunities are concerned. Once you set up a monitoring process, it is important to use it.

Acting Roles

One job opportunity that needs special explanation is the "acting role." This is a situation in which you assume a temporary role or responsibility without an official title or commitment. There are advantages and disadvantages to accepting an acting role. As long as you understand both components clearly, you can make a good decision.

First, keep in mind that an acting role is not the real thing. It is considered "acting" because the supervisor is not in a position or not ready to commit the job to you in total. Being asked to take a job is seductive, and you can easily be caught up in the glamour and drama of perceived advancement, when in reality the advancement is not permanent.

The issue of permanency is at the heart of the problem when considering an acting role. Although you may gain valuable experience and may actually be an official candidate, there is always the risk that you will not get the job. Not being selected for the job on a permanent basis means you must return to your former job, if it is still there, and become a peer once again to persons who were for a time subordinates.

This is difficult. In addition, the person who has acquired the job on a permanent basis may resent you because you still retain some of the characteristics of supervisor but have moved back to a subordinate position. That places you at great risk with the new person who is himself struggling to assume power.

Therefore, when assuming an acting role, be sure you know what is to be gained and what is to be lost. You may acquire experience, a chance to prove yourself, and another level of visibility. However, you may have to leave the setting when the acting role is over, or you may find you liked the role so much you do not wish to return to your former status. If you assume an acting role, determine how long you are to fill the role (eg, for 6 months or 1 year), so that the supervisor will have a time frame and impetus to hire a permanent person.

If you do assume an acting role, you cannot view every decision as if it were temporary. Expand your resource base, nurture new contacts, and visibly do the job well. Be sure you negotiate the title you will use and any compensation changes you desire. Once you accept the acting role, your ability to negotiate options diminishes dramatically.

When You Quit

Quitting a job is a highly sensitive and political act. Never think that the quitting process is any less important than the hiring process. The way you behave at the end of a job will be what persons will remember about you. Plainly put, no matter what the reason for your leaving, the process should be professional, discreet, and well thought out.

Often, a person who quits a job is in the midst of great emotional turmoil. It is immaterial whether this is a result of disappointment, rage, or righteous indignation. No matter how "right" you are about leaving, the only memory among coworkers will be the style with which you depart. Keep in mind the old adage that "the organization will survive." Although you may feel that "they can't survive without you," in fact, they will. Whether you view your departure as positive or negative, conduct the process in such a manner that you are viewed as a professional, well-mannered person.

Review the personnel policies carefully and understand the procedures to follow for severance of employment. Such details as the required number of days' notice and required actions are important and may determine your future eligibility for rehire. Keep in mind that organizations change. Although you may not think you would ever rejoin that organization, you never know. So do not burn bridges, and carefully meet the termination requirements.

You will need to submit in writing a note to your manager indicating that you will be leaving, the exact date, and a brief explanation stated in a positive manner. A positive statement about your time on the job or your reluctance to leave is appropriate. Do not make the mistake of using the letter of resignation as a place to vent your litany of complaints. After all, this letter goes in *your* personnel file and could be used adversely in the future.

If you want to air your concerns, do so in an exit interview. Make an appointment with the appropriate persons to discuss your reasons for leaving and share your feelings. In this way, you have your say, you inform them of issues, but you do not place the problems in your permanent file.

EVALUATION OF CAREER PROGRESS

Evaluation is a critical part of career success but is usually the area in which you tend to spend the least amount of time. Evaluation is important because it reminds you of how well you are doing and where you need improvement and keeps you cognizant of needs for additional development.

Evaluation takes place at many points and should be consciously recognized as such. For example, each time you update your resume, look it over carefully for gaps and needs. Arrange to round out your experiences, so as to round out your resume. In your annual employee evaluation, you have an opportunity to consider your strengths and needs and to discuss them candidly with your supervisor. As you review your career map annually, the areas for development should be quite clear.

Additionally, you may want to review your accomplishments and aspirations with mentors, colleagues, and superiors. Talk with your teachers and other professionals about opportunities. Never assume you can build a career by yourself. A career is ultimately the result of your contributions to a bigger entity; assistance from others will support your career growth.

Your career evaluation should take place at least annually in a formalized and comprehensive manner. If you do not do so, the years are likely to slip by and you will find yourself looking back and wondering how time got away from you. Career success requires strategizing and restrategizing. It is the evaluation process that allows you to keep on track in terms of your work roles and your time frame.

SUMMARY

Most careers, no matter how carefully planned and executed, include a number of surprises, both pleasant and unpleasant. Most persons tend to attribute the happy events, promotions, and rewards to their own capabilities; they place the blame for unpleasant happenings such as job problems, demotions, or dead-end positions on circumstances beyond their control or on the actions of others. Nurses must begin to see that most career developments reflect their performance, their relationships with other persons, and their particular circumstances.

Career advice usually focuses on keeping your options open and being prepared to take advantage of promising opportunities. For a successful career, however, a strong commitment must be made to the task at hand. Sooner or later, a heavy investment of intellectual and emotional energy will be needed.

The sooner a new nurse gains a positive perspective of her career, the better. Early planning can result in better outcomes. Although nurses know that all careers have ups and downs, the intent of career strategizing is to maximize the ups and minimize the downs. With the overwhelming amount of change and turmoil in health care today, it is important that new nurses begin to develop a clear vision of where they are headed. Otherwise, the chances of becoming a victim of the confusion are great.

Career strategizing is a formal, informal, and methodical process. It takes time, energy, and commitment. But if you consider the alternative of being adrift in an uncertain environment, the time is well spent. New nurses who understand this concept can do a good deal in charting their careers. The chances of success are phenomenal. After all, isn't that the goal of every nurse? Success is no accident; it is planned every step of the way.

DISCUSSION QUESTIONS

1. Develop a one-page resume that emphasizes your strengths as a professional nurse.
2. Design a career map for one career option you might like to pursue.
3. Describe the benefits of career management as a means to achieve professional goals.

REFERENCES

Brody, M. (1985, November). Meet today's young American worker. *Fortune* 120(22).

Ginsburg, S. (1983, May). Evaluating job offers: Seeking the seven C's. *Nursing Management* 14(5).

Lewis, H. (1985, June). The best career path? *RN* XII, 40.

McEwan, B. (1984, January). The risk management approach to career planning. *Supervisory Nurse* 15(1).

SUGGESTED READING

Coleman, J., Dayani, E., & Simms, E. (1984, January). Nursing careers in the emerging systems. *Nursing Management* 15(1).

Driscoll, D., & Goldberg, C. (1993). *Members of the club.* New York: Free Press.

Galinsky, E., Bond, J.T., & Friedman, D. (1993). *The changing workforce.* New York: Families and Work Institute.

Networking Strategies

Catherine A. Robinson

> *A hundred times every day I*
> *remind myself that my inner and outer*
> *life depends on the labors of other men,*
> *living and dead, and that I must exert*
> *myself in order to give in the measure as*
> *I have received and am still receiving.*
> *Albert Einstein*

LEARNING OBJECTIVES

This chapter will enable you to:

1. Understand the skills, challenges and benefits of professional networking.
2. Identify the three types of networking.
3. Develop action steps for networking.

Vestal, K.W. Nursing Management:
Concepts and Issues, 2 ed.
© 1995 J.B. Lippincott Company

Although Einstein didn't know it as such, what he was stating was a rather elegant definition of what today is commonly known as networking. Since 1980, when Welch first used the word to describe "the process of developing and using your contacts for information, advice, and moral support as you pursue your career," networking has gained widespread acknowledgment as a legitimate career-building strategy.

Not that it is a new or novel approach. Networking has been around for centuries. In the traditional male-dominated business and career world of the past, it was known as the "good old boy" system. Notice that Einstein "depends on men...", not people or women.

Times, of course, have changed. Such political incorrectness would not be tolerated today by persons of either sex, both of which are successfully using networking to advance their careers. Indeed, business leaders have estimated that half of all positions are filled by word-of-mouth contact—a percentage that is probably even higher in the nursing profession.

THE BASIC PURPOSE OF NETWORKING

The basic purpose of networking is to improve one's personal and professional effectiveness. Networking itself refers to a system of interconnecting and cooperating individuals. When applied to nursing, networking (or the utilization of contacts for information and advice) is an essential part of the process of developing and expanding a tested base of knowledge, which then constitutes and governs professional nursing practice. Networking has the potential to become a vital link in the quest toward advancement of nursing practice. Basic to successful networking is the knowledge and understanding of the various categories of networks, the advantage and disadvantages of alliances, and the process of information brokering.

Networking in nursing falls into three categories: personal, political, and research. Within each of these networks, three types of networking relationships are possible. Nurses can network among nurses in their own institution, they can network outside the home institution but still within the nursing profession, and lastly, they can network with people in other disciplines and professions outside the home institution. The major focus of this chapter is to describe the challenges of developing a personal network. Additionally, it discusses the status of political and research networks in the nursing profession and offers practical strategies for increasing one's personal power.

PERSONAL NETWORKING CHALLENGE

The process of networking successfully is only one strategy for personal and professional success. While you should develop sincere, trusting, supportive relationships with your nurse colleagues and with people in other disciplines, you shouldn't rely solely on this activity. The current interest in networking serves to remind us that, yes, we are indeed our brothers' and our sisters' keepers. However, a concentrated effort to develop a personal support network may or may not be successful. It is difficult to relate to someone who has not experienced successful networking how the traditional network really works. Network relationships are like friendships. Just as friendships require attention and care, so do networking relationships. A personal network is not an object that can be seen, yet it is a very real, although intangible, structure. Network relationships are not preordained; they develop according to one's natural needs and interests. The entire process is almost always informal, complete with all the nuances of any other interpersonal relationship. The challenge is to gain an awareness of networking opportunities by being sensitive to and knowledgeable about those individuals who have the power, influence, and direction to assist you as you seek to improve your personal and professional effectiveness.

The current interest in networking among nurses is both a source of pride and a cause for concern. The heightened interest in nurses helping nurses to succeed and to achieve career goals is a source of pride. The naivety with which it seems to be undertaken is a cause for concern.

Bonnie Garson (1977) captured the essence of this concern when she wrote:

> You can't assume that the successful woman in an organization is going to be on your side. You can't assume that the liberal male manager is going to be on your side. Assumptions like that get you into a lot of trouble. . .if you can find a good person, male or female, that can set an example for you, you are very lucky.

Nursing administrators, colleagues, and faculty can assist new nurses in using the informal support process that exists in the nursing profession as well as in individual organizations; however, caution is urged. You cannot assume that every successful nurse wishes to assist the novice. One also cannot assume that merely joining a networking group or organization will lead to a clear understanding of how networks really function.

Networks, like relationships, develop out of mutual goals, needs, and desires. And just as relationships have the potential for positive and negative results, so do the contacts formed through the process of networking. Anyone participating in such an endeavor is cautioned to be aware at all times that other participants are constantly evaluating the risks and benefits of opening up their world of contacts or their personal network to the newcomer. How interested others are in networking with the newcomer will always depend on their perceptions of what the newcomer has to offer. The benefits and costs of entering into a new networking relationship are certainly being measured by all involved parties.

The novice may ask a colleague or faculty member for guidance in this process. The nurse colleague or the individual faculty person considers the benefit/cost ratio in the decision of whether or not to extend one's self to the newcomer. Individuals differ in their willingness to help others and in their actual ability to assist others in launching a successful career. Merely attending a class on power or networking conveys on the person attending the class neither power nor a powerful networking relationship. The subtlety of mutual needs expressed through informal support networks is captured in part in the following description:

> Being aware of the informal world is being aware of the changing (interpersonal)...relationships, the person-to-person sensitivities, the informal political values and taboos and the informal understandings between functions and among people within the function as well as knowing what thou shalt and shalt not do. Arrangements within the unstructured world are seldom written down; there are no descriptions of the informal interpersonal credit bank — in fact, the entire power dimension is never fully described. You must gain your awareness by tuning in to the arrangement to sense who has the clout, power, influence, direction. (Silber, 1974)

By keeping the mutual needs in mind and by always serving to give more than one gets, the staff nurse's chances for success will be greater.

FORMING NETWORKS

For most staff nurses, a distinction exists between a personal support group made up of friends from outside work, family, or neighbors, and a professional support network. Throughout the country networks are forming generally for the purpose of providing professional information and support to colleagues. As the new nurse matures and advances, joining such a group may be beneficial. The challenges of networking bring a wealth of benefits, though it is not undertaken easily or without cost. Some of networking's challenges are:

Building your web of support and friendship will not happen quickly or without effort. It will require your *patience,* your *sustained energy and attention,* and your *follow-up.* For example, you may need to attend meetings of a particular group repeatedly before you begin to realize your ambitions in the group. Persevere—it will be well worth it.

As you interact with individuals from cultures, backgrounds, and lifestyles that are different from yours, you will need to cultivate and maintain an attitude of *openness and sensitivity.* You will need to *suspend judgment,* since your new friends may have goals and values different from yours. Their agendas and their needs may not necessarily correspond with yours. Yet their viewpoints need to be considered and valued, as you would have them do with yours.

Rejection of your initiatives should not be taken personally, nor should it necessarily be discouraging. As you become assertive in stating your interests, such as obtaining a certain job, earning a higher rate of compensation, or initiating a professional relationship, it is important to respect the rights of others to say no. And it is important to accept their decisions without having those decisions unduly affect your considered path.

NETWORKING GUIDELINES FOR THE NEW NURSE

In addition to developing an understanding of networking relationships, certain organizational strategies can increase the likelihood of successful networking, which requires planning and follow-up. Identify individuals who have the potential to assist you and who can give you the information you need for success. Keep records (names, addresses, and phone numbers) regarding people who may be able to help you obtain the information you are likely to need.

Attend presentations given by individuals whom you have identified as potential resource persons. Introduce yourself to the individual, follow up with a call or letter, and always be appreciative of any help given to you. The recommendations or components of successful networking listed below can assist you in evaluating the present status of your personal network. Your network includes all of the individuals, students, employees, and employers who have influenced your personal and professional life. In part, your success will depend on how competently you use your personal network.

One means of systematically keeping track of the individuals you meet is to exchange business cards. The cost of having business cards printed is minimal. Although the actual cost may vary from place to place, 1000 cards usually can be purchased at a minimal price. When

DISPLAY 16-1. STEPS IN SUCCESSFUL NETWORKING FOR THE NEW NURSE	
OBJECTIVE	**ACTION PLAN**
Join American Nurses Association	Attending local and state meetings will provide opportunities to meet nurses in leadership positions.
Join specialty organizations such as NAPNAP, AACN, ENA.	Involvement can lead to relationships with other nurses in your specialty area.
Volunteer for committee memberships in your workplace.	An outstanding performance brings you to the attention of nurse leaders in your organization.
Demonstrate commitment and competence in staff nurse role.	A work record characterized by competence and integrity is an essential base for future career advancement.
Attend national ANA or NLN conventions or specialty conventions.	This provides an opportunity to keep your knowledge current and allows you to know who's who in nursing and in your area.

you meet persons at conferences or other meetings, you can ask them for a business card and give them one of your cards.

Business cards should always be printed on good-quality paper similar to that of a fine wedding invitation. White cards are acceptable, as are off-white and cream. At no time should business cards be printed on cheap paper or colored paper; such choices indicate poor taste on the part of the cardholder. The information to be printed on business cards varies with personal preference; however, the following is one example for the staff nurse.

Keep the cards you receive in an organized fashion. Most office supply stores have an assortment of folders designed to assist in the organization, storage, and easy retrieval of business cards. It is important to invest early in a handy folder for business cards and other names and addresses that could be important to future success. Be sure to ask

Karen Jones
Registered Nurse–Critical Care

Mercy Hospital
110 Summerset
Someplace
USA, 28433
919-441-9262

for business cards from key persons you meet at conventions or other meetings. When attending conventions and conferences, try to be present at *all* sessions, including cocktail hours, luncheon meetings, and dinner meetings. Successful networking requires organization, commitment, and time. A list of networking do's and don'ts compiled in part by Puetz follows:

- Do learn how to ask questions. Don't be afraid to ask for what you need.
- Do follow up on contacts. Don't pass up any opportunities.
- Do report back to your contacts. Don't tell everything to everybody.
- Do try to give as much as you get. Don't share personal information.
- Do keep in touch with your contacts. Don't ask personal questions.
- Do be businesslike as you network.

The long-term goal in building a personal network is to increase one's base of contacts and one's personal power. According to Josefowitz (1980), there are two views of power. The first refers to the traditional, finite idea of power, that is, there is just so much power and no more. The second view of power, referring to effectiveness, is more elastic and relates more to the nurse's potential personal power. In this sense, power can spread out or change its shape depending on the needs of the individual or organization. The derivation of the word power is "pouvoir," a French word meaning to enable. In order to empower others, the new nurse must first acquire some power of his or her own.

DISPLAY 16-2. COMPONENTS OF SUCCESSFUL NETWORKING

Record keeping:
Keep organized files amd business cards of people who can assist you in the future.

Follow up:
Write letters after workshops amd conferences expressing your apprecia- tion for a suggestion or a contact.

Extend yourself to others:
Assist your colleagues when they need help.

The health care industry increasingly is going to need and value nurses who know what they want and where they are going with their careers—nurses who can develop goals, action plans, and timetables for implementing the goals. Few nursing education programs have concentrated on helping students set professional and personal goals. Institutions such as hospitals need nurses who can balance the competing demands of work and personal responsibilities.

Establishing professional and personal goals is one way of determining where you want to go with your career. According to Carr-Ruffino (1985), the process of developing clearly stated goals involves all of the following:

> ... understanding the difference between goals and activities, learning to state goals in specific terms, brainstorming a comprehensive set of goals, refining and ranking them, categorizing them according to career, personal development or family orientation, and recognizing the relative importance of these categories for you.

The next consideration is how to attain these goals. An action plan that is clear, simple, and realistic is an action plan that is likely to work. An action plan that is ambiguous, complex, and beyond the scope of the resources available is an action plan on a collision course with failure. This is not to suggest that the plan cannot be an ambitious one nor is it to suggest that it be one absolutely guaranteed to succeed. There undoubtedly should be some challenge involved, but the challenge must be a reasonable one.

Dividing the action plan into specific activities with a realistic timetable increases the likelihood of accomplishing one's goals. Avoid becoming a fanatic over the planned timetable. Persistence and flexibility are ingredients that most often lead to success.

MENTORING AND SPONSORING RELATIONSHIPS

Young nurses often establish mentoring and sponsoring relationships with their nursing faculty, head nurses, supervisors, and clinical nurse specialists. The young staff nurse looks to these relationships for support and advice. Generally the relationships terminate when the nurse changes jobs. The relationships are probably not true mentor relationships, but fall more into that of the young nurse seeking a role model.

POLITICAL NURSING NETWORKS

With more than 2 million nurses in the United States, political and health analysts have commented on the potential power of the profession, based on the fact that one out of every 44 voters is a nurse.

Effective political involvement and influence require additional development of all types of political networks. Political networks offer two opportunities for advancing the nursing profession. The value of "connections" or access to the right person is a well-known political strategy; however, political networking also requires the deliberate use of politics or the use of influence and interpersonal relationship to achieve some planned goal or purpose.

These political networks are of three types. The first one resembles an "old boy network," in which older, more experienced nurses assist younger, less experienced nurses in the political process. The second type of political network is a system designed to put expert nurses in contact with legislators. Committee staff and legislators themselves have long relied on this type of contact for advice and information as they seek to make technical decisions. The third type of political network is a grassroots organization designed to allow for the rapid deployment of letters, calls, and telegrams when nursing issues arise. The political clout of nurses and the nursing profession depend in large part on the profession devoting more resources to this process. Unless we do so, nurses will continue to be omitted from health policy decision-making process.

Political networking has generally resulted when a group of nurses become very polarized in support of or in opposition to an issue or cause. To date, networking in nursing seems to have had the greatest potential when it was used as a vehicle creating a united effort on behalf of a cause or when a vital issue in the profession of nursing was at stake.

A call to arms such as the one described in Hauser's description of the Cape Girardeau incident is an excellent example of a nurses' political network. In this example, nurses joined together to protest a court decision involving nurses who were accused of practicing medicine without a license. The issue—the use of protocols and standing orders—affects nurses in multiple settings, from home health care and the administration of an enema to the critical care nursing administering lidocaine for a life-threatening arrhythmia.

Still another example of successful nurse networking occurred when the membership of the Virginia Nurses' Association sought to block the introduction of Chelsea beer into the marketplace. An initial television advertisement portrayed teenagers seated around a table drinking Chelsea beer and eating peanut butter sandwiches. Although the beer had an alcoholic content approaching that of regular beer, the market strategies had targeted traditional soft drink markets. Through the efforts of the involved members of the Virginia Nurses' Association, plans to market Chelsea beer as a soft drink were dropped and, in fact, Chelsea beer was dropped from the Anheuser-Busch Company's product list and resulted in an estimated loss of $5 million in company revenues.

RESEARCH NETWORKS

Another example of a successful nursing network is in the area of research. The networking process can provide nurses the opportunity to exchange ideas about research, initiate new projects, and collaborate on ongoing research activities. Opportunities for nursing research exist on local, state, regional, and national levels. Collaboration can advance the quality of nursing research and assist in the dissemination of findings. Multiple approaches and solutions are more likely to be forthcoming when the research process has included the opportunity for extensive collaboration within the profession.

Networking also has the potential to help alleviate the sense of isolation that often accompanies the conduct of independent research projects. Careful, sensitive networking has the potential to improve not only your personal effectiveness but also your professional effectiveness.

PRACTICAL APPROACHES

What are some of the most effective key skills and approaches to use as you integrate networking into your professional and personal growth? Here are several:

Develop and focus upon your goals. We've all heard the adage "You can't get there from here if you don't know where you're going." You can't get help to get there either if you don't know what you want. Networking is a way to get help to achieve your plans and ideals. Having a *clear sense of self* is probably the single most important ingredient in realizing the many benefits of these alliances. Your connections will be more meaningful with a clear sense of direction.

Show up. A wise colleague once said that 80% of life is simply *showing up*. After you have identified your priorities, act on them. Attend meetings, events, and functions of your choosing. Go to the parties to which you receive invitations and participate in activities that interest you. Make your selections based on your interests and goals, and then *show up*. There are always reasons why we can't do something—those who are successful will find a way.

Be at ease with yourself and others. Sincere connections with other people are much easier to form from a position of strength and personal integrity. Feeling comfortable with who we are inside radiates outward, and others feel more comfortable and more forthcoming in our presence.

Be assertive. Don't wait to be discovered. As you develop a clear vision of your personal and professional goals, you can begin to achieve them with intentional acts of choice. Others may or may not notice and heed you or your interests. It is up to you to *seek those ideas, resources and people that can enhance your professional goals and ambitions.* Developing and finely tuning your abilities to be direct and ask for what you want are key qualities of successful personal and professional relationships.

As you practice these intentional acts to seek what you want, remember that others are often shy. They may actually appreciate your direct and natural approach. At the same time, it is important to allow others to say no. You may understand that someone else is able to help you or serve your interests in some way. Yet the other party to your assertive and positive position may not wish to participate. It helps to remember that the other person is exercising the right to be assertive as well.

Know how to develop "win-win" networks. Networking emphasizes positive self-interest. This is best achieved in an atmosphere of *mutual* gain and benefit. Know how to give something back in your exchanges with other people, and be aware of how you may be able to help another, whether or not that person has helped you.

There are many dimensions in which this principle succeeds in collaborative efforts, beginning with the very simple exercise of sincerely listening to others. This is a seemingly obvious practice, yet it is so easily brushed aside when we are busy formulating our next remark. As you learn of information or resources that will be useful to you, it is vital that you are cognizant of your benefactor's interests as well.

Recognize opportunities. With clear goals and an alert mind, you can begin to see the opportunities that present themselves as you evolve. There are many, but recognizing them requires an awareness of ourselves, our intentions, our needs, and our potential.

Participate in professional and community activities that interest you. It is easy to get caught up in the demands of daily living and family and professional life. Yet, we are foregoing the short- and long-term benefits and pleasures of outside professional or civic involvement. Participation according to your interests and your available time will benefit you immeasurably, for you will gradually build your personal network *and your options* as you become more involved and known to others.

Broaden your professional viewpoint. Try to focus beyond the specifics of nursing practice today. What we consider discrete professions in health care are becoming increasingly interdependent. In the future, successful individuals will be more interdisciplinary in their training and in their orientation. You can achieve that outlook by beginning today to read not only nursing journals but also broader health care and business literature. Empathetically listen to your colleagues, friends, and associates who are in the nursing profession and outside it.

Follow up. This is an important aspect of successful networking—perhaps the most important. When you make agreements with people, you should follow up. But this principle also applies in many other situations. When you meet someone who truly enriches you in some way, a personal note of acknowledgment or thanks is always welcome. If you have learned of someone's key goals and you later discover a resource that may be useful to them, pass it on. If a friend is moving to another locale and you have contacts that may be of help, share them. These seemingly small gestures can be very meaningful to others, and, in turn, to you when the favors are returned.

BENEFITS OF NETWORKING

There are many benefits to enhance our professional lives to be gained from networking. Some will last for a short time; others will last for a lifetime. There are significant *long-term* gains to be made from networking over a lifetime. Maintaining your professional relationships as you change jobs, locations, and careers will provide you with rich resources throughout your personal and professional life. With consistent effort, you will meet new friends and colleagues through your original network of peers and be in a better position to maximize and achieve your career goals.

It is highly likely your network will be *geographically dispersed.* If you begin actively connecting with others in your profession and in your community while you are still in school or just finishing, your class-mates and instructors will tend to move far and wide. These people can form a base of friendship and support that you can add to and draw from throughout your life. When you travel to new destinations, you will have people you can call. When you move to a new spot, you will already have the beginnings of a professional network. And, if you rise to positions of leadership, you will already have a broad base of professional support.

From your network of peers and associates, you may identify a *mentor*. Mentors are supremely important to your professional growth and development over the course of your career. Through their role modeling and counsel you may learn and emulate the obvious as well as the more subtle aspects of superior performance in your chosen endeavors. Your mentor may already be part of your current network of colleagues.

Finally, one of the richest benefits of this activity is the *knowledge and awareness* we develop from knowing one another. We need to work together, as a nursing profession, as a health care profession, and as a society. We need to understand each other's perspectives, particularly as

---

DISPLAY 16-3. STEPS IN THE ANALYSIS OF A PERSONAL NETWORK

1. Identify individual(s) who have had most influence on your career.

2. Identify successful mentor-protégé relationship(s) during your career.

3. Whom would you use as references in appling for a new position?

4. Where do you go for career guidance and counseling?

5. Who are the individuals in your life who share your successes and your failures?

6. Reverse the perspective in questions 1–5 and answer the questions again.
   Whose career have you influenced?
   Whom have you mentored successfully?
   Who uses you as a reference for a new position?
   Who turns to you for career guidance and counseling?
   Who shares her successes and failures with you?

The list of persons generated from answering these questions forms the core of your personal network.

valuing diversity becomes a greater and greater part of our professional mandate and our society's evolution.

SUMMARY

The most successful networking in the nursing profession to date has centered around nurses uniting for a common purpose involving a political cause or some fundamental issue affecting the profession. Networks of nurses organized around the goal of fostering nursing research interests and activities have also been successful in achieving limited goals. It is in the area of forming individual nurse networks for the purpose of improving personal and professional effectiveness that the greatest attention needs to be focused. This attention must be both supportive and encouraging to young nurses, but also must be realistic and incorporate the subtleties of all aspects of human relationships, including the human support relationship that is the essence of the networking concept. Some steps to help you analyze your own personal network are outlined in Display 16–3. Finally, a challenge to all nurses: Strive to be the kind of nurse who does not have to put out another person's light so that your own may shine more brightly.

DISCUSSION QUESTIONS

1. Describe opportunities for networking that exist within your peer group, work setting, and community.
2. Develop a plan for networking over the next year, focused on professional networks.
3. Discuss the multiple networking requirements to establish yourself as a successful professional nurse.

REFERENCES

Bunkers, S. (1992). The healing web. *Nursing and Health Care* 13(2).

Carr-Ruffino, N. (1985). *The promotable woman.* Washington, DC: Wadsworth Publishing.

Chalich, T. & Smith, L. Nursing at the grass roots. *Nursing and Healthcare* 13(5).

Davis, C. K. (1992). New leaders needed. *Nursing and Healthcare* 13(1).

Driscoll, D. & Goldberg, C. (1993). *Members of the club.* New York: Free Press.

Einstein, A. (1983). In Wallis, C. L. (Ed): *The treasure chest,* San Francisco: Harper & Row.

Garson, B. (1977). *Views from women achievers.* New York: AT&T Corporation.

Houser, P. (1983). Networking: Tactic for the Supreme Court Case. *Missouri Nurse* 52(3):12.

Josefowitz, N. (1980). *Paths to power*, Reading, MA: Addison-Wesley.

Maraldo, P. (1990). The nineties: A decade of search of meaning. *Nursing and Healthcare* 11(1).

Puetz, B. (1983). *Networking for nurses*. Rockville, MD: Aspen.

Silber, M. B., Sherman, V. C. (1974). *Managerial performance and promotablity*. New York: American Management Association.

FOCUS ON CONTEMPORARY NURSING ISSUES

Health Care Policy Issues:
Nursing, Politics, and Power

Carmella A. Bocchino
Nancy J. Sharp

LEARNING OBJECTIVES

This chapter will enable you to:

1. Describe the role of nursing in influencing social and health policy development.
2. Review the governmental process of enacting new legislation.
3. Compare the congressional budget process to an organizational budget process.

Vestal, K.W. Nursing Management:
Concepts and Issues, 2 ed.
© 1995 J.B. Lippincott Company

The nursing profession, too often called the "sleeping giant" in the health policy field, may finally have awakened to realize its full potential. Nursing has recognized the importance of influencing policy decisions that affect nursing practice and nursing's commitment to expand quality care to underserved populations. This recognition has broadened nursing's involvement in the public policy arena (Mason, Talbott, & Leavitt, 1993). The link of policy and practice, although often misunderstood, is increasingly important to all practitioners, especially as health care becomes a more dominant social issue.

Successful involvement in the political process depends largely on recognizing periodic opportunities for change and turning those opportunities into results. The rise or fall of ideas, recommendations, and opinions are interlinked with a public policy process that nursing has enjoined in some fashion since the passage of Medicare and Medicaid in the mid-1960s. The enactment of these two major social programs marked the last comprehensive reform of the United States health care system. Then, nursing stood tall as the only professional group to actively support the passage of these two new federal entitlement programs serving the poor, disabled, and elderly. But never before has the nursing community stood to gain more than today, as the comprehensive reform of the U.S. health care system is being debated. The need for nurses' involvement in the political process has never been greater.

HEALTH CARE AS A DOMINANT SOCIAL ISSUE

Varying dominant social issues have directed the action of the federal government and the United States Congress. The 1990s has seen health care reform become a major domestic issue, if not "the issue of the 90s." Our health care system is on the brink of collapse because it is burdened with escalating costs, expanding populations of uninsured and underinsured, and a questionable quality of care.

During the 1960s, concern for the poor, elderly, and disabled saw an increase in federal spending for the development of public social welfare programs. Public social welfare programs provide direct benefits to individuals and their families and are designed to address such issues as health care, education, Social Security, and welfare.

With strong Presidential leadership, Congress passed the first significant health care legislation creating the Medicare and Medicaid programs in 1965. Medicare is a nationwide program that provides health insurance to most individuals aged 65 and over, to persons under 65 who are disabled and meet the eligibility criteria for Social Security or railroad retirement, and to individuals and their dependents who require kidney transplantation or dialysis to sustain life. The Medicare program is financed by employer and employee contributions through payroll taxes and beneficiaries copayments and premiums. Medicaid is a jointly funded federal and state program that provides medical assistance for certain low-income individuals or members of families with dependent children who are aged, blind, or disabled. Each state assumes administration of its respective state medical assistance programs according to federal eligibility and service requirements. States have some flexibility to expand services offered and populations served (Health Insurance Association of America, 1990). Both programs are administered by a federal agency, the Health Care Financing Administration, within the Department of Health and Human Services.

The social programs of the past addressed the problems and needs of specific populations. The debate today centers on how to improve the existing health care system for *all* Americans and how to recognize health care as a "right" of every American. National polls and repeated surveys clearly show that the American public, fearful of losing insurance coverage or anxious over meeting the cost of a catastrophic illness or long-term care, is demanding comprehensive, sweeping changes in our health care system (Schmid, 1991). It is this massive public outcry that will have the greatest impact on Congressional members and state legislators. Constituent power can set, alter, or move any political agenda.

The demographic, social, and economic changes in the 1990s are affecting the policy decisions of this country. American society is aging and living longer, with the average life expectancy now at 75 years of age. The increase in the elderly population brings with it another highly contested debate, the ethical dilemma of prolonged medical care, especially in terminal cases. This dilemma will be complicated by the continued development of more sophisticated medical technologies and procedures that extend life.

The economic recession of the past several years has resulted in increased unemployment and reduced capital investments, leaving the American public pessimistic about the future of the economy. Economic constraints have affected the middle class and have increased the number of low-income or near-poverty families. Legal and illegal immigration to the United States continues to rise. The increase in social problems, such as illegal immigrants, the rising number of single-parent families, a weakening social structure, growing community violence, and epidemics such as AIDS have combined with economic restraints to place new burdens on the health care system. The increase in social problems has broadened the health care needs of individuals to include services such as homemaking, nutritional support, and extended social services. Medicare and Medicaid were designed and financed to pay for health care, not social services. However, it is these broader social changes that have intensified public support for reform.

These changes have also placed nurses in an advantageous position to advance their practice. Over the last decade, nurses have provided primary care services in rural and urban areas for populations often at high risk and who otherwise would not have received care. However, direct reimbursement for these services has continued to evade nurses because repeated analyses by government agencies have shown that expanding reimbursement to advanced practice nurses would add to rapidly escalating health care costs. Striving to gain direct payment for nursing services is a goal that has been unreachable because of well-recognized barriers.

The opposition of organized medicine to the goal of direct payment for nurses continues to be effective. This opposition, the rapid increase in health care costs, the uncontrolled federal deficit, and the lack of public understanding of advanced practice nursing have all contributed to the failure of reaching this goal (Mittelstadt, 1993). However, just as effective lobbying by organized medicine succeeded in opposing federal and state legislation to extend direct reimbursement to advanced practice nurses, active participation by nursing in the political process will counter their efforts and hopefully advance nursing's agenda.

Therefore, it is imperative that the nursing community understand policy debates and how nurses can influence the political process effectively. No proposal put forth by Congress or the Administration will be perfect, but the introduction of a legislative proposal or bill is a process, not a one-time event. As this process moves forward, it will be widely debated in the nation's capital, in local town meetings, and by media and policy experts alike, thus providing ample opportunity to critique the proposal and suggest ways to modify or change it.

Major health care reform requires that the general public and lawmakers recognize the need for fundamental change, agree on a direction to achieve change, and have strong political leadership committed to ensure enactment. Timing is a crucial element in the legislative process. Establishing relationships and beginning dialogues early in the process will enable you to recognize allies and opposing views. It is important to realize that like medicine, government and the public policy arena have a vocabulary and jargon that is not familiar to the general public. Therefore, nurses must fully understand all proposals submitted for consideration and present a clear and concise description of their role as practitioners and what they seek to achieve.

Understanding the process and the players and recognizing the opportunities within the framework of any public policy debate will enable all of us to be responsible professionals and citizens.

THE STRUCTURE OF GOVERNMENT

Although often criticized as displaying partisan rivalry and being self-serving and weak, the United States Congress is the most democratic of government institutions ("How Our Government Works," 1985). Our forefathers strove to create a government "for the people." Therefore, they developed a system of checks and balances to prevent a return to a tyrannical rule like that of England. This balanced system involved three branches of government, each with separate responsibilities: the executive branch, the legislative branch, and the judicial branch. This fundamental division of power—the President with limited executive authority, the Congress with responsibility for enacting laws, and the judiciary with responsibility for interpreting the Constitution and the thousands of state and federal laws—prevents the return of authoritarian power and historical oppression.

The power of the President allows for public appointments, reprieves and pardons, and the authority to veto legislation passed by Congress. However, even that executive power is limited by the ability of the Congress to override such action with sufficient approval or votes. It is the Congress, the so-called "people's branch of government," that has served as the "battleground of social change" and has the broadest authority of all three branches ("How Our Government Works," 1985).

The 100 senators and 435 members of the House of Representatives rely on staff, advisors, and constituents for new ideas and information. Federal laws, new programs, expanded entitlements, and even new taxes all begin in discussions with a member of Congress. These discussions become the framework for new ideas and solutions for recurring problems. Few of these elected officials have firsthand knowledge of many of the tough issues addressed by Congress. And yet, the decisions made by these elected officials result in expenditures of billions of dollars. The process for enactment of laws is similar for state and federal governments. However, because the process is different in each state, this chapter focuses on defining activities at the federal level. A better understanding of the legislative process will make clearer one's ability to influence that process.

THE LEGISLATIVE PROCESS: AUTHORIZATION AND APPROPRIATIONS

THE AUTHORIZATION PROCESS

There are two basic types of legislation: authorization and appropriations. Authorizing legislation creates or expands existing programs and may provide for a maximum level of funds to be expended for implementation. New program ideas may arise due to an interest of a Congressional member, staff member, advisor, or representative of a special interest group who has gained the support of a congressperson to introduce a legislative proposal. Because of the expanding duties of Congressional members, staff members often assume many of the responsibilities of the member. This may include drafting the legislation for a particular bill.

Any proposal or bill can be introduced by any member of Congress, either a senator or representative. A bill is introduced by the member in the respective chamber of Congress to which the member was elected—either the House of Representatives or the Senate. Once introduced, the bill is given a number dependent on the order filed and is referenced to the particular chamber where the action occurred. For example, "H. R. 1" denotes a bill introduced in the House of Representatives, whereas "S. 1" denotes a bill introduced in the Senate. At the time of introduction, the bill is also referred to a committee of Congress that has jurisdiction for the issue within the bill.

Both the House of Representatives and the Senate share legislative duties but are elected separately and function by different governing rules. The House has approximately 180 committees and subcommittees, while the Senate has 132. But each of these committees is responsible for a designated area of public policy (eg, armed forces, public health, taxes, Medicare and Medicaid). In the Senate, most health-related authorizing legislation falls under the jurisdiction of the Finance Committee or the Labor and Human Resources Committee. In the House, the Energy and Commerce Committee and the Ways and Means Committee have jurisdiction over similar health issues.

Other committees may have responsibility for authorization of specific health programs that fall within their jurisdiction. For example, the House and Senate Veterans Affairs Committee considers bills that establish or continue health programs for veterans including jurisdiction over legislation that would affect nurses who work in veterans hospitals. Public and private housing falls under the jurisdiction of the

House or Senate Committee on Banking, Housing and Urban Affairs and directs efforts to resolve the problem of homelessness throughout the United States.

It is this maze of committees and subcommittees that serves to complicate the legislative process and to confuse the public. The complexities of the legislative process and the "mystique" of the Washington power base have served as obstacles to many professionals, limiting their involvement in the policy arena. As the role of government grew, new congressional committees evolved. Each committee is assigned responsibility for carefully evaluating and analyzing proposed legislation and recommending subsequent actions.

Once a bill is referred to a committee, public hearings are usually held. These hearings enable key supporters of the bill and those in opposition to provide testimony. Verbal testimony is requested from expert witnesses, administration officials, and special interest groups. Anyone wishing to submit written testimony may do so following the directions set by each committee. All testimony is considered part of the hearing record.

After sufficient information is received by way of hearings and ongoing meetings between members on the committee, the member's staff, and the committee's staff, the bill progresses to a "markup." A "markup" session is held for all committee members to review each provision in the bill and to amend, revise, or delete sections by a majority vote of the committee. Once the revised bill is approved by the committee, the bill is sent to the full chamber—the House or Senate—for approval.

In the House, most bills approved by committee first go to the Rules Committee, which determines how a bill will be handled on the House floor and in debate before all members of the House. For example, decisions are made about the amount of time allotted for debate and whether amendments will be permitted. This key committee and its chairman have an extremely important function—deciding which bills will move and which will be delayed.

The majority leader in the House, in conjunction with the House Speaker—two leadership positions elected by the majority party in each chamber—determines when to call a particular bill for action. Debate on each piece of legislation is set, and members are given a limited amount of time to speak for or against the proposal. After a bill is passed by one chamber, it is sent to the other chamber for continued action. If the House and Senate enact different versions of the bill, a conference committee composed of key members of both the House and Senate resolves the differences. The compromise bill must then be approved by both chambers of Congress before being sent to the Presi-

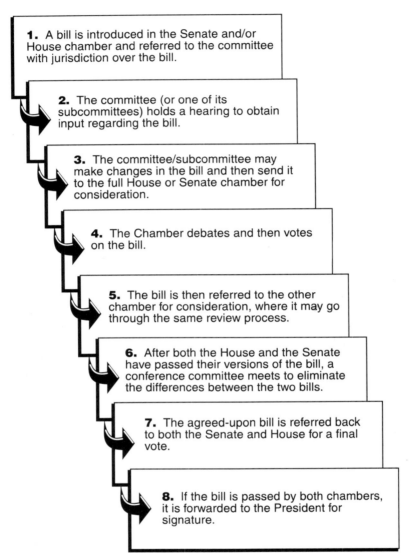

1. A bill is introduced in the Senate and/or House chamber and referred to the committee with jurisdiction over the bill.

2. The committee (or one of its subcommittees) holds a hearing to obtain input regarding the bill.

3. The committee/subcommittee may make changes in the bill and then send it to the full House or Senate chamber for consideration.

4. The Chamber debates and then votes on the bill.

5. The bill is then referred to the other chamber for consideration, where it may go through the same review process.

6. After both the House and the Senate have passed their versions of the bill, a conference committee meets to eliminate the differences between the two bills.

7. The agreed-upon bill is referred back to both the Senate and House for a final vote.

8. If the bill is passed by both chambers, it is forwarded to the President for signature.

FIG 17-1. The legislative process.

dent for signature. Passage and subsequent approval by the President authorizes the new or expanded federal program. Authorization for federal programs may occur at any time during the congressional year.

Once programs are established, reauthorization may be required every 3 to 5 years. This reauthorization process allows for reexamination and evaluation of the program and modification as needed. For example, the

National Health Service Corps, which was created to expand the placement of physicians and nurses in rural and urban medically underserved areas, must be reauthorized every 3 years to remain a federal program. A similar example is the Nurse Education Act, which provides federal funding for baccalaureate and graduate nursing education. Without reauthorization, these programs would be eliminated.

In the course of a 2-year session of Congress, nearly 15,000 bills may be introduced, with only several hundred enacted into law. Passage depends on numerous factors: the political environment, competing bills, the time of introduction, the national importance of the issue, and whether there is broad support from Congressional members, the White House, and the public. Wide diversity in political views and regional interests, the influence of special interest groups, and political caution often keep Congressional members from reaching agreement and enactment. In fact, many of the bills sent to committee receive no further action after referral and "die" or stall as the result of inactivity. Consensus is more easily reached during a national emergency or crisis such as war or natural disasters.

Special interest groups such as those representing nursing and medicine have demonstrated their ability to provide the expertise and in-depth understanding of many of the issues before Congress. However, vast knowledge about a particular issue is not the only resource provided to Congressional members by special interest groups. Additionally, as the cost of conducting a successful political campaign increases, members are often swayed with another vital resource—money. Therefore, both information and financial resources make some groups more highly visible and resourceful advisors. Nurses are learning how to be more savvy in both arenas.

THE APPROPRIATIONS PROCESS

Once a program is authorized (or reauthorized), it cannot be implemented until funds have been "appropriated" from the federal budget. However, only those programs that have been authorized previously by legislation can receive funding through the appropriations process. By constitutional mandate, the House Committee on Appropriations initiates all appropriations bills (National Health Council, 1991). The appropriations committees in the House and the Senate are responsible for allocating federal funds to specific government programs and approving new spending authority. Unlike the number of authorizing committees with jurisdiction for an issue, there is only one appropriations committee in each chamber. However, each appropriations committee has 13 subcommittees responsible for a specific domestic issue: agriculture, commerce, judiciary, defense, energy/water development, foreign operations, interior, labor/health/human services, legislative, military construction, transportation, general government, and independent agencies.

For example, the Subcommittee on Labor, Health and Human Services, Education and Related Agencies has the responsibility for funding recommendations for the National Institute of Nursing Research (NINR), the National Institutes of Health (NIH), and the Division of Nursing, which is part of the Health Resources and Services Administration (HRSA), one of the major departments of the Public Health Service (PHS). Both the NINR and Division of Nursing annually award federal scholarships, traineeships, and grants to schools of nursing equal to congressional appropriations, now in excess of $100 million.

Given the power of these subcommittees, the political jockeying by Congressional members for these committee assignments is fierce on both the House and Senate sides. The subcommittee recommends specific funding levels to the full appropriations committees in the form of a bill. Once approved or modified by the full committee, the bill is forwarded to the full House and Senate for a floor vote. Unlike authorizing legislation, appropriations bills follow a time schedule and are expected to be implemented by October 1, the beginning of the new federal fiscal year.

The House generally begins consideration of appropriations by June 30. Between July 1 and October 1, the Senate is expected to complete their work on similar legislation. Conference committees resolve any differences in the legislation before being sent for approval by both chambers. If disagreement occurs on a particular bill, the deadlines may not be met. If the appropriations bill fails to be enacted by October 1, Congress must pass a continuing resolution (CR), which allows the government to fund the continued operation of federal programs until legislation can be passed. In addition to appropriating funds for the new fiscal year, Congress also has a mechanism to allocate supplemental appropriations for unexpected emergencies. Supplemental appropriations bills can be passed at any time by Congress. The appropriations subcommittee with jurisdiction for the issue—or an emergency—would introduce a bill seeking financial support. Natural disasters such as hurricanes, floods, or earthquakes are examples in which supplemental appropriations for relief funds are enacted.

THE BUDGET PROCESS

It would appear that the excessive spending of the last decade and the embarrassing federal deficit has caused the administration and

Congress to refocus its attention on the need to balance the federal government's budget. For too long, Congress, which has the responsibility for this nation's "tax and spend" activities, has ignored the annual budget shortfall in favor of expanding or creating new programs. The federal deficit, now at $4 trillion, has resulted in the interest paid on the deficit being a major federal outlay each year, second only to spending on entitlement programs. Monies spent on interest for the federal deficit reduce funds available for domestic and other programs.

The budget process begins in January, when the President submits a budget to Congress. Given the veto power of the President, the Administration's budget is considered a blueprint around which the congressional debate ensues—granting serious consideration to the President's proposals. The House and Budget Committees each draft their budget documents and, as with any committee, hold hearings and meetings to debate the merits of the various proposals. Other congressional committees review the President's budget and provide their opinions and estimates on appropriate spending levels for those programs within the jurisdiction of their respective committees. The congressional budget process is governed by several major legislative statutes that set deficit targets, ceilings on budget authority for specific programs, the payment mechanism for new or expanded programs, and automatic spending cuts to prevent deficit growth.

Pursuant to the Congressional Budget Act of 1974, the Congressional Budget Office (CBO) was created. The CBO was intended to serve as a nonpartisan organization that advises Congress on budget-related information and provides analyses of alternative fiscal and budgetary issues and the cost of all proposed legislation. Each bill when introduced is sent to the CBO for a cost estimate. In regard to the annual federal budget, the CBO submits a report to the budget committees, analyzing budget requests, options, and the overall economic outlook of the country.

As the federal deficit remains out of control, Congress continues to change the rules of the budget process. These changes, in particular spending limitations, are necessary to avoid any net increase in the federal deficit. As Medicare and Medicaid and other entitlement programs represent the largest growth segment of the federal budget, these programs continue to come under congressional scrutiny to control costs. In addition, economic forecasts remain dismal, due in part to an unstable economy and the costs associated with the savings and loan crisis (Wakefield, 1990). Monies for new programs, increased funding levels, and reauthorization of existing programs depend on the ability to identify clear benefits and to gain broad constituent support. Programs that are less protected or appear to offer less direct benefits to society as a whole will be trimmed or reduced.

If the recession remains, with no sound economic growth over the next year, revenues supporting federal programs will remain restricted. Rising unemployment, the increase in failing businesses, and other factors have resulted in federal trust funds becoming depleted due to their dependency on tax dollars. In the process, consideration is given to shifting the burdens and costs of some federal programs onto the private sector. For example, funding for nursing education could be shifted to hospitals, universities, or other partners in education rather than continuing to receive federal support.

Nurses need to remain vigilant throughout the budget process to ensure that health care services receive adequate funding. The need for nurses to remain proactive and vocal in pursuing health care funds is at an all time high.

THE REGULATORY PROCESS

After legislation is enacted, the administrative responsibility of implementing or modifying the program falls to the executive agency or department with jurisdiction for the program. The legislation usually authorizes the agency to formulate regulations and defines how the law will be implemented. Congress continues to retain oversight.

Most health-related legislation becomes the responsibility of the Department of Health and Human Services (DHHS) and will be written by several divisions within DHHS: the Public Health Service, the Health Resources and Services Administration, the Health Care Financing Administration, and so forth. Under the Administrative Procedures Act, a two-part procedure was established for rulemaking or producing regulations. Draft regulations are developed by the respective agency with jurisdiction and published in a federal publication, the *Federal Register*.

The *Federal Register* is published every federal working day and informs the public about the activities of the federal agencies. It includes agency regulations, legal notices, presidential proclamations, executive orders, and other administrative orders. Initially, the federal agency must publish a *notice of proposed rulemaking (NPRM)* defining the legislative reference, a description of the subject and issues involved, a projected timetable, and a call for public comment on the proposed regulations. Public comments may include a request to submit written comments on the proposal, to testify at a public hearing held by the agency, or to respond to inquiries included in the notice of proposed rulemaking.

A response to most written comments received is usually included in the final rulemaking and published in the *Federal Register*. The final rule will provide a date for implementation if different from the date set in legislation. Many laws are passed by Congress but implementation may be delayed due to the extensive time needed to develop, review, and analyze comments received and publish a final regulation. Congress has been highly critical of the extensive delays by federal agencies in releasing regulations and frequently includes language enacting specific provisions about the publication of regulations. The public comment period is another opportunity for nurses and nursing organizations to provide their opinions or opposition to the proposed rule. Relationships with staff at the federal agencies assigned to health care legislation should be established by nurses during the legislative debate so that nurses, whether as individuals or a group, can easily convey ideas and opinions in the earliest draft stages of the proposed rulemaking.

EDUCATING YOUR MEMBERS OF CONGRESS

If one is to negotiate the maze of political procedures and protocol, two characteristics are essential: flexibility and perseverance. The increased complexity of relationships and the steady building of networks designed to influence the direction of proposed legislation demands early involvement in the process. Trade-offs, negotiations, and compromise are the core of political action. Being able to overcome numerous obstacles, changes in the political environment, and modifications by special interest groups demands flexibility.

Perseverance in looking for opportunities to influence the process leads constituents to recognize the importance of professional relationships with Congressional members, particularly those who serve on the authorizing committees for health care issues. These members then become an essential linchpin that is needed to introduce new legislation or modify existing programs. Nurses who learn of important legislation that will have an impact on their clinical specialty or health care facility must determine who they can reach to express their views, either favorable or unfavorable.

Nursing's growing concern for adequate federal support for nursing education, research, AIDS treatment, maternal and child health, or any other health care issue overcame the inertia or noninvolvement of these professionals. Congressional decision makers respond to what they see and hear. Individual contact with members of the state's Congressional delegation serves as a educational experience for both the nurse and the member of Congress and heightens the role of nurses as an integral and critical component of the health care system.

Congressional members who are not assigned to committees with jurisdiction over health care programs should still be contacted because all members vote on all the issues when they come before the full House or Senate. The collegial relationships among members also provide a broad base of support for important issues. Members consult with each other on issues with which they are less familiar.

The most important rule is to start early. Timing is crucial throughout the process. Therefore, the relationships established with members of Congress before the heat of a controversial debate will be a resource for information and opinion. Nurses who volunteer as workers on senators' and representatives' election campaigns provide a head start on establishing early relationships. Nurses seen at regular intervals, speaking knowledgeably about health care reform issues and clearly describing their role as care givers and their professional practice, will heighten the visibility of nursing in the political arena.

NETWORKING AMONG NURSES TO AFFECT HEALTH POLICY

Political savvy is now a nursing skill! Networking is a fundamental and basic component of political savvy. Networking applies to all nurses in all areas of nursing practice, education, research, and administration. It is individual nurses who will decide to what extent they wish to use the techniques of networking.

Although networking is sometimes perceived negatively, it is not necessarily a "commitment to a larger cause, the adoption of a militant posture toward an issue, or the unhealthy manipulation of others to get one's way" (Puetz, 1983). Networking allows nurses to take advantage of those contacts already established and to expand those contacts to meet future goals for themselves, the nursing profession, and their community. Networking is largely a process of exchanging information between individuals (Puetz, 1983).

As a new nurse studying management concepts, the lessons of teamwork on patient care units and projects in the classroom emphasize the importance of a cohesive team effort. Ambivalence and disjointed agendas only serve to confuse all participants and block goal achievement. As a professional, the structure provided by one or more of the professional nursing organizations will provide ample opportunities for networking. The American Nurses Association is recognized as the major nursing organization, but the growth in specialized nursing organizations has further advanced the nursing community in the health policy arena.

No amount of book learning can substitute for actually seeing, hearing, and feeling firsthand the intensity and the urgency that accompanies the legislative process on Capitol Hill. Every nurse in the United States should have the opportunity to experience it. It personalizes the immense need for nurses to involve themselves in the legislative process and shows the impact that nurses can have on the process of health policy formulation. Local and state agencies, in an effort to increase involvement in public policy, offer legislative conferences, fellowships, and internships that provide an excellent training ground for future nurse leaders.

Another opportunity for networking is found among the pages of *The Nurses' Directory of Capitol Connections*. This is a directory of positions and opportunities for nurse participation in health policy development in Washington, DC. There are more than 400 nurses listed. The directory is designed as a resource tool to be used to access information about the Washington health policy world from nursing colleagues within the policy arena. The goal is to increase the number of nurses in the infrastructure of the Washington health policy circle.

Coalitions, networks, roundtables, and regular nursing organizations are all important to your career development, whether your career takes you on a clinical, educational, research, or administrative path. Begin early to build long-term relationships with your nursing colleagues, keep in touch throughout the years, meet as often as you can, and share your successes. Or, perhaps even more importantly, enlist their support and advice as you go through difficult times in your professional career.

Political decisions will continue to shape nursing practice. Nursing has been far more effective on the state level of government where amendment of the nurse practice act must occur. Achieving consensus and seeking to reach a compromise position on many issues has enabled nursing to amend state practice laws to allow for prescriptive authority, direct third-party reimbursement by private payers, and, to a limited degree, admitting privileges. These gains, achieved by working the state political process, have advanced nursing practice. As nurses continue to struggle for autonomy and independence, their role in the policy arena will be heightened if the challenge to do so is accepted.

The successful recognition of nursing as a participant in this process is further substantiated by the appointment of nursing leaders to state and federal leadership positions. In the early 1980s, nursing was honored to have Carolyne K. Davis, PhD, RN serve as Administrator of the Health Care Financing Administration. This trend continues with the appointment of Kristine Gebbie, MSN, RN as the AIDS Policy Coordinator and member of the Domestic Policy Council in the White House. The broadening of nursing's role in public policy will serve to increase recognition of the profession and advance nursing's influence on legislative decisions.

SUMMARY

If nurses are to continue to advance their practice, to secure adequate funding for nursing research and education, and to remain effective practitioners, their participation in the political environment is essential.

The extensive time and complex process in enacting legislation often intimidates many individuals. Yet, an organization's lack of response only serves to enable others to effect change without open debate and full exploration of the potential outcome. Therefore, it is critical that our nursing organizational representatives become students of this process and be given the authority to act quickly on behalf of the nation's 2.2 million nurses when legislation affects the practice of nursing—either as a potential threat or a benefit. Our organizational representatives must be extremely vigilant about the entire legislative process and have an expansive network of local nurses ready to respond when a massive grassroots show of support is needed.

Because the reform of the United States health care system emphasizes primary and preventive care, the opportunities for nurses to advance nursing's agenda have become intensely focused on long-established goals and outcomes. But only if nursing remains an active participant in the process. The reform of the U.S. health care system has reemphasized the importance of primary and preventive health care services, and nursing has clearly demonstrated its successful role in providing these services. If achieved, reform will advance nursing's role toward broader independent practice — but only if nursing remains focused and active. Remember, "silence is *not* golden."

DISCUSSION QUESTIONS

1. Develop an overview of a networking initiative to have an impact on health care policy development.
2. Outline the legislative process.
3. Write a letter to your congressperson stating your opinion on a current health care issue.

REFERENCES

Barnes, F. (1993, May). What health-care crisis? *The American Spectator*, 20–23.
Health Insurance Association of America. *Source book of health insurance data: 1990.* Washington, DC: U. S. Government Printing Office.

How Our Government Works. (1985, January 28). *U. S. News and World Report.*

Mason, D. Talbott, S., Leavitt, J. (1993). *Policy and politics for nurses: Action and change in the workplace, government, organization and community.* Philadelphia: WB Saunders.

Mittelstadt, P. (1993). Third-party reimbursement for services of nurses in advanced practice: Obtaining payment for your services. In M. D. Mezey, & D. O. McGivern (Eds.), *Nurses, nurse practitioners* (pp. 322–341). New York: Springer.

National Health Council. (1991, April). *Congress and health: An introduction to the legislative process and its key participants.* Washington, DC: National Health Council, 4–242.

Puetz, B. (1983). *Networking for nurses.* Rockville, MD: Aspen.

Schmid, G. (1991). Demographic, social and economic changes in the 1990s. In R. J. Blendon & J. N. Edwards (Eds.). *System in crisis: The case for health care reform* (pp. 31–51). New York: Faulkner & Gray.

Sharp, N., Biggs, S., & Wakefield, M. K. (1991). Public policy: New opportunities for nurses. *Nursing and Health Care 12*(1), 17–19.

Sharp, N. Nurses in public policy. (1993). *Nursing Management 24*(11), 22–24.

Wakefield, M. K. (1990). Perspectives on health policy: Influencing the legislative process. *Nursing Economic$, 8*(3), 188–190.

Wakefield, M. K. (1991). Capitol commentary: If you don't like the score, just change the rules. *Nursing Economic$, 9*(2), 122–123.

Ethical Issues

Deborah A. Proctor

LEARNING OBJECTIVES

This chapter will enable you to:

1. Outline the history of the bioethics movement.
2. Identify ethical principles most frequently involved in health care dilemmas.
3. Describe a process for resolving bioethical dilemmas.
4. Distinguish between legal and ethical issues in clinical care delivery.
5. Discuss the use of ethical clinicians, ethical consultants, or bioethics committees in multiple delivery settings.

Vestal, K.W. Nursing Management:
Concepts and Issues, 2 ed.
© 1995 J.B. Lippincott Company

Johnny G. was admitted to St. Katherine's Hospital with pneumonia and chronic renal failure. His renal disease required dialysis 3 times a week on an outpatient basis, but a recent bout with a cold had progressed to pneumonia, resulting in this hospitalization. Johnny was well known to the nurses on 4 East who had cared for him during many acute episodes over the past several years. During that time, as his renal failure progressed, Johnny often spoke to the nurses of his wish not to be "kept alive" if he were to arrest. After discussions with his nephrologist, Dr. M., his family, and the hospital chaplain, a do not resuscitate (DNR) order was placed on his chart. The order was rewritten with each hospitalization.

This morning, Sherry J., RN made a serious medication error that resulted in Johnny becoming semicomatose and experiencing cardiac arrhythmias. Dr. M. was notified immediately, along with Johnny's wife, Glenda. The 4 East nurse manager explained to Glenda that the change in his condition was a direct result of the medication error. Glenda expressed her immediate concern that nothing be done to resuscitate Johnny if the arrhythmias worsened, and the manager assured her that everyone was aware of the DNR order on Johnny's chart.

While Glenda and the nurse manager were meeting, Dr. M. phoned in an order to remove the DNR from Johnny's chart until further notice. When the nurse receiving the order reminded Dr. M. of Johnny's adamant stand on resuscitation, he replied, "Johnny expressed the wish not to be resuscitated if he were to arrest as a result of his renal disease. This condition is temporary and has nothing to do with those wishes. Besides, I know Johnny well enough to know that he would not want Sherry to feel directly responsible for his death. I am confident that if he were alert enough for me to discuss this with him, Johnny would want everything done for this short period of time."

The case of Johnny G. illustrates some of the many ethical dilemmas that arise in health care delivery settings as a result of technology advances, emphasis on individual rights, conflicting values, increasing demands for fair distribution of resources, and changing relationships among health care professionals. Traditional ways of handling these problems no longer work for patients, families, and health care organizations. Medical questions still respond nicely to medical answers, but many of the most complex issues health care professionals face are no longer exclusively medical in nature. They are questions about individual values, about the personal meaning of life and death, and about fairness and justice.

Nurses alone are not responsible for ethical decisions in the care of their patients. Each nurse is, however, accountable for understanding his or her personal value system and the impact it has on the decision-making process. Nurses are also accountable for bringing an understanding of ethical principles and problem-solving methodologies to their delivery of care, to minimize the difficulties in very complex situations. Presenting a reasoned approach to very emotional issues enhances the nurse's ability to assist the patient, family, and other care givers to arrive at decisions in the best interest of the patient.

By understanding the ethical theories that have shaped the bioethics movement and by applying a realistic process for dealing with such dilemmas, nurses can arrive at the "best"—if not necessarily the "right"—answer. If we could figure out the "right" answer, there would be no dilemma.

ETHICS IN HEALTH CARE: A BRIEF HISTORY

During the past 20 years, the health care industry has made many advances in dealing with bioethical issues. Decisions made by physicians alone, ignoring patients, families, or other health care worker's input, are now rare. Open and honest discussions of patient treatment or more often, withdrawal of treatment, use a broader array of the medical, social, and legal facts necessary to make quality decisions. Frequently, health care workers, patients, and families can seek the assistance of ethical experts or committees who have been trained to assist in ethical problem solving. Understanding the appropriate use of these additional resources is important for the new practicing nurse.

In the late 1950s and early 1960s, the United States saw a rapidly unfolding emphasis on individual rights. Beginning with a focus on race, the issue of civil rights soon was applied to other disenfranchised groups, including mental patients, children, and even the "sick." Everyone was called to recognize that individuals deserve respect as human beings. Part of that respect was the right to make their own informed decisions about medical care.

Technological advances resulted in questions we had not yet thought to ask, much less answer, and they required a new dimension to medical decisions. New technologies (eg, organ transplantation and artificial breathing apparatus), the abortion rights movement, and changes in medical research practices forced health care workers to examine traditionally held beliefs and often left them unprepared for the conflicting emotions and thoughts they evoked. Faced with increasing consumer awareness and patients' rights activists, professionals could no longer afford to act on once trusted medical protocols. Instead, they were forced to open discussion of the *right* way to approach patient care.

From these difficulties arose the field now commonly referred to as *bioethics*. So new is this field that the word describing it is not included in dictionaries of the early 1960s. Today's *Webster's Unabridged Dictionary*, however, defines bioethics as "the study of ethical problems arising from advances in science, especially in the fields of biology and medicine." Although there have been many advances, several stand out as having great impact on the emergence of this field, including concerns about medical research and the development of transplant, hemodialysis, and artificial respiration technologies.

MEDICAL RESEARCH

Although medical research may be viewed as essential for continuing success, it has not been without its difficult questions. These issues came to the attention of the public over the course of the late 1960s and early 1970s as questionable research practices were revealed. Three such situations illustrate the key concerns arising in the research arena:

Elderly patients with chronic illnesses were injected with live cancer cells in an effort to discover whether the cells would survive in a person who was ill but did not have cancer. Neither patients or their families were asked for their consent to participate in the study because researchers hypothesized that the cells would not survive and that there was therefore no threat to the patient.

Hepatitis was given by injection to mentally retarded children to find a way to reduce the damage done by the disease. Since hepatitis was endemic in most institutions at this time, it was believed that each subject would eventually contract the disease. Parents did consent to the study, but the issue here was one of coercion because children who were placed in the study were accepted into the institution ahead of a long waiting list.

A group of poor, uneducated black men with syphilis were involved in a study in which, as a control group, they did not receive penicillin, even though the beneficial effects of the drug in the treatment of this condition had been known for many years.

As a result of projects like these, the National Commission for the Protection of Human Subjects was created in 1974. The most notable outcome from this group was the mandate to establish an institutional review board (IRB) in any institution receiving federal funds for research. These boards were to review all biomedical and behavioral research proposals to ensure they met ethical standards and protected the rights of the potential subjects.

TECHNOLOGICAL ADVANCES

Although research practices fueled the fire of the IRBs, technological advances led to the development of "medical-moral" committees in hospitals. It is difficult to pinpoint a particular advance that resulted in the bioethics movement as we know it today. Several key events, however, brought the new conflicts to the forefront.

The ability to transplant hearts, as pioneered by Christiaan Bernard in 1967, forced the development of criteria for brain death. Previously, a patient was pronounced dead when his heart stopped beating and when he stopped breathing. However, physicians had already recognized that the brain might quit functioning before this ultimate cessation of vital functions. The diagnosis of brain death allowed physicians to declare a patient dead while continuing to support these vital functions with the use of a respirator and maintaining critical organ function for transplant.

The development of hemodialysis brought two different dilemmas that are still very much a part of bioethical debates today. Initially, the issues focused on the fact that treatment was not widely available and as such was a scarce resource. Decisions had to be made about who would receive dialysis and whether everyone needing it was entitled to it. The question of allocating this treatment was answered when the Social Security Act was amended to include medical coverage for all end-stage renal disease patients.

However, a new question regarding the right to refuse treatment developed as patients began to experience "being tied to a machine" for the rest of their lives. The ability to restart stopped hearts through the use of cardiopulmonary resuscitation (CPR) and the advanced life support techniques of intubation and drug therapy raised the question of "just because we can, should we?" Over time it became clear that it was becoming increasingly difficult to die in a hospital because almost any life-threatening condition could be prolonged by some technological advance. Decisions that were once left up to fate or God were now becoming decisions of personal choice. Terms like "quality of life" and "right to die" became commonplace on patient units.

The legalization of abortion and the development of in vitro fertilization capabilities raised a set of questions surrounding the beginning of life that could not have been anticipated before the active use of these techniques. Fetal rights issues have grown more complex as technology allows for fetal surgery and experimentation. Parental rights questions are now complicated by the development of surrogate parentage. Although many of the dilemmas raised by these advances continue, they will be replaced as newer technologies are created and social priorities change.

As the field of bioethics continued to grow, the President's Commission for the Study of Ethical Problems in Medicine and Medical and Biobehavioral Research was established in 1978 and began work in 1980. Charged by Congress to study and report on a number of topics, the commission published nine reports in 1984 addressing issues such as the definition of death, informed consent, withdrawal of life support, and allocation of scarce resources. These reports became the foundation for the ethical regulation of the health care industry and are frequently cited in legislation and judicial findings.

ETHICAL THEORY AND PRINCIPLES

Sara A. was on duty the night that Sam was admitted to the intensive care unit. Sam was working the late shift at a doughnut shop when two armed men entered, robbed Sam, and shot him in the head as they left. On arrival in the unit he was on a respirator, comatose, and not expected to live through the night, although he did. Over the next 2 months Sarah cared for Sam and his family, who were devastated by the senselessness of this crime against their son. Last week, Dr. T., the neurologist, met with the family and reviewed the prognosis. Sam was in a persistent vegetative condition from which he would not recover. Having had time to adjust from the initial shock, Sam's family openly discussed the situation with the nurses, social workers, and other family members in the waiting room. Finally they met with Dr. T. and shared with him a discussion they had with Sam while watching television one night. Sam had made it clear that he would never want to be kept alive if he couldn't "be himself." After several gut-wrenching discussions, the family and Dr. T. agreed to remove the respirator. The family wanted to wait until their older son arrived at the bedside, so Dr. T., who was needed to evaluate an emergency room trauma patient, wrote an order for Sarah to disconnect the tube when the son arrived. Although she had great compassion for the family's dilemma, Sarah refused to remove the respirator.

Although Sarah's decision may or may not be the one we would make, what is useful to consider at this point is why Sarah arrived at this decision. We are probably safe to assume that, using whatever cultural, religious, and professional influences that formed her beliefs, Sarah determined that removing the respirator was a *wrong* action. Our processes for arriving at the idea of *right* or *wrong* actions are often invisible to others and sometimes so deeply ingrained we can't even explain them. Sarah's argument for not removing the respirator might have gone something like this: The respirator is keeping Sam alive. Therefore, if I remove the respirator I am killing Sam. I believe it is morally wrong to intentionally kill an innocent human being.

In one of the classic biomedical texts, *Principles of Biomedical Ethics,* Beauchamp and Childress (1983) describe how our ethical reasoning progresses through a thought hierarchy. Sarah's decision not to participate in removing the respirator is "a judgment that expresses a decision, verdict, or conclusion about a particular action." Her statement that killing is wrong can be thought of as an ethical rule, which generally states that actions of a certain kind ought (or ought not) to be done because they are right (or wrong). If pressed further, Sarah might justify this ethical rule by her belief in the sanctity of life, an ethical principle that is more general and fundamental than ethical rules and may support several ethical rules. Finally, the principle, the rule, and the judgment may all be justified by an ethical theory, "a collection of principles and rules that are systematically related" (Beauchamp & Childress, 1983).

There are two principal ethical theories: deontology and teleology. Deontology explains the rightness or wrongness of an action based on the act itself. That is, the act is inherently right or wrong. In deontology, taking a human life is wrong in principle, not because it hurts people or because it makes the living unhappy. It is inherently wrong, intuitively wrong, or wrong because God has forbidden it. Exceptions are not generally granted in deontology. Therefore, if I thought about killing from a purely deontologic view, I would not accept it under any circumstances as a right action.

Teleology determines the goodness of an act based on the consequences of the act. The rightness (or wrongness) of the act will depend on what happens as a result of the act. From a teleological point of view, I may believe, in general, killing is wrong. However, I would be willing to look at the consequences of the killing to determine the true rightness or wrongness of it; killing one to save many may be justified even if the one is innocent. Most of us do not use purely one theory or the other. We may at one time believe strongly in a principle and at another time believe in looking at the consequences of an action.

Understanding our thought processes and the existence of these different ethical theories can be helpful in explaining why the resolution of biomedical issues is often a complex challenge. Conflicts may arise within my own principles; I may value life highly but also adhere to the prevention of suffering. When faced with the dying patient whose suffering is prolonged by tube feedings, I may feel quite confused. Conflicts also arise when multiple decision makers are using different ethical theories to determine what is right for the patient. The nurse who believes in truth telling may feel angry when confronted with a family who want to minimize their loved one's suffering by not revealing the terminal diagnosis.

In their *Handbook for Hospital Ethics Committees*, Ross, Bayley, Michel, and Proctor (1990) point out that moral development must be considered to understand why conflicts occur. Based on the work of Lawrence Kohlberg, who identified six stages of moral development, the authors illustrate an additional potential for misunderstanding. If you asked the same question of someone at each of the six stages, the answer might be the same, but the explanation for the decision would be different. The authors use the example of a terminally ill man in great pain who asks the doctor or nurse for enough barbiturates to commit suicide.

The Stage 1 health care provider might reply, "No, because I could lose my license if anybody found out I had done that." The decision is based on the thought "I will be punished" if I do this act.

The Stage 2 doctor or nurse might answer, "No, because if I became known as a doctor or nurse who did that kind of thing, other doctors and nurses might not refer patients to me." The decision is based on what will come of the action for me in relation to others.

The Stage 3 doctor or nurse could reply, "No, because that's against the law and professionals should obey the law." The decision is based on the idea that others whom I care about (my colleagues in the profession) have taught me that this is what a good person does.

At Stage 4 the reply could be, "No, because if everyone did that, then doctors and nurses would no longer be trusted to save lives." Explanations at this stage demonstrate understanding of our role in society and how decisions further the social order.

At Stage 5 the decision might be "No, even though the patient might suffer less, we need to be faithful to our respect for life because otherwise we might lose our standards and abuse our authority." This justification explains that acts will contribute to social well-being, and that each member of society has an obligation to every other member.

A Stage 6 decision might be explained as "No, because I personally believe that no one has a right to take his or her own life and thus I cannot be a party to such an action." The decision here is justified by appeals to personal conscience and universal ethical principles.

These stages help illustrate why discussions about the right course of action often become frustrating. Individuals approaching problems at different stages can feel as if they are speaking another language. Frequently in these discussions, if someone states the legal facts, it is felt that the problem has been solved. However, this is generally Stage 4 thinking, and clinicians are often well served to reason beyond the legal facts of the issue.

Finally, it is important to remember that ethical decisions and the questions we use to arrive at these decisions may differ depending on the perspective from which we are thinking of the issue. We might ask different questions to determine our action on the issue of surrogate motherhood depending on whether we were considering it on an individual, institutional (eg, hospital), or societal level.

Most dilemmas in health care arise from our presumption that there must be respect for persons. Based on this presumption, there are three ethical principles which encompass most issues: autonomy, beneficence/nonmaleficence, and justice.

AUTONOMY

The word *autonomy* comes from the Greek for "self rule" and is used to describe a person's right to choice and control in relation to him or herself. Autonomy means that the person has all the necessary information to decide on a course of action, which he or she is free to choose. Respecting autonomy requires that I recognize that the individual's choice is based on his or her values and that those values do not have to be shared by me. We must be careful to recognize that not all individuals are in a position to act autonomously, including infants, medically or psychologically compromised individuals, or those society has chosen to restrict, such as prisoners. In health care, autonomy is the principle underlying informed consent, the right to refuse treatment, and the right to appoint a surrogate decision maker (eg, a durable power of attorney).

BENEFICENCE OR NONMALEFICENCE

Although beneficence (doing good) is sometimes distinguished from nonmaleficence (causing no harm), in health care the term *beneficence* is generally used to incorporate both concepts. When taken as the encompassing principle, however, some ethicists propose that beneficence consists of four concepts:

1. Do not cause harm to another.
2. Prevent harm to another.
3. Remove sources of harm to another.
4. Promote good.

According to Frankena (1973), these concepts are listed in rank order; that is, if you must choose between not causing harm or doing good, then one should choose not to cause harm.[4]

JUSTICE

Justice is a broad principle and as such incorporates many ethical rules. In health care, however, we most often find ourselves concerned with distributive justice, that is, deciding how to distribute benefits and burdens. Distributive justice is called into action when there are scarce resources to be allocated among those in need. Principles of distributive justice might include the following (Beauchamp & Childress, 1983):

- To each person an equal share
- To each person according to individual need
- To each person according to individual effort
- To each person according to societal contribution
- To each person according to merit

Questions of justice often arise at both macroscopic and microscopic levels of allocation. *Macroallocation* refers to decisions at a societal level, such as the debate taking place over health care reform. How much of the gross national product should we spend (distribute) on health care? How much should be spent on different populations, diseases, research, and so forth? *Microallocation* refers to decisions of who will receive scarce resources, as described in the earlier history of dialysis treatment.

When working with individual patient care decisions at the clinical level, autonomy is usually considered to be the most important principle. Arguments for the right to privacy and the doctrine of informed consent are frequently played out in the media and are based on the principle of autonomy. As we move from the individual to the institutional or societal level, beneficence and justice may take priority.

Ethical principles frequently come into direct conflict with each other. For example, autonomy conflicts with beneficence, which takes precedence when we decide to hold someone involuntarily because we determine the person to be a danger to him or herself or to others. Beneficence and nonmaleficence are frequently in conflict as new technologies allow us to promote good through the extension of life but result in extreme pain or suffering.

BIOETHICAL LANGUAGE

As with any discipline, bioethics has developed a language of its own. The clinician must be careful in the use of language because ethical conflicts are often highly emotional and volatile. Thoughtful decisions require a clear understanding of the ethical theories and principles at the base of all individuals' decision making. Equally important is the need to be sure everyone is using the same words to mean the same things. Frequently, health care professionals use the many terms associated with neurologic dysfunction as if they were interchangeable. However, terms such as *persistent vegetative state, permanent unconsciousness, brain death,* and *irreversible coma* are not synonymous. The terms *living will, durable power of attorney,* and *natural death act directive* are frequently used interchangeably, although they may have different meanings in different states.

Our use of language may confuse patients or families if we are not careful. If we inform a family that the patient is brain dead and then speak of removing the respirator to allow him or her to die, we are merely adding to the family's difficulty in comprehending brain death. Language such as this may serve to alienate the family or to prevent them from working collaboratively with the health care team as they move forward.

Among the concepts that often give professionals and patients difficulty are euthanasia, suicide, and assisted suicide. *Euthanasia* literally means "good death." The term is usually applied to death that comes early and has been hastened or not prevented. Generally, experts distinguish between active euthanasia (or "mercy killing") and passive euthanasia. *Active euthanasia* refers to a death as the result of an action taken by a person other than the patient with the intention of ending the patient's life. Active euthanasia is still, as of this writing, considered murder. *Suicide* is a direct action on the part of the individual to end his or her life. *Assisted suicide* refers to someone providing the patient with the means to end his or her life and is illegal in most states.

If a nurse intentionally gives a dying patient a lethal dose of morphine, it is active euthanasia. If a nurse cares for the dying patient and adjusts a morphine drip within specified medical guidelines and does not resuscitate the patient when he stops breathing, it is passive euthanasia. If the dying patient collects her pain killers and takes them in one massive dose, it is suicide. If the nurse provided the patient with the medication, but the patient administered it to himself, it is assisted suicide.

Other terms that can cause confusion are *withholding treatment* and *withdrawing treatment.* In the late 1970s and early 1980s, the issue of withholding a treatment versus withdrawing a treatment already started was prominent in hospitals around the country. However, in The President's Commission Report (1983), the term *foregoing treatment* was used to encompass both terms. Since that time, courts have upheld the consensus that there is no appreciable difference between withholding and withdrawing treatment.

The difference between the terms *suicide* and *refusing treatment* is less clear cut than in those terms already discussed. Ethicists and courts have struggled to make clear distinctions, but the line remains hazy. Albert Jonsen (1984) suggests that the patient who refuses treatment acknowledges that there is help available but refuses that help based on the overriding burden of their condition. The person committing suicide, however, takes the position that there is no help available and therefore that there is no choice. The most renowned case in which this distinction was brought to the public's attention was that of Elizabeth Bouvia, a young quadriplegic woman who asked that she be allowed to die in the hospital while refusing food but receiving pain medication. Because there was no imminent threat of death in Ms. Bouvia's condition, much of the discussion in the highly publicized court case centered around the critical issue of suicide and assisted suicide (see discussion later in this chapter).

Other confusing terms include *ordinary treatment* and *extraordinary treatment.* The idea of ordinary versus extraordinary treatment developed in the initial stages of the bioethics movement as patients, clinicians, and courts tried to determine what treatment must be provided. Initially, the terms helped to clarify reasonable actions. It was reasonable and expected that ordinary treatment must always be provided, but extraordinary treatment was optional. These terms became limited in their usefulness as patients, families, and clinicians began to question the appropriateness of what were previously considered ordinary treatments, such as antibiotics and nutrition and hydration. This argument was initially revised to distinguish *proportionate* from *disproportionate treatment,* but these terms also were found to be unclear. Ultimately, the standard of *beneficial* versus *nonbeneficial* or *burdensome treatment* was used to assist in making treatment decisions.

DECISION-MAKING PROCESS

R. J. is a 23-year-old male admitted to ER in acute respiratory distress due to *Pneumocystis* pneumonia. He was intubated and placed on a ventilator. This hospitalization is his third in 6 months as his AIDS has progressed rapidly. Although he was conscious and coherent on admission, his condition rapidly deteriorated and he was no longer able to communicate with the staff. As his prognosis worsened, the physicians alerted his family that there was little hope at this stage of the disease. Although he could not be certain, he felt R. J. would not recover from this acute phase.

Mike, R. J.'s lover, requested a meeting with the care team to express his wishes that R. J. be allowed to die peacefully. He shared with the team his discussions with R. J. on many occasions about his aggressive resuscitation.

R.J.'s parents learned of this discussion and became very angry. They insisted that everything possible be done for their son. When asked what discussions they had had with R. J. regarding his treatment, they admitted they had not specifically discussed his treatment. In fact, R. J. had not been in direct communication with his parents for 3 years before this hospitalization, due to their disapproval of his homosexual life-style. Recognizing the seriousness of R. J.'s condition, Mike had called his parents and asked them to come to the hospital.

Jonathan has cared for R. J. in prior hospitalizations. During previous admissions, R. J. discussed with Jonathan his hope for a peaceful, dignified death. When he mentioned this to R. J.'s parents, they adamantly stated that everything must be done for their son or they would sue the hospital, physicians, and nurses.

As previously discussed, ethical dilemmas arise when there is a conflict between rights, duties, or values, all of which are good in themselves, but not all of which can be satisfied. These dilemmas require that a variety of medical, ethical, legal, and interpersonal factors be considered. In today's team environment, collaborative decision making is preferred to individual or ad hoc approaches. Collaboration, however, often increases the complexity of the issues. To facilitate the best decision making, professionals need a systematic process for addressing the issues.

One such process uses four critical steps (Ross, Bayley, Michel, & Proctor, 1990). Although the steps are outlined sequentially, professionals often find themselves working through one or more steps simultaneously. Clear decision making, however, is best facilitated by a reasoned progression through each of the four steps:

1. Assess the facts.
2. Name the dilemma.
3. Identify an alternative course of action.
4. Implement and follow up the decision.

ASSESS THE FACTS

Although this step may appear obvious, it is generally the most overlooked due to the highly charged, emotional atmosphere surrounding most dilemmas. A thorough examination of facts in key areas will assist the health care team in moving beyond assumptions, myths, and misconceptions.

Assessment should begin with an examination of the patient's medical condition and treatment. Although this area is the most comfortable for the health care team to examine, professionals often have difficulty with this stage. Most problems arise when the time moves quickly from clarifying these medical facts to expressing their values regarding these facts. A skilled facilitator can often help a care team by refocusing them on the objective of this step: clarifying all pertinent facts related to the medical condition.

The following outline will guide you in assessing key factors:

Medical Condition and Treatment
    What is the patient's current condition?
    What is the expected prognosis?
    What treatments are possible?
    What are the benefits/risks of treatment/nontreatment?

Patient Preference
    Is the patient competent to make a decision?
    Does the patient have the information necessary to make an informed decision?
    Has the patient made previous statements regarding his or her preference?
    Has the patient prepared a written statement (advance directive) about his or her preference?
    If patient is incompetent to make a decision, did he or she appoint a surrogate decision maker?

View of Family and Friends
  Who are the family and friends involved with the patient and
    are they informed about the patient's condition?
  What are their positions relative to the dilemma?
  Does anyone have legal custody of this patient, that is, conser-
    vatorship or guardianship?
  Has one person emerged or been identified as the surrogate de-
    cision maker?

View of Care Givers
  Do care givers have all the facts?
  What are their views and on what are these views based (ie,
    their values or patient's wishes)?
  If care givers disagree, what is the disagreement based on?

Legal, Administrative, and External Factors
  Are there state statutes or case law that apply?
  What potential liability may be present for the hospital, provid-
    ers, or family?
  Are there hospital policies or guidelines applicable in this situ-
    ation?
  Are there similar issues reported in the literature that may help
    the decision making?

When providers are uncomfortable with a situation, often the easiest "answer" is to suggest an action is *illegal*. It is crucial that providers spend adequate time seeking clarity about the legal issues. Many providers have misconceptions about the legalities related to ethical issues.

NAME THE DILEMMA

This step focuses on identifying the underlying values in conflict. If the values are not ethical ones related to principles, the dilemma may not be an ethical dilemma. As the team explores the facts, providers often discover that the problem is a communication gap or an adminis-trative uncertainty.

If the values are ethical in nature, the team should focus on finding a spe-cific name for the issue. For example, the issue may be described as "patient autonomy versus doing good for the patient." As principles come into con-flict, providers need to establish priority or precedence of these values. This step, although difficult, is often made easier by the process of naming the di-lemma. As mentioned earlier, patient autonomy is usually given priority. If the competent patient has made a clear statement regarding his or her wishes, the patient's autonomy should be respected. If the patient is not competent but has previously made clear his or her wishes, court precedence generally has supported patient's wishes, although exceptions occur, as in the case of a patient demanding assisted suicide.

IDENTIFY ALTERNATIVE COURSES OF ACTION

As dilemmas arise in a clinical setting, health care providers often focus on one or two courses of action, usually polar opposites. Rarely, though, are there only two alternatives. The essence of this step is spending adequate time considering all possible actions that might be appropriate. Frequently, care teams have used the technique of brainstorming to generate a complete list of options. Once identified, options are then prioritized to determine the most appropriate fit.

IMPLEMENT AND FOLLOW UP

It is tempting to release a sigh of relief when the patient care team reaches agreement on the best course of action. Many good decisions, however, have been compromised by lack of planning regarding how the action will occur. Providers must spend adequate time outlining the implementation steps. On rare occasions, teams have found that their carefully thought through decision does not feel comfortable when they begin implementation planning. It should be clear to all members of the health care team what conclusions have been reached and what action is required. For example, if a decision is reached to remove a patient from a ventilator, implementation planning may address issues such as the following:

Who will discontinue the ventilator?
Will the family be present with the patient?
Will the patient require medication to ease difficulties of breathing?

BIOETHICAL EXPERTISE

As the field of bioethics progressed, hospitals began to see the need for bioethical experts. Medical ethics committees trace their history to the development of dialysis. In the face of scarce resources, Dr.

Belding Scribner and the University of Washington formed a treatment committee. The committee's job was to review the cases of patients who were medically qualified for dialysis and select the one or two people who would receive treatment. In 1976, almost 15 years after the development of Scribner's treatment committees, the New Jersey Supreme Court suggested the use of a hospital ethics committee. In the case of Karen Ann Quinlan, the justices were faced with the question of removing Quinlan's ventilator. In their landmark decision, the court stated that if Quinlan's attending physician determined that there was not a reasonable hope of recovery and "if a hospital ethics committee agreed with the prognosis," then the ventilator support could be withdrawn (70 NJ 10, 1976).

Although these committees examined prognosis more than ethics, the idea of developing ethical expertise to support physicians began to grow slowly in hospitals across the country. In 1983, The President's Commission for the Study of Ethics Problems in Medicine and Biomedical and Biobehavioral Research issued its report, *Deciding To Forego Life Sustaining Treatment.* The report suggested that hospitals themselves should provide effective decision making for incompetent patients.

The development of ethics committees and clinical ethics specialists should not be seen as relieving the direct care providers from critical decision-making accountability. Instead, these committees have three key functions: education, policy development, and case review.

Education. Committees assist providers in understanding issues, remaining current regarding statutory and case law, and developing confidence in the decision-making process. Education is focused on all key audiences including physicians, clinical staff, patients, families, and the community.

Policy Recommendation. Committees develop appropriate policies and guidelines for professionals regarding decisions making in problematic cases. Policies may address allocation of resource issues.

Case Review. Committees assist providers in determining the best decision through both prospective and retrospective review.

LANDMARK CASES AND STATUTES

Although there have been many important court cases over the past 20 years, several have had critical effects in shaping the field of bioethics. Below is a brief summary of a few of these cases. Nurses should take time to understand and familiarize themselves with others that are well detailed in the literature.

FOREGOING TREATMENT: INCOMPETENT PATIENTS

In the Matter of Karen Ann Quinlan, 1976

Quinlan is significant because it was the first case to deal specifically with the question of withdrawing ventilatory support from a permanently unconscious patient. Karen Quinlan was unconscious when she arrived at the hospital. Her physicians believed that there was no probability of her regaining consciousness. Her father asked to be granted guardianship and to be allowed to discontinue ventilatory support because her physician refused to do so.

Physicians testified that under current medical standards, treatment could not be discontinued as long as the patient was not brain dead. The New Jersey Supreme Court decided the decision was not strictly medical and thus did not need to be held only to medical standards. The Quinlans were ultimately named as guardians. The ventilator was removed, and although everyone had expected Quinlan to die, she lived until June of 1985.

Barber v. Superior Court, 1983

In this highly publicized case, doctors Barber and Nedjl were charged with murder and conspiracy to commit murder following the death of a patient under their care. In consultation with the family, Barber and Nedjl discontinued the ventilator from a patient who did not recover consciousness after a postsurgical cardiac arrest. When the patient continued to breath on his own, the family agreed to discontinue intravenous therapy, food, and fluids.

The California Second District Appellate Court dismissed the charges on the grounds that physicians have no duty to provide treatment that is ineffective. The court used a standard of treatment that is proportionate versus disproportionate. Barber was an important case for several reasons:

It involved criminal charges against the providers, which must be acknowledged as a risk.

It established that the state must not always preserve biological life and that family members are appropriate decision makers.

The case evolved to its public and criminal status because of poor communication between physicians and nurses. Physician treatment decisions were not developed collaboratively or adequately explained to nursing staff, resulting in concerns regarding adequacy of care.

In the Matter of Claire Conroy, 1985

The ruling in this case allowed a guardian of Claire Conroy to remove a feeding tube, although Ms. Conroy died prior to the resolution of the case. This ruling was the first Supreme Court (New Jersey) ruling on the withdrawal of artificial feeding from incompetent but conscious patients. The court did, however, establish strict guidelines under which feeding could be discontinued.

In the Matter of Nancy Cruzan, 1990

This case attracted great public attention and was the first to reach the United States Supreme Court. The case was brought forward by the State of Missouri, which claimed its obligation to protect life. Nancy Cruzan's parents sought the right to discontinue feeding their daughter based on her previously expressed wishes. A *New England Journal of Medicine* article (Annas, G.J. et al, 1990) on September 6, 1990, explains the results of the Crugan decision as follows:

1. It affirmed the right of competent patients to refuse treatment.
2. It did not treat the foregoing of artificial nutrition and hydration differently from the foregoing of other forms of treatment.
3. It said the state of Missouri could require continued treatment of a patient in a persistent vegetative state unless there was clear and convincing evidence that she had explicitly authorized the removal of the treatment before the incident.
4. It did not require other states to adopt the Missouri standard of proof.

It is the general feeling that the Crugan case did not alter the laws, ethical standards, or clinical practice permitting the foregoing of life sustaining treatment that have evolved in the United States since the Quinlan case.

FOREGOING TREATMENT: COMPETENT PATIENTS

In *Bouvia v. County of Riverside* (1983), Elizabeth Bouvia, a patient with severely debilitating and painful effects of cerebral palsy, requested the ability to refuse feeding and be kept comfortable in a hospital in California. The hospital announced its intention to force-feed her or transfer her when Ms. Bouvia sought recourse from the courts.

The court did not find in her favor, concluding that she did not have the right to ask the hospital to assist in her suicide. The Bouvia decision demonstrates the court's concern about value judgments, on the part of society or the patient, regarding the worth of a handicapped life. Later, an Appellate Court held that Ms. Bouvia was entitled to refuse the tube feedings. The case was appealed to the Supreme Court, which declined to review it.

INFORMED CONSENT

Cobbs v. Grant, 1972

This case is clearly the driver for all current practices regarding informed consent. In deciding this case involving a patient who did not receive an explanation of the risks of surgery, the California Supreme Court outlined how the issue of informed consent should be handled. The court held that the patient's right to exercise control over his or her body and to make reasonable decisions was primary.

PATIENT SELF DETERMINATION ACT OF 1990

As a result of many of these cases but most specifically the Crugan case, the Patient Self Determination Act was passed in 1990. This act requires hospitals, nursing homes, home health agencies, and others to:

Inform all adults on admission of their right to accept or refuse treatment and to execute an advanced directive (eg, living will or durable power of attorney).
Explain their policies and procedures on implementation of this right and to document the patient's decision in their medical record.
Provide education for their staffs and community on advanced directives.

The act also states that hospitals are not required to discontinue treatment or otherwise discriminate on the basis of whether a patient has executed an advanced directive and they must comply with state laws regarding advanced directives.

JOINT COMMISSION ON ACCREDITATION OF HEALTH CARE ORGANIZATIONS

The Joint Commission's *Accreditation Manual for Hospitals* requires accredited hospitals to have in place mechanisms for the consideration of ethical issues arising in the care of patients. Hospitals must also provide education to care givers and patients on ethical issues in health care. Nurses should familiarize themselves with the available ethical resources to address difficult situations.

SUMMARY

Professional nursing presents a myriad of challenges. As nurses assume the role of care manager, the ability to engage in clear, rational decision-making processes will become a critical competency for success. Even the best among us can find it difficult to reach a decision when the issues are ethical in nature.

As technology continues to challenge the limits of our social standards and as pressure for health care reform continues to result in economic pressures and therefore allocation issues, our ability to reason effectively is seriously tested. Professional nurses must:

Familiarize themselves with basic ethical principles.
Identify clinical situations that might become highly emotional.
Assist the health care team in a logical problem-solving process that establishes value priorities.
Identify all available resources to assist in decision making.
Explore their value sets and recognize the role of those values in the decision-making process.

Ethical dilemmas remain an uncomfortable issue for health care providers. Whenever we are faced with decisions that have no clear *right* answer, our discomfort increases. Our task is to make the *best* possible decision that supports the underlying ethical principles of highest value.

DISCUSSION QUESTIONS

1. What can the nurse do to ensure patient autonomy during hospitalization?

2. How will the health care team make a decision regarding care when the values of the patient, family, nurse, and physician conflict?
3. Should the health care team always follow a recommendation from the hospital attorney that minimizes risk of legal action?

REFERENCES

Annas, G.J. et al. (1990). *Bioethicists' statement on the U.S. Supreme Court's Cruzan decision (occasional notes).* N Engl J Med 323 (10), 686–687.

Beauchamp, T. L., & Childress, J. T. (1983). *Principles of biomedical ethics.* New York: Oxford University Press.

Frankena, W. K. (1973). *Ethics.* Englewood Cliffs, NJ: Prentice-Hall.

Jonsen, A. (1984). Address made at Conference on Emerging Issues in Bioethics. Los Angeles, November 9, 1984.

President's Commission for the Study of Ethical Problems in Medicine and Biomedical and Behavioral Research. (1983). *Deciding to forego life sustaining treatment.* Washington, DC: Library of Congress.

Ross, J. W., Bayley, C., Michel, V., & Proctor, D. (1990). *Handbook for hospital ethics committees.* Chicago: American Hospital Association.

Webster's Unabridged Dictionary. (1983). New York: Simon and Schuster.

SUGGESTED READING

Pence, G. E. (1980). *Ethical options in medicine.* Oradell,: Medical Economics.

Veatch, R. M. (1977). *Case studies in medical ethics.* Cambridge: Harvard University Press.

Winslade, W., & Roth, J. (1986). *Choosing life or death.* New York: Free Press.

Legal Issues

Patricia T. Driscoll

LEARNING OBJECTIVES

This chapter will enable you to:

1. Identify legal issues nurses may encounter in caring for patients and supervising others.
2. Describe specific ways in which nurses can minimize potential liability for malpractice.
3. Discuss the application and implications of Nurse Practice Acts.
4. Recognize the role of law in clinical decision making.
5. Describe the elements of effective documentation.

Vestal, K.W. Nursing Management:
Concepts and Issues, 2 ed.
© 1995 J.B. Lippincott Company

In the cost-conscious, collaborative, and competitive environment of health care, nurses are expected to act quickly and appropriately in confronting varied and complex practice situations. They cannot do so if they lack the knowledge and skill to formulate defensible judgments. The law permeates the practice of nursing. Therefore, knowledge of the legal issues inherent in a given situation is an essential element of the decision-making process. Nurses who have a solid understanding of legal issues can logically and systematically incorporate them to enhance the quality and effectiveness of the services they deliver.

THE LAW

The provision of health services is heavily regulated by law. Nurses often misconstrue the application of legal principles and therefore resent the "intrusion" of law into practice. This is not a defensible position because legal rules, however imperfectly constructed, reflect societal values, which should and must be considered in professional decision making. The dilemma for nurses is to recognize the appropriate relation between law and nursing in everyday practice. To appreciate how law affects professional decision making, it is important to understand what the law is and is not.

Contrary to popular belief, the law is not analogous to the Ten Commandments, written in stone and providing strict rules of conduct. Furthermore, although the legal profession has long been surrounded by a quasi-mystical aura, lawyers are not Moses or "lawgivers" in the sense that they can, with certainty, provide answers to complex practice problems that involve professional, technical, ethical, and legal components.

In a world fraught with uncertainty, most of us cling to the desire that law be simple, immutable, and eternal. Unfortunately, human conduct and human knowledge do not allow it to be that way. The law is sometimes contradictory, often complex, and almost always vague. There are vast gray areas between the black and white.

A simple example: Out of every formalized religion, there comes a simple rule of law—THOU SHALT NOT KILL. Four simple words.

THOU SHALT NOT KILL. It sounds good, it is easy to say, it certainly has morality and goodness in front and behind it. And that is the warning to all of us—simple laws, like simple answers, do not usually work.

THOU SHALT NOT KILL. Except when? Except perhaps when somebody tries to kill me? Yes, we call it "self defense," and it is morally and legally acceptable.

If someone tries to kill a person that I depend on or that depends on me, can I go to their defense and kill to prevent that loss of life? Yes, we call that "defense of others."

Can I kill if I am ordered to by lawful authority, whatever that authority may be? Not only can I, in some instances I must, or I may risk being killed.

Can I kill to defend my property? Yes, because property is essential to life and if you take my property I may not survive.

And can I kill if I think I am in peril of losing my life to an assailant, when in fact I am not in danger but I honestly and reasonably think so? The answer is yes.

We took a simple four-word law and opened it up to all those other words that in turn need interpretation. Beware of the simple, easy phrase that is offered as law, because life is not simple nor would we want it to be. Law is man-made and reflects the ever-changing needs and expectations of a given society. Therefore, it is dynamic and fluid. Law, like health care and nursing, is not an exact science but rather an ongoing, organized system of change in response to current conditions and public expectations.

SOURCES OF LAW

The laws applicable to the issues surrounding the delivery of nursing services stem from many different sources, including the United States Constitution, the constitutions of individual states, statutes, administrative regulations, various local laws and ordinances, and federal and state court decisions. Although most people understand that statutes and constitutions are laws, it is not always clear that regulations are also law for those who are subject to them. All regulations emanate from a statute providing authority to an agency or official to give detail and substance to the law. An example is the State Board of Nurse Examiners, which is empowered by the Nurse Practice Act to regulate the practice of professional nursing in each state.

Another form of law that is often confusing is common law, which is based on judicial opinions. Judicial opinions can be described as interpretations of laws and as laws in and of themselves. However, before we play the popular game of "Have you heard about the case" and grant a case or judicial opinion the force and effect of law, it is important to understand the doctrine of *precedent* or *stare decisis*. This doctrine, which literally means to "let the decision stand," is applied in cases with similar fact situations to those previously decided. The court looks at the current dispute and applies the same rules and principles used in the previous case. This doctrine has significance for nurses because it provides insight into ways in which the court has previously fixed liability in given situations.

Precedent is binding, or law, *only* in courts of lower jurisdiction within the same jurisdiction. In other words, a case decided in California is not binding in Texas. A case decided by a state district court in one city has no binding effect in another city in the same state. Judicial decisions in other jurisdictions (states) may be of interest for their predictive value, but they should not be interpreted as law in our jurisdiction.

All laws, regardless of origin, are not static. Constitutions can be amended. Statutes may be repealed, amended, or expanded. Administrative bodies can be dissolved, expanded, or redefined. Judicial decisions may be modified or overturned. At its most basic level, law is an expression of public policy. It is the way society views a given matter at a particular time. Consequently, it is subject to human foibles and must be evaluated in that context.

Law provides merely one component of the nurse's professional decision-making process. Professional, technical, moral, and ethical factors must also be weighed. Law should never be used to shorthand or circumvent the need for sound professional decision making. To act contrary to professional judgment on the mistaken belief that "the law made me do it" is never an appropriate interpretation of the law.

PROFESSIONAL LIABILITY—MALPRACTICE

The most common exposure to potential liability for nurses is in the area of negligence or malpractice. Nurses and the public frequently interchange the terms *malpractice* and *negligence.* Although the distinction is technical, there is a difference. *Negligence* is a general term that denotes conduct lacking in due care. Anyone can be liable for negligence. *Malpractice* is a more specific term and looks at the professional status of the care giver and the professional standards of care. Malpractice is the failure of a professional person (eg, physician, nurse, or lawyer) to act in accordance with the prevailing professional standards or failure to foresee consequences that a professional person, having the necessary skills and education, should foresee. To be successful in a malpractice cause of action, the injured party (or plaintiff) must prove the following:

1. Duty owed to the patient (eg, a nurse–patient relationship exists that gives rise to the duty to perform according to the standard of care).

2. Breach of the duty owed to the patient (ie, failure to conform to the standard of care as established by expert testimony, learned treatises, and institutional policies and procedures).
3. Injury (ie, the patient must suffer compensable injury or damage as a result of the breach; pain and suffering or emotional distress are considered compensable injury only if they accompany a physical injury).
4. Proximate cause (ie, the injury must have been incurred directly because of the breach of duty owed to the patient).

The plaintiff has the burden of proving each and every one of the four elements. Therefore, if the patient expired while in the hospital (injury and duty) and no nursing documentation was present on the chart (breach), the plaintiff must prove that the lack of documentation actually caused the patient to die.

Even if all the required elements of a cause of action for malpractice are present, that does not necessarily mean that a lawsuit will be filed. The fifth element of the cause of action is a *willing plaintiff,* that is, someone willing to invest the time and financial and emotional expense involved in a lawsuit. Whether or not an injured party becomes a willing plaintiff is usually related to the strength of the professional–patient relationship and the patient (family) expectation. As a rule, patients and their families lack the technical sophistication to recognize whether a bad outcome is an unavoidable complication or an iatrogenic injury. Lacking this knowledge, care is judged on the basis of two criteria: (1) Was the outcome consistent with the perceived seriousness of the original condition? (2) Was the care delivered in a professional manner (ie, did the nurse appear competent, and was the nurse responsive to the patient's needs)?

This realization has enormous implications for practice. No matter how diligent, we are all subject to the possibility of making a mistake, so we cannot always prevent malpractice. What we can do is be sensitive to the quality of the professional relationship we have with patients and their significant others. It is important to keep families involved and informed of the various facets of treatment and prognosis to reduce the likelihood of a lawsuit. If the patient dies, the family becomes the potential plaintiff. Remember, it is people who sue, not the action or event that triggered a bad outcome.

NURSING PRACTICE LITIGATION

It is a common misconception that most lawsuits against nurses arise from the highly technical, sophisticated aspects of care. In reality,

---

DISPLAY 19-1. GUIDELINES FOR AVOIDING MALPRACTICE

1. "Love thy patient as thyself." Treat patients and their families with respect and honesty. Communicate in a truthful, open, and professional manner.
2. Use nursing knowledge to make appropriate nursing diagnoses and to implement necessary nursing interventions. Nurses have an affirmative duty to make correct assessments and to take the actions required to implement those assessments.
3. The primary duty is to the patient. If the physician is hesitant to order necessary therapy or to respond to a change in the patient's condition, call your supervisor or follow hospital procedure to contact another physician.
4. Question physician orders if they (1) are ambiguous or unclear, (2) are questioned or refused by the patient, and (3) are inappropriate, such as when a major change occurs in the patient's status and orders remain unchanged. Do not provide secretarial services for physicians; that is, don't take verbal orders when the physician is present and capable of writing the order.
5. Remain current and up-to-date in your skills and education. Keep abreast of new developments in the field in which you practice and be familiar with published guidelines for care and treatment of patients.
6. Refuse or seek help to perform skills or procedures with which you are unfamiliar.
7. Base nursing care on the nursing process model; this reduces the likelihood of inadvertently overlooking vital parts of required care for a given patient.
8. Document the nursing care plan and the patient's responses to interventions. Express yourself clearly and completely. Record entries as soon as possible while the facts and observations are clear in your mind.
9. Readily seek consultation with colleagues. Be familiar with your organization's policies and procedures, and help to update those that do not reflect current practice. Ensure that those personnel whom you supervise are aware of policy and procedure.
10. Delegate patient care wisely, and know the scope of practice for yourself and those whom you supervise. Never accept or allow others to accept more responsibility than can be handled.

---

errors in basic care are usually at the root of malpractice lawsuits. Many of these errors occur when a nurse is tired or distracted by personal concerns. Areas of potential risk can be classified in various ways. Caffee (1991) suggests using the categories of assessment errors, planning errors, and intervention errors.

Assessment errors include such things as failing to adequately gather and chart information about the patient, or failing to recognize the significance of information such as laboratory values, intake and output measures, vital signs, or patient complaints that require immediate action. To avoid these assessment errors, a comprehensive baseline initial assessment is essential.

Planning errors include (1) failing to record patient problems and neglecting to address them in the plan of care, (2) failing to communicate effectively (eg, using language in the plan of care that other nurses cannot understand), (3) failing to provide continuity of care because of poor communication or the lack of a plan of care, and (4) failing to give discharge instructions that the patient understands. To avoid these errors, do not underestimate the value of a plan of care that is well thought out. If it is well written, it will provide a clear approach to the patient's problems. Modify the plan as new assessment data is gathered. The plan should be realistic, based on prevailing standards, and include patient input. Communicate clearly, both orally and in writing. Follow the plan through with careful discharge instructions that include the family. Don't take anything for granted; validate your assumptions.

Intervention errors include failing to interpret and carry out physician orders, failing to perform nursing tasks correctly, failing to pursue the doctor if you do not get a response to telephone calls, or failing to notify your supervisor if the doctor is unavailable. Classic intervention errors involve basic nursing tasks such as reading written orders, identifying a patient before performing a procedure, administering medications, and applying restraints. The most common and therefore most dangerous area seems to be the administration of medications. Breakdown of communication (eg, sloppy writing or lack of charting) often leads to errors. Don't guess if you have a question about medications. Continuing education can help reduce intervention errors.

DOCUMENTATION

Complex medical problems, along with the multiplicity of personnel involved in the care of patients in today's health care organizations, demand accurate, effective, and up-to-the minute medical record keeping that coordinates and communicates patient care activities. Unfortunately, the focus on the medical record as a legal document has reduced its legal and medical effectiveness. Nurses and other health care professionals, repeatedly told that the best defense to allegations of malpractice is a good medical record, often forget that the record is valuable only to the extent that it documents the actual rendering of good care. A poor record may prevent providers from establishing the good care that was given to the patient, but a good record is not a substitute for good care. The misunderstanding of the purpose of the medical record as simply a legal tool has led to the inclusion of so much data in the record that it is often impossible to retrieve necessary information in a timely manner.

The primary purposes of the medical record are to ensure continuity of care, to provide relevant information about the patient's condition, and to serve as a tool to evaluate and bill for the care rendered. The record should be structured to accomplish these objectives. If this is done, it will automatically provide legal protection. Any method of charting that facilitates the comprehensive and factual documentation of patient care is appropriate. Simple narrative charting does not usually meet the communication needs of the complex hospital patient and should not be retained if outmoded. Long narrative paragraphs should be used infrequently and only in exceptional circumstances. Grafts, logs, checklists, flow sheets, and other methods of abbreviated communication are appropriate and in fact facilitate the transmission and understanding of relevant data.

It is important that these documentation aids be used consistently and in such a way that a reviewer (court or attorney) can ascertain that proper consideration was given to the elements of care listed or contained on the form. A simple slash or N/A reinforces that an item was dealt with and not simply overlooked. Avoid duplication of this information elsewhere on the chart. It is unnecessary, negates the need for the form, and, if not done consistently, may give rise to an inference that the abbreviated form is unreliable.

The entries in the medical record must be legible, complete, and accurate. A record that cannot be interpreted because of illegible entries, abbreviations that have no standard means of interpretation, gross misspelling, incomprehensible grammar, or obvious lapses of time casts doubt not only on the record but on the credibility of those providing the care. All entries should be relevant, concise, objective, and factual. Statements such as "patient's condition deteriorating" or "patient uncooperative" or "resting comfortably" provide no relevant information. Qualifiers such as "appears to be" and "seems" should be avoided.

The record should represent the actual care the patient received. No attempt should be made to obscure information from the record. The filing of an incident report, which should never become a part of the chart, does not preclude the need to document the facts relative to the patient's diagnosis, care, and treatment in the medical record.

CONFIDENTIALITY

The right of privacy encompasses two separate and distinct concepts: (1) the constitutional right of personal privacy, and (2) the common law or statutory right of informational privacy. The constitutional right of personal privacy protects the individual's interest in autonomy and self-determination. Issues such as the right to choose in private matters, the right to refuse treatment, and the right to terminate life-prolonging treatment arise from this doctrine.

Informational privacy is directly related to the concept of confidentiality. Informational privacy addresses the person's "right to be left alone," that is, to be free from unwarranted publicity and unwanted disclosure of information (*Olmstead v. U. S., 1972*). When individuals are admitted to a hospital or otherwise access the health care system, they retain their right of privacy. The intimate and sensitive nature of health care requires that patients disclose personal, financial, and medical information about themselves. Once the information is revealed, the patient is exposed, vulnerable, and dependent on the health care providers to use the information judiciously and effectively.

The law supports the legitimate expectation that the information that is obtained through this process will be kept confidential. Therefore, nurses have a responsibility to ensure that case discussion, consultation, examination, and treatment are confidential and conducted discreetly. Those not involved in the care of the patient should have the patient's permission to be present. All communications and records pertaining to the patient are confidential (American Hospital Association, 1972).

Although the hospital owns the medical record, that ownership is subject to the patient's interest in the information in it. As discussed previously, the medical record and its contents are considered confidential. Therefore, release of information that has not been authorized by the patient (or parent or legal guardian) or is not made pursuant to statutory, regulatory, or other legal authority constitutes a violation of the patient's right to privacy and can give rise to liability.

The rise of consumer rights activism and increasing concern over possible compilation of expansive dossiers made possible by computer technology without the knowledge or consent of the individual concerned have prompted increased judicial and legislative activity in this area. The concern for protection of privacy relating to treatment for substance abuse and AIDS also has had an impact. It is important to be aware of relevant federal and state statutes and regulations that create a positive duty not to disclose information except as specified.

The practical dilemma of how to preserve the confidentiality of patients presents a major challenge. Even with reasonable diligence, it is difficult to ensure that inappropriate disclosure of information does not occur. Nurses should be sensitive to the fact that the less confidential information that is recorded in the chart, the fewer the opportunities for unintentional or harmful disclosure. Nurses tend to record far more detailed information than is needed for either documentation or the provision of care. Only relevant and necessary data should be recorded, and only to the degree necessary for therapeutic and communication purposes.

This caution may appear to contradict previous admonitions to ensure that charting is "complete." That is not the intent. Nurses should be cognizant that the medical record is a permanent document that often is reposited outside the control of either the patient or provider. The patient's interest in having privacy maintained can best be ensured by careful discrimination on the part of health care providers in determining what is written and the manner in which it is stated.

NURSING PRACTICE REGULATION

The practice of nursing is regulated in all states by statutes referred to as *Nurse Practice Acts.* Nurse practice acts are intended to protect the public at large from unsafe practitioners; they accomplish this objective by defining the practice of nursing, developing criteria for admission into the profession, and enacting rules and regulations that implement, maintain, and enforce the standards of nursing practice. Because the "police power" or authority to legislate for the public safety and welfare is a state right, every state has enacted its own nurse practice act and its own definition of nursing. Consequently, there is no nationally recognized legal definition of nursing practice, and the scope of practice that the law regulates can vary from state to state. Perhaps this accounts for the diversity and confusion surrounding nursing education and the scope of nursing practice.

The board of nursing is the state agency responsible for interpreting and enforcing the nurse practice act in most states. As a state administrative agency, it generally has both legislative and adjudicatory power. That means that the board has the authority to develop rules and regulations that govern nursing licensure and practice and to hear and decide cases involving violations of the standards, rules, and regulations contained in the nurse practice act.

In conjunction with the adjudicatory power, the board can enforce licensure requirements through disciplinary actions. Most acts provide the board with the authority to impose a range of disciplinary actions, depending on the gravity of the violation, including (1) private reprimand or warning, (2) public reprimand, (3) stipulations or practice restrictions, (4) probation, (5) suspension, (6) refusal to renew license, and (7) revocation of license.

A nurse who is charged with violating the nurse practice act is entitled to due process rights, including the right to adequate notice of the alleged misconduct, an opportunity for a full and fair hearing on the issues, and the right to appeal the decision before sanctions are imposed.

Most nurse practice acts enumerate grounds for discipline that may in turn be expanded by the board through regulation. According to Northrop (1987), the most common categories are:

1. Fraud or deceit.
2. Unfitness, incompetence, and malpractice.
3. Substance abuse.
4. Mental incompetence.
5. License revocation in another state.
6. Violation of the provisions of the act.
7. Unprofessional conduct.

The unprofessional conduct category is broad and gives the board latitude to address a wide range of behaviors. Because of the concern for notice under due process and the differing interpretations of courts, many boards are further defining unprofessional conduct in their rules and regulations. The clarification usually consists of a list of behaviors deemed unacceptable and is preceded by a warning that unprofessional conduct includes, but is not limited to, the acts indicated.

Most conduct that gives rise to an allegation of malpractice (ie, failure to practice at acceptable standards) would also be grounds for disciplinary action. In the regulatory context, however, all four elements of malpractice need not be present. The board could impose sanctions whether or not the breach caused injury. An example would be a medication error or series of medication errors that caused no injury to the patient involved. In that case, the patient who received the wrong medication but suffered no ill effects could not recover for malpractice against the nurse. However, to protect future patients from harm, the board could discipline the nurse. It is essential for nurses to acquire current and accurate knowledge about the state nurse practice act and the rules, regulations, and standards promulgated by the board.

Most nurse practice acts contain provisions that require reporting of violations of the act. Knowing how and when to report a coworker is difficult. The concern may involve unprofessional conduct, extended scope of practice, substance abuse, or some other conduct. It may be easier to "look the other way." Reporting mechanisms are available through the organizational structure (chain of command) in most health care institutions. Alternatively, reports can be made directly to the board. Although this process seems straightforward, the following scenario emphasizes the potential dilemma for nurses:

> One of your best friends, Nancy K., RN works at another hospital in town. You have known each other since college, where you both majored in nursing. You see each other frequently at social events and professional meetings. Recently you have noticed that Nancy seems to be drinking more than you would consider appropriate at social functions. In fact, on one occasion when you told her she was too drunk to drive, Nancy confided to you that she needs to drink to face her problems and has started to use cocaine as well. Will you report Nancy to the board of nursing? Would you report her to her employer? Would your decision or concerns be different if Nancy was a colleague at your hospital? Would you report Nancy if she were not working in a hospital but did chart review for a lawyer?

THE NURSE AS EMPLOYEE

DOCTRINE OF PERSONAL LIABILITY

Nurses rarely function in isolation; they usually work as part of a team. Nevertheless, the doctrine of personal liability makes each individual responsible for his or her own actions. The law will not allow a person to avoid legal liability merely because a third party or entity also has responsibility. For example, if the nurse carries out an inappropriate doctor's order, the nurse is answerable for the results of that conduct, even though the physician is also liable for his or her order.

On the other hand, the mere fact that another member of the team is liable does not mean that liability is conveyed to others because of the relationship. For example, as a team leader you assign a staff member to care for an uncomplicated patient. The staff member delivers care in a negligent manner and causes harm to the patient. As team leader you would not be liable, even though you assigned the patient's care to the negligent staff member. As a team leader you have a right to expect that staff are capable of performing functions within their area of expertise. The situation changes, however, if the staff member expressed to you at the time of the assignment a lack of knowledge or competence necessary to perform the assignment. In that case, you can incur liability for negligently performing supervisory responsibilities. The staff member would not be excused and would also incur liability.

RESPONDEAT SUPERIOR

Respondeat superior, meaning "let the master respond," is a form of substitute or vicarious liability based on the employer–employee relationship. The effect of the doctrine is that the hospital (employer) is responsible for the negligent acts of its employees if they are acting within the scope of their employment. The rationale for this approach is one of allocation of risk. Employers are able to select, control, and direct the actions of their employees and benefit from their labor; they are also in a better position to sustain a loss than an employee or injured plaintiff. In essence, it is a method of shifting costs to the public or community at large.

A nurse functioning in a supervisory capacity is an employee of the hospital and not the employer. Therefore, a nursing supervisor may be liable if there is a negligent act by an employee, but that supervisor's liability could be incurred only because of a failure to perform supervisory duties in a competent manner, *not* because of the supervisory relationship or the doctrine of respondeat superior. Broad statements such as "the charge nurse is responsible for all the patients on the unit" or "the head nurse is responsible for the unit 7 days a week, 24 hours a day" are often seen in nursing literature and hospital policies and have led to a misunderstanding of the legal responsibilities.

STAFFING ISSUES

Liability issues related to short staffing involve a number of legal principles. First, the doctrine of personal accountability specifies that every employee is responsible and accountable for his or her own actions. This principle must then be viewed within the context of the hospital's liability under respondeat superior and the doctrine of corporate liability (the hospital is responsible for its own acts).

In general, accountability follows control, and the staff nurse clearly is not in a position to resolve short-staffing problems. Therefore, Politis (1988) suggests that nursing accountability should not extend beyond the scope of nursing decisions within the framework of the nurse–hospital relationship.

In two cases dealing with short staffing, the courts focused on the reasonableness of the nurse's actions or professional judgment and reached opposite results. In one case, the nurses were found not liable because they acted reasonably under the circumstances (*HCA Health Services of Midwest Inc. v. National Bank of Commerce,* 1988). In the other case, the nurses were found liable based on inappropriate professional judgments (*Horton v. Niagara Falls Memorial Medical Center,* 1976). The exercise of reasonable professional judgment, the establishment of priorities, and the communication of problems to the nursing supervisor will place the staff nurse in a defensible position in any claim involving short staffing.

"Floating" to patient care settings to which the nurse is not primarily assigned can also cause consternation. Unless the nurse has a contract that specifies work only in agreed areas, there is no legal protection for refusing to cover another nursing unit that is understaffed. Most hospitals are within their legal right to suspend or terminate the nurse who refuses to float. Guido (1988) offers the following guidelines for nurses temporarily assigned to another unit:

1. Before accepting a patient assignment, communicate any hesitancy that you might have about it to appropriate persons (direct supervisor, charge nurse, or team leader). Make your objections clear and specific. Suggest actions for making you feel more comfortable in the reassignment, such as attending an orientation period of learning about nursing routines.
2. State your qualifications and skills concerning assessment, performance of routine procedures, and so forth to the appropriate charge person. Thoroughly understand the patient assignment before accepting it; once accepted you are legally accountable for the nursing care and cannot simply walk away from the patients before the end of the shift.
3. Identify your immediate resource person, and ask any questions you might have about the assignment, routine procedures, and so forth.
4. Recognize and give yourself credit for your strengths while remaining aware of your weaknesses. Ask for help when truly needed.
5. Remember that much of the case law concerning float nurses involves the broad area of medications. Double check references, call the pharmacist, or contact your direct supervisor before administering any medication about which you are unsure. If there are numerous unfamiliar medications to be given to several patients, try to arrange a trade-off to perform more routine procedures while another nurse who is familiar with the unit administers all medications (Guido, 1988).

PROFESSIONAL LIABILITY INSURANCE

In today's medical–legal climate, it is surprising that a debate exists concerning whether nurses should carry their own professional liability insurance. Although well-meaning hospital administrative staff and some lawyers may assure nurses that they can depend on their employer's insurance coverage, the truth is that if they do so, they will not be adequately protected. Institutional liability policies have limited coverage and cover employees only while they are performing as employees.

For example, suppose a nurse is in the hospital solely to visit a hospitalized coworker. During the visit, the nurse assists the other patient in the room to the bathroom. The nurse slips and falls on top of the patient, causing serious injury. If that patient sued, it is possible that the institutional insurance carrier could argue that the nurse is not covered because she or he was not "performing as an employee."

Further, the hospital's insurance policy is designed to protect the interests of the institution. If these interests conflict with those of the individual nurse, the needs of the hospital will prevail. For example, the hospital may elect to settle a case rather than contest liability. This may not be in the nurse's best interest, particularly if disciplinary proceedings are pending, and the nurse will be left with the expense of preparing and defending her actions in that forum. Also, should the hospital decide to bring a claim against the nurse for the incident that triggered the lawsuit, the hospital policy will not provide coverage nor will it pay for representation.

Finally, the current economic environment coupled with the fact the many hospitals are self insured (at least to a certain point) make claims for indemnification by employers against nurses more likely whether or not the nurse has personal liability coverage. The frequently heard argument that nurses are more likely to be named as defendants in a lawsuit if they have insurance is not persuasive. Nurses are named in lawsuits to ensure their attendance and participation and to provide a conduit for the employer's liability coverage through respondeat superior. When the injured party originally files suit, existence of insurance is not known. Therefore, nurses are advised to carry their own liability insurance.

Guido (1988) provides the following guidelines regarding professional liability insurance:

1. Read the policy carefully before purchasing it and ask for explanations as needed. Make sure the policy will augment a basic employer policy.
2. Make sure that the dollar coverage for both claims and aggregate coverage is adequate for your specific nursing needs. This will depend on the litigation climate in your geographic area.
3. Check information that relates to malpractice claims in your area. Resources include the local law library, insurance carriers, health claims arbitration boards, and hospital attorneys.

4. Make sure that the policy gives you optimal coverage. It should be occurrence-based coverage and ideally will include protection for both your direct professional actions as well as your involvement with those you supervise.
5. Understand the exclusions of the policy. Will you still be covered if you float to a different area in the hospital? If the exclusions also include your job description, negotiate for a rider to supplement the basic policy.
6. Above all, remember that you are a member of a profession with the potential to have lawsuits filed against its members. Don't go without the protection provided by liability insurance.

SUMMARY

The practice of professional nursing is complex and challenging. Unfortunately, nurses often view the legal implications of practice with fear and misunderstanding. Although the legal issues confronting practicing nurses today are many, the nurse should view the law as a helpful adjunct to defining nursing practice and arriving at appropriate decisions. To do this, the nurse must be aware of the relation between law and the other aspects of professional decision making. An awareness of legal rights and responsibilities is essential. To limit potential liability, the nurse must be cognizant of relevant legal doctrines and prevailing professional standards and incorporate this knowledge and sound professional judgment into everyday practice.

DISCUSSION QUESTIONS

1. How do the legal aspects of delivering nursing care affect the routine performance of a nurse?
2. What steps can the nurse take to ensure adequate documentation of care?
3. Discuss legal issues of delegating care to others.
4. Describe the major elements of your state's Nurse Practice Act.

REFERENCES

American Hospital Association. (1972). *Patients' bill of rights*. Chicago: Author.

Caffee, B. E. (1991). Protecting yourself. *Nursing 91*, 34–39.

Guido, G. W. (1988). *Legal issues in nursing*. San Mateo, CA: Appleton & Lange.

HCA Health Services of Midwest Inc. v. National Bank of Commerce, 745 SW2d 120 (Ark. 1988).

Horton v. Niagara Falls Memorial Medical Center, 380 NY S. 2d 116 (NY, 1976).

Northrop, C. E., & Kelly, M. E. (1987). *Legal issues in nursing.* St. Louis: CV Mosby.

Olmstead v U. S., 277 U. S. 438, 478 (1972).

Politis, E. K. (1988). Nurses' legal dilemma: When hospital staffing compromises professional standards. *University of San Francisco Law Review, 18,* 110.

SUGGESTED READING

Bergerson, S. (1988). More about charting with a jury in mind. *Nursing 88, 18*(4), 50–56.

Caffee, B. (1991). *Staying out of court: A self-assessment guide for nurses.* Beachwood, OH: Author.

Clark, A. P., & Garry, M. B. (1991). Legal implications of standards of care. *Dimensions of Critical Care Nursing 10*(2), 96–102.

Cournoyer, C. P. (1989). *The nurse manager and the law.* Rockville, MD: Aspen.

Feutz, S. (1989). *Nursing and the law* (3rd ed.). Eau Claire, WI: Professional Education Systems.

Fiesta, J. (1988). *The law and liability: A guide for nurses* (2nd ed). New York: John Wiley & Sons.

Labor Relations Issues

Diane M. McDonald

LEARNING OBJECTIVES

This chapter will enable you to:

1. Distinguish between the characteristics of a union and nonunion environment.
2. Describe the evolution of the labor movement in nursing.
3. List the steps in the collective bargaining process.
4. Understand the negotiation process.

Vestal, K.W. Nursing Management:
Concepts and Issues, 2 ed.
© 1995 J.B. Lippincott Company

Labor relations, the relationship between management and employees within the work environment, includes communication, remuneration, job security protocols, and other conditions of employment. This relationship depends on the extent to which labor and management can agree on the conditions necessary for meeting each other's general employment requirements.

The goals of management reflect the desire to produce a profitable product or service through the efforts of employed workers. Labor desires safe working conditions, reasonable tangible and intangible remuneration, job security, and opportunities for growth and advancement.

The most desirable circumstance is for labor and management to communicate, interact, and problem solve to achieve mutual agreement. When this is impossible, our democratic society acknowledges and provides for the employees' right to organize and bargain collectively with management directly or through a representative. The power of an organized collective group is inherently stronger than the singular actions of an individual when dealing with unacceptable employee working conditions. In fact, management that is not competent, responsive, and economically strong is usually a weak match for organized employees. Conversely, a union will never be successful in an organization where management is strong, understands the employees, communicates effectively, and provides for the responsible fulfillment of employee needs and wants.

In the health care industry and particularly in professional nursing, unions have had an interesting and recent evolution. The unionization process (collective bargaining) is inherently complex because a wide range of appropriate and inappropriate behaviors is specified by law. Further, the unionization process is highly charged emotionally because collective bargaining issues always relate to one's work environment and personal security.

Individual considerations are compounded in health care by global concerns about the care giving process, the essential dependence of the client on the care giver, society's view of health care as a right, the obligation of the care giver to intervene appropriately, and the moral and ethical ramifications of unionization and collective bargaining activities. Each staff nurse must make judgments and decisions about participation in collective bargaining based on a knowledge of the process and careful consideration of the circumstances of each situation.

338

OUR LABOR RELATIONS HERITAGE

The American labor movement began in the nineteenth century. Extremely poor working conditions existed for those who were uneducated and helpless against the power of state and economic capital. Craftsmen's guilds were the earliest form of unions but experienced limited success, although they still exist today. Industrial unions did not become a practical, powerful reality until long after the rise of factory systems and the development of mass production (Beal & Begin, 1982). Nevertheless, the size and success of unions have fluctuated with economic conditions and the World Wars.

The history of unionization in nursing is fairly recent and is rooted in the early working conditions for nurses in America. Before 1930, student nurses provided most of the nursing care for patients in the hospital. "Graduate nurses" practiced independently as private duty nurses in homes, community agencies, and other health care organizations. The depression of 1929 brought a reduction in personal health expenditures including the hiring of private duty nurses. Coupled with the decline in nursing school enrollment during this period, hospitals found it economically feasible to hire "graduate nurses" for little more than room and board. Thus, hospitals became the primary workplace for nurses (Bullough, 1971).

Hospital employees were permitted to engage in collective bargaining under the National Labor Relations Act (Wagner Act) of 1935. Two years later, the American Nurses Association (ANA) drafted its charter, which included provisions for improving "every phase of [nurses'] working and professional lives" (Pointer, 1972). However, it was not until 1946 that the ANA officially initiated its Economic Security Program (Berneys, 1946). The ANA received a mandate from its membership to act as the bargaining agent for nurses to improve the economic conditions and status of the profession. Thus, in 1946, the ANA began its first collective bargaining programs for nurses (Ballman, 1985).

The "Brown Report" titled *Nursing for the Future* was published in 1948 and described the working conditions at that time (Alexander, 1978). Essentially, staff nurses had little freedom in making clinical nursing judgments and had no participation in solving the simplest of problems. The environment was highly authoritarian and unrewarding.

The Department of Labor's Survey of the Economic Status of Nurses (1946–1947) found that nurses worked longer hours, did more shift work, and received less pay and fringe benefits than most workers in industry or in comparable occupations. The average annual salary was

$2100, well below the level of female industrial workers, teachers, secretaries, and social workers.

Despite the apparent need to improve working conditions and concomitant rewards for nurses, wide-scale attempts at collective bargaining were complicated by the Labor-Management Act of 1947 (Taft-Hartley Act), which excluded nonprofit hospitals from its jurisdiction and protection. During congressional debate on exclusion of nonprofit hospitals from the protection of the act, Senator Taylor of Idaho expressed concern that the amendment would bar nurses from organizing:

> I have in mind that nursing is one of the most poorly paid professions in America . . . it is perhaps the poorest paid, in proportion to the service rendered to humanity. I do not want to place the nursing profession under any handicap in their efforts to obtain an improved standard of living.

The senator withdrew his objection when he was assured by legislative colleagues that the amendment ". . . will [not] affect them in the slightest way . . . they can still walk out" (Gershenfeld, 1970).

Finally, during the 1960s, the collective voices of professional nurses began to ring out. Federal and state employees were protected in collective bargaining by several statutes, including President John F. Kennedy's Executive Order No. 10988 of 1960. Nurses participated in demonstrations, picketing, sit-ins, call-ins, and slow-downs. Typical of the era was Cook County Hospital in Chicago, which lacked basic resources such as toilet paper and suction machines in addition to having inadequate staffing ratios. The nurses' attempts to make known the seriousness of these problems were futile. They therefore resorted to stronger tactics and initiated a unionization drive. The nurses emphatically stated that their main goal was the improvement of nursing care through improved working conditions and increased salaries (Mauksch, 1971).

In 1974, Congress amended the National Labor Relations Act to include nonprofit hospitals and other health care institutions (Zimmerman & King, 1990). The Taft-Hartley Amendments of 1974 extended the legal protection of nurses for collective bargaining to 2 million employees in 3300 nonprofit hospitals (Stickler, 1990). These amendments were eagerly supported by unions because of the decline in union membership in the traditional manufacturing industries. The Service Employees International Union (SEIU), for example, designated the 1980s as the decade in which every nonunion health care worker would be the focus of an organizing drive (Rectz & Rectz, 1984). In keeping with this overall strategy, union attempts to organize hospital employees steadily increased from 1974 to 1980. However, health care unionization activities reached a zenith in 1980 and have been declining since (Stickler, 1990). The reason for the decline can be found in the 1974 Taft-Hartley Amendments and the National Labor Relations Board (NLRB) activities under these amendments.

Although the Taft-Hartley Amendments opened the possibility for many nurses to bargain collectively, they left the NLRB with the responsibility to determine what was an appropriate bargaining unit in size and composition. All NLRB decisions are subject to review by the 12 federal Circuit Courts of Appeal. In early decisions under the 1974 amendments, the NLRB found for a separate bargaining unit for registered nurses. Over time, however, the Courts of Appeal began rejecting the Board's approval of RN-only units. The conflict over an appropriate unit for nurses continued for 15 years (Zimmerman & King, 1990). Labor activity gradually declined as the NLRB issued conflicting decisions about what constitutes an appropriate bargaining unit. The decisions divided health care employees into smaller, more fragmented groups, but such decisions were quickly overturned by a Circuit Court of Appeals.

In response to the mounting criticism, the NLRB made a landmark decision in 1984 in *St. Francis Hospital II,* 271 NLRB 948 (1984). The Board stated that it would recognize two broad units of professional and nonprofessional employees (Stickler, 1991). The decision dealt a serious blow to union organizing efforts because large, highly disparate units are difficult to meld into a consensus force for collective bargaining. Over time, the Federal Court of Appeals overturned *St. Francis II.*

In 1987, The National Labor Relations Board took a bold step to resolve the issue of bargaining unit appropriateness. It announced that it would use its rulemaking power to establish circumscribed appropriate bargaining units, thereby discarding its case-by-case adjudication approach. In its 55 years, the Board had never used rulemaking to establish collective bargaining units in any industry (Zimmerman & King, 1990). The NLRB proposed rules for hospitals only, designating eight bargaining units (Stickler, 1991):

- Registered nurses
- Employed physicians
- All other professionals
- Technical employees
- Skilled maintenance employees
- Business office and clerical staff
- Security guards
- All other nonprofessional employees

Nursing homes, psychiatric hospitals, and rehabilitation facilities were considered exempt. These rules were to be implemented in 1989, and unions began preparing for enhanced unionization activity.

However, in May of 1989, the American Hospital Association obtained injunctive relief against the rules, and on July 25, 1989, the Chicago Federal District Court issued a permanent injunction against the rule (Zimmerman & King, 1990). It appeared that union expansion in health care was again stalled. But on April 11, 1990, the United States Court of Appeals for the Seventh Circuit reversed the lower court's decision and set aside the injunction. The stage was now set for a decision by the Supreme Court.

In the meantime, the NLRB had developed a backlog of labor petitions and unit clarification decisions. Both hospitals and labor unions were pressuring for a final decision in the matter. In April 1991, the United States Supreme Court unanimously upheld the original NLRB ruling stating that unions can organize as many as eight separate groups of hospital employees (Stickler, 1991). A 15-year controversy surrounding the appropriateness of hospital bargaining units was over, and the way was now paved for an aggressive assault by unions on a minimally unionized health care industry.

CURRENT STATUS OF LABOR RELATIONS

Most nurses (1,120,000) in the United States work in nonunionized environments (Ballman, 1985). Many staff nurses are satisfied with the way their organizations manage labor relations and do not feel the need for union representation. Some nurses do not believe that union representation reflects the professional level of representation they prefer. Still another group of nurses may not recognize that union representation is an alternative method for problem resolution when management and labor relationships are fractured.

Nevertheless, as of the early 1990s, there were more than 333,000 nurses organized for collective bargaining purposes. The ANA's economic and general welfare program is the largest of these organizations and represents 139,000 registered nurses in 841 bargaining units in 27 states. The SEIU and the American Federation of Teachers (AFT) are the next largest, representing 42,000 and 35,000 registered nurses respectively ("Labor Unions Ready," 1990).

The geographical distribution of union activity has been historically concentrated in the northeastern States (New York, New Jersey, Massachusetts, and Pennsylvania) along with California and Michigan (Kilgour, 1984). This reflects the fact that collective bargaining has not been a national phenomenon. The larger unions have established an aggressive agenda to alter the present geographical concentration significantly by targeting key cities and "vulnerable organizations" throughout the country. Recently, the National Union of Hospital and Healthcare Employees voted to affiliate with SEIU (Hepner & Zinner, 1991). The creation of such "super unions" could strengthen the impact of unionization activity, particularly in areas where unions have had minimal success.

More than 30 unions have attempted to organize health care workers since the 1974 Taft-Hartley Amendments, with varying degrees of success (Hepner & Zinner, 1991). The success of a union campaign generally depends on a complex set of issues, including the employee's perception of management's effectiveness and the union's ability to surface and represent those issues most crucial to the employee group. The general economic environment of the health care industry strongly influences the issues deemed most important by nurses. It has been suggested that in collective bargaining, the settlement with regard to wages has a 99% correlation with the inflation rate (Yanish, 1985).

Wages were an important issue during the early period of collective bargaining. On average, union nurses earned salaries 6% higher than their nonunion counterparts (Wilson, Hamilton, & Murphy, 1990). However, by the mid-1980s nurses were becoming increasingly concerned with job security, cross-training for clinical and job diversity, shift rotations, health care benefits, and the general organizational wage structure (Abelow, 1985). Additionally, because of the deep concern regarding escalating health care costs, many unions elected to form health care coalitions to control costs (Powills, 1985).

The nonunion organization met the economic environment demands of the mid-1980s and early 1990s by maintaining open communications with employees during periods of fiscal belt-tightening. Hospitals that maintained two-way communication with employees regarding cost effectiveness and productivity measures avoided the threat of unionization. Careful and sensitive planning for strategic downsizing, forewarning of impending employee cutbacks, providing counseling services, and assisting employees with job placement efforts eased the challenge of streamlining staff levels to fit decreased client census and utilization patterns.

Principles of continuous quality improvement applied to the workplace in the form of quality action teams, self-managed work teams, and employee-driven work restructuring and redesign are excellent techniques for ensuring communication and employee enfranchisement. However, these approaches, if not managed properly, can be construed as violating the National Labor Relations Act (Flarey, 1989).

Current labor relation practices within health care organizations have emanated from the 1974 Taft-Hartley Amendments and the 1991 Supreme Court ruling supporting eight separate bargaining units. Since that time, health care administrators have examined their approaches to employees and have attempted to establish successful employee relation programs to maintain their nonunion designation status. Along with attitude changes, most administrators routinely examine compensation packages for equity within the organization and the marketplace. The successful nonunion environment provides effective labor relations training for management, surveys employees on a regular basis regarding critical work environment issues, and conducts periodic management audits (Stickler, 1991). Thus, the enhancement of labor relations in the work environment of the industry as a whole is directly attributable to the efforts and successful unionization of a small portion of its workers.

THE COLLECTIVE BARGAINING PROCESS

The work of a staff nurse is highly demanding. It requires physical stamina, emotional commitment, and psychological health and robustness. Therefore, the environment and conditions under which staff nurses work must be supportive and in concert with their activities. If they are not, problems and conflict will emerge that can escalate, fester, and lead to unionization efforts. Usually problems in the areas of job security, compensation, benefits, and leadership and direction that cannot be resolved through normal procedures can lead a unionization effort. (See Display, Reasons Employees Join Unions, for more detail.)

Under the provisions of the Taft-Hartley amendments, nonprofit hospital workers have the right to choose a representative (union) that will speak on their behalf in negotiations with their employer. The employees join together to operate in concert and form a labor organization. The National Labor Relations Act defines a labor organization as an organization "of any kind including an employee committee that exists for the purpose, in whole or in part, of dealing with employers concerning grievances, labor disputes, wages, rates of pay, hours of employment or conditions of work" (Flarey, 1989). The process of unionizing is initiated by the employees as follows (Henry, 1984):

1. Employees sign a petition or cards demanding an election for union representation. The minimal number of signatures needed is 30%, but most unions will not move forward without at least 50%.

DISPLAY 20-1. REASONS EMPLOYEES JOIN UNIONS

- **Security**
  Fair Treatment of all employees is lacking.
  Favoritism is shown to specific employees.
  Opportunity for advancement is not available.
  Recognition as a person is rarely extended.
  Working conditions are perceived as unsafe.
  Training is not provided.
  Economic security is not perceived by employees.

- **Benefits are not measurable, adequate, or competitive.**
  Hours of work (number and shift)
  Wages
  Opportunity for overtime
  Rate of overtime pay
  Shift differential
  Career ladder/professional stratification systems
  Vacations
  Sickpay
  Retirement coverage
  Medical insurance
  Life insurance
  Holidays
  Severance pay
  Funeral pay
  Jury duty
  Educational/training subsidies

- **Poor Leadership**
  Inappropriate executive, middle, and first-line supervision
  Ineffective grievance adjustments
  Ineffective communications and employee feedback
  Opportunity for self-expression is not present
  Toleration of poor-quality performance
  Inconsistent treatment of all

---

2. A preliminary hearing is held to determine if the employees are under the jurisdiction of the NLRB and to set the date, hours, and place of the election.
3. Appropriate employee placement into bargaining units is achieved. Employees are grouped according to the eight bargaining groups discussed earlier in this chapter.

4. Preelection behaviors are observed to ensure compliance with the law. A summary of unlawful activities is outlined below.
5. The election is conducted by the NLRB in the workplace, with the outcome determined by the simple majority of those who vote. Observers are usually present from both management and the union.
6. The election results may be appealed. If the election is won by the employees, the NLRB issues a certificate to the labor organization reflecting its right to represent the employees.
7. Both parties, management and union, prepare to negotiate the collective bargaining agreement. Subjects to be negotiated include wages, hours, and other terms and conditions of employment.

This unionization process proceeds swiftly and is usually completed within 45 days. The general atmosphere of the preelection process is one of confusion and turmoil as the opposing forces—management and union—jockey for the employees' votes and support. Often, the employer is not aware of the union's activities on behalf of the employees until the requisite number of cards are signed and the petition presented. In an effort to forestall unionization, management may hire a labor relations consultant, whose job it is to ensure that the employer wins the election. On the other hand, the union will send its group of consultants to meet with employees and ensure a winning strategy for

---

DISPLAY 20-2. UNLAWFUL ACTIVITIES DURING THE UNION CERTIFICATION PROCESS

MANAGEMENT
1. Management cannot promise pay increase, promotion, improved benefits, betterment, or special favor for voting against a union.
2. Management cannot say the organization will close if unionized.
3. Employees cannot be fired, laid off, given a less favorable job, or otherwise discriminated against because of union activities.

UNION
1. The union cannot use threats or actual violence against employees who refuse to participate or cooperate.
2. Union members cannot interfere with, restrain, or coerce employees in forming, joining, or assisting labor organizations.
3. The union cannot use surveillance or questioning concerning employee interest or activities related to unions.

labor. The short intensive campaign can be highly volatile and usually polarizes employees against management and against each other. Regardless of who wins the election, time is always needed to settle emotions, resolve unanswered questions, and minimize further conflict.

THE UNION CONTRACT

The collective bargaining agreement is known as the *contract*. It defines rights, responsibilities, and benefits to both management and the union. The agreement usually gives the union rights related to a grievance procedure, dues check-off, and access to a bulletin board. Most agreements grant the hospital a Management Rights provision and a no-strike clause for the duration of the contract. The Management Rights provision allows management residual rights, that is, control of any issue not in the contract. The contract is valid for an agreed-upon number of years, although specific portions of the contract may be negotiated within the life of the original agreement. For example, a 3-year contract may allow for the wages portion to be reopened for negotiations after the first year.

A contract for unionized health care organizations usually contains a clause stating that management shall not discharge or take other disciplinary action without just cause. This clause effectively limits the organization's authority to discipline and fire employees. "Just cause" may be defined as "substantial reasons to justify the actions taken" and is open to interpretation and potential arbitration for a final decision. This forces the organization to adopt and uniformly administer personnel policies.

Each collective bargaining agreement seeks to establish an effective grievance procedure outlining the method for handling employee complaints and providing for a continuous relationship between the parties. It is meant to cover the gaps and ambiguities in the contract. Thus, the contract becomes a living document in that the parties continue to interpret the language through the grievance procedure. Usually the grievance procedure consists of at least three steps or stages of appeal. Such procedures are also frequently outlined in personnel manuals.

The first step is usually a presentation of the grievance or alleged wrong to the immediate supervisor. If the manager at this level is unable to resolve the conflict or right the alleged wrong, the employee may take the grievance to the next step. This step is usually a review by a higher level manager who can overturn the previous decision. In a unionized organization, the contract defines the time parameters for reviews at each step, and the employee is represented by a union "steward." In the event the grievance is not resolved in an earlier step, many contracts specify a final step of binding arbitration. Both parties are usually eager to settle the conflict before the final step because arbitration can be costly and may mean adherence to a decision that neither party desires (Fay & Morril, 1985).

One of the most important tenets of unions is the adherence to the concept of seniority. Seniority defines each individual employee's longevity or length of continuous service in an organization, a job class, or a specific department. As a concept, seniority is deeply ingrained in our society, and long service usually relates to benefits and security. A nonunionized organization, however, is under no obligation to consider employee seniority. In fact, recent human resource approaches tie rewards and benefits to measurable and achieved goals and outcomes. Nevertheless, the seniority clause in a contract offers protection against untimely layoff and may create a preferred status for vacation periods, shift assignments, overtime opportunities, and promotion.

The negotiation of a new contract occurs on or before the termination date of the present contract. Both parties send representatives to the bargaining table with demands for changes in the contract. These changes are usually called *proposals,* and the other side's response is called a *counterproposal.* The proposals usually reflect the current national and industrial economic status, competitive shifts in the marketplace (real and anticipated) since the last contract negotiation, and those changes desired in professional practice and care for patients. The negotiation period can be very brief or can go on for many months, as long as it is deemed that the parties are negotiating in good faith.

The costs of unionization are incurred by both management and labor. Management loses flexibility in job assignment, promotion, and rewarding superior individual performance. The salary and benefit packages may result in higher costs to the organization and diminished flexibility in quoting salaries or adjusting them to maintain a competitive position. Finally, management is forced to work through a third party (the union) to resolve problems and initiate some types of changes. This can cause unwanted delays and complexity.

The unionized employee pays dues and fees to the union for the maintenance and activities of the union. Most contracts require an agency fee for those individuals who do not wish to join the union officially. The fee is usually equivalent to the annual dues and fees. The employee, like management, uses the union as a third party to resolve conflict and grievances. In the event of a strike, participation is required and at times advancement can be constrained by seniority.

Although the above conditions are described as costs, it is clear that an individual may choose to view the conditions as gains. This typifies the nature of collective bargaining and the divergence it can engender.

NEGOTIATION DIFFICULTIES

The law specifies that the contract negotiations must proceed in a timely manner with substantive results. This obligation to negotiate in good faith is actually a state of mind that is difficult to measure (Henry, 1984). Behaviors have been identified, however, that characterize failure to bargain in good faith:

1. Failure to participate meaningfully.
2. Issuing unreasonable demands or conditions.
3. Postponing negotiating sessions repeatedly.
4. Rejecting proposals without reasons.
5. Engaging in dilatory conduct.
6. Making no real effort to reconcile differences.

Strikes are not a desirable way of resolving labor disputes, but they can and do occur, with varying success. The various types of strikes include economic strikes, strikes over unfair labor practices, sympathy strikes, jurisdictional strikes, and recognition strikes. The union must provide 10 days' notice to management before striking. The purpose of giving notice is to ensure the continuity of client care, or at the very least to lessen the impact of the work stoppage on continuity of care.

A total of 43 major strikes occurred at health care institutions between June 1954 and March 1982, each involving 1000 or more employees (Metzger, Ferentino, & Kruger, 1984). These strikes averaged 18.8 days and ranged from 1 to 95 days. Strikes occur less frequently when the unemployment rate is up and inflation is down. Southern states experience less strike activity, and nursing home strikes generally last longer.

Striking is costly to both parties. The organization loses patient revenues and incurs costs related to overtime, security, and legal counsel. It also incurs a loss of public confidence. Striking workers lose pay and can be replaced (Metzger, Ferentino, & Kruger, 1984). Striking causes considerable stress to all involved. It is not easy for the staff nurse to face the ethical dilemmas associated with striking. However, when one or both parties are unable or unwilling to reach agreement, striking has a definite effect on the positions of both labor and management.

SUMMARY

Labor relations in its optimal form ensures that the needs and wants of the organization and the employees are met responsibly. A match between the values and behaviors of the employer and employee creates a stable corporate culture that promotes job satisfaction and security for the employee and competitive advantage and profitability for the organization. More importantly, in health care, the quality and cost of patient care is optimized. There are a number of variables that significantly favor the spread of unionism in the current health care environment:

- The emphasis on cost cutting
- The competitive labor market
- The desire of the nursing profession for a collective voice
- The NLRB ruling authorizing eight separate bargaining units
- The trend toward creation of "super unions"
- A 90% nonunionized labor pool in health care
- The current emphasis on productivity with employees' perception of marginal quality.

DISPLAY 20-3. TYPES OF UNION STRIKES

Economic strikes	Employees are attempting to compel their employer to accept their demands by withdrawing their services.
Unfair labor strikes	A strike that is caused or practice prolonged by the unfair labor practices of an employer or a union.
Sympathy strikes	Employees of one employer or craft strike in support of workers of another. Employees can also refuse to cross the picket line of another.
Jurisdictional strikes	A work stoppage because a dispute between two or more unions over the assignment of work. Unions will strike because the employer will assign a particular job to another union.
Recognition strikes	Work stoppages to enforce an employer to bargain with a particular organization.
Illegal strikes	Examples of illegal strikes include violent strikes, secondary or boycott strikes, and wildcat or unauthorized strikes.

Employees expect and should receive competent supervision, equitable and consistent treatment, adequate compensation and benefits, written rules, policies, and procedures, personal recognition, and a reasonable amount of job security. Nurses should be able to practice their profession with autonomy and participation in the administrative process. Conversely, organizational management expects and should receive the best performance an employee can offer, professional conduct, compliance with rules, policies, and procedures, loyalty, and a commitment to fiscal constraint and profitability in the delivery of quality client services.

Occasionally, irreconcilable differences between management and labor will result in the unionization of employees. Unionization creates an environment in which management and employees are in a more balanced power posture; however, their positions tend to be adversarial, and represented and modulated through a third party, the union.

The new staff nurse has multiple roles with regard to labor relations. The first is that of individual practitioner who has the responsibility to ensure the quality and efficacy of the care provided to the patient.

Another role is that of a recipient of an organization's management programs and culture. Associated with this role is the responsibility to provide direct feedback to management or the union representative. The third role is that of extender of labor relations when working with nonprofessional personnel. Each staff nurse must make a considerable personal contribution to positive labor relations if quality patient care is to be provided.

DISCUSSION QUESTIONS

1. Describe the working conditions that employees desire to have in their organization.
2. Discuss the differences professional nurses experience in practicing nursing in union or nonunion settings.
3. List the steps of a union campaign.

REFERENCES

Alexander, E. (1978). *Nursing administration in the hospital health care system.* St. Louis: CV Mosby.

Ballman, C. (1985). Union busters. *American Journal of Nursing, 29,* 963–966.

Beal, E., & Begin, J. (1982). *The practice of collective bargaining.* Homewood, IL: Richard D. Irwin.

Berneys, E. L. (1946). How to influence your own future. *RN, 12,* 42–44.

Bullough, B. (1971). New militancy in nursing. *Nursing Forum, 11,* 273–288.

Fay, M. S., & Morril, A. K. (1985). The grievance-arbitration process: The experience of one nursing administrator. *Journal of Nursing Administration, 6,* 11–16.

Flarey, D. L. (1989). Quality circles and labor relations issues. *Nursing Economic$, 7,* 266–269.

Gershenfeld, W. (1970). Hospitals. In A. L. Wolfbein (Ed.), *Emerging sectors of collective bargaining.* Braintree, MA: DH Mark.

Henry, K. (1984). *The health care supervisor's legal guide.* Rockville, MD: Aspen Systems.

Hepner, J. O., & Zinner, S. E. (1991). Nurses and the new NLRB rules: Implications for healthcare management. *Health Progress, 72,* 20–22.

Kilgour, J. (1984). Union organizing activity in the hospital industry. *Hospital and Health Services Administration, 29*(6), 79–90.

Labor unions ready big push to organize nurses, counting on courts to uphold new bargaining rule. (1990). *American Journal of Nursing, 90,* 151–153.

Mauksch, I. G. (1971). Attainment of control over practice. *Nursing Forum 11,* 232–238.

Metzger, N., Ferentino, J., & Kruger, K. (1984). *When health care employees strike.* Rockville, MD: Aspen Systems.

Pointer, D. (1972). Organizing of professionals: Associations serve union functions. *Hospitals 46*(5), 70–73.

Powills, S. (1985). Labor: A growing force in controlling health costs. *Hospitals,* November 16, 82–85.

Rectz, R., & Rectz, J. (1984). Collective bargaining in the health care industry: Implications for the long term care administration. *Journal of Long-Term Care Administration,* 11–19.

Stickler, K. B. (1990). Union organizing will be divisive and costly. *Hospitals, 64,* 68–70.

Stickler, K. B. (1991). The cost of unionization. *Health Progress, 72,* 18–19.

Wilson, C. N., Hamilton, C. L., & Murphy, E. (1990). Union dynamics in nursing. *Journal of Nursing Administration 20,* 35–39.

Yanish, D. (1985). Nurses' unions lower sights on wages to make gains in non-economic areas. *Modern Healthcare, 76,* 88.

Zimmerman, D. A., & King, G. R. (1990). Union elections and the NLRB: The healthcare industry continues to challenge bargaining unit determinations. *Health Progress, 71,* 96–101.

SUGGESTED READING

Blanchard, K., Carew, D., & Parisi-Carew, E. (1990). *One minute manager builds high performing teams.* New York: William Morrow.

Block, P. (1987). *The empowered manager: Positive political skills at work.* San Francisco: Jossey-Bass.

Dawson, R. (1992). *The secrets of power persuasion.* Englewood Cliffs, NJ: Prentice-Hall.

Francis, D., & Young, D. (1992). *Improving work groups.* San Diego: Pfeiffer.

Jandt, F. E. (1985). *Win–win negotiating: Turning conflict into agreement.* New York: John Wiley & Sons.

Nanus, B. (1992). *Visionary leadership.* San Francisco: Jossey-Bass.

Yates, D. (1985). *The politics of management.* San Francisco: Jossey-Bass.

Managing Cultural Diversity

Mary Elizabeth Mancini

LEARNING OBJECTIVES

This chapter will enable you to:

1. Understand the changing demographics of patient and employee populations.
2. Identify issues related to working with a culturally diverse patient population.
3. Identify issues related to working in a culturally diverse work force.

Vestal, K.W. Nursing Management:
Concepts and Issues, 2 ed.
© 1995 J.B. Lippincott Company

Whether taking care of patients or interacting with other health care workers, managing diversity is an essential element of every nurse's daily activities. The changing demographics and the shift to patient-centered, patient-focused care and an employee-centered, employee-focused work environment requires nurses to be knowledgeable about and skillful in dealing with issues related to cultural, gender, and age diversity.

PATIENT CARE SCENARIOS

A Cambodian-American nurse says that in her culture women are prohibited from making eye contact with men. If such contact occurs, it means that the woman is having, or is open for, an affair. Her colleagues find it very difficult to deal with her not looking them in the eye, which indicates a lack of truthfulness in American culture.

A nurse from India notes that Americans seem to place great importance on greeting one another in the mornings or on the first encounter of the day. Initially, when she fails to respond in a similar fashion, she is accused of being unfriendly, although in reality she is following an age-old Indian custom. Women from India rarely speak out.

A visiting nurse from England walks into a patient's room and sees a bouquet of long-stemmed red roses. To most Americans, the red roses are a symbol of love, friendship, or wishes for a speedy recovery. But in England, red roses are a signal of death. She thinks it is terrible that someone would "actually send a death signal" to a sick patient.

The United States was once considered a great "melting pot" in which people from all cultures came together and somehow formed a new and cohesive "American culture." Yet each of us brings to this culture a heritage of customs and values that does not always fit into someone else's expectations. We assume that we understand where others are "coming from." However, our template for "acceptable" or "appropriate" behavior is often limited to our own beliefs, values, and traditions. We must reorient our thinking to understand and use cultural difference as a positive force. One way to do this is to replace the cultural metaphor of a "melting pot" with that of a "mosaic" of many different colors and hues.

Nurses do not provide care for homogenous patient populations, nor do they work in isolation. The demographic picture of the population from which our work force will be chosen is changing dramatically. Labor projections indicate that by the year 2000, 24% of the work force will be African American, Hispanic American, and Asian American. With the emphasis on cross-functional teams, collaborative practice, and case management in health care, nurses must be skilled in dealing with a diverse work force.

UNDERSTANDING OTHERS

The challenge for all people living in the increasingly diverse population of this country is to learn how to understand and respect cultural differences of people of diverse backgrounds. Health care workers must want to be culturally sensitive. They must be motivated to change. Hopefully, the motivation is a desire to achieve quality patient care.

Understanding diversity is particularly crucial for nurses, who must deal with patients, families, and coworkers in a way that values each individual and recognizes his or her unique contributions to the wellness and healing processes. However, care must be taken when managing these uniquenesses. Managing diversity is becoming a contradiction in terms, for it is important to be focused on the characteristics common to a culture, race, gender, or age. Yet at the same time, employees and patients with these characteristics should be treated as individuals.

To best serve patients, the concept of *patient-centered care* needs to be expanded to incorporate each patient's values. This is the philosophy of Parkland Memorial Hospital in Dallas, Texas, as expressed by Ron J. Anderson, MD, President and Chief Executive Officer (Boumbulian et al., 1991):

> It is not enough for a health care professional merely to 'do good' or to try to 'avoid evil,' although these goals remain vitally important within the ethical foundation of the provider/patient relationship. We must analyze what is good from within the value system of the patient, moving beyond medical or epidemiologic outcomes that may primarily reflect the caregiver's values. Without being paternalistic, we must understand more of the cultural, religious, ethnic, and class differences that separate clinician from patient, and that affect the clinician's approach to medical practice. Further, we must recognize the uniqueness of each individual while we continue to strive to understand those things that provide a common bond. Above all, the care that we render must respect the patient's autonomy and desire for wholeness.

> After all, illness is the experience of disease through an individual patient's world view and personal circumstance, including the patient's values and beliefs; emotional, intellectual and financial resources; hopes and

dreams. We must consider these values, beliefs, and anxieties as much a part of the patient's history as is the traditional review of organ systems. This helps us move beyond merely treating disease to considering and managing the patient's illness.

NURSING CARE

For nurses, the challenge is to integrate respect for cultural diversity and individual value systems into the care of patients and the management of staff. Even simple physical contact can have significant cultural impact. Although most Americans don't give a second thought to offering a hand upon meeting someone, in Cambodia it is wrong to touch someone else's hand or skin, especially a woman's. A Cambodian would offer a smile and nod. But Americans might consider this rude or unfriendly. Although the intent is not to intrude into private space nor to be unfriendly, in dealing with culture it is very difficult to undo everything you believe. How aware are we, as health care providers, of how our patients perceive the "laying on" of our hands, the touching we do without asking for permission or without consideration of the cultural implications?

Even children are often caught between cultures. On the one hand, they are living in the United States and have adopted the American way of life. On the other hand, they are a reflection of their cultures. Again, in Cambodia, once a child reaches the age of 4 or 5, there is no more "baby talk" or hugging and kissing. It can be very difficult for a Cambodian child living in the United States who sees her friends being hugged and kissed by their parents. She may come to the conclusion that her own parents don't love her, although nothing could be further from the truth. In addition, such actions, guided by culture, may even be misunderstood as signs of child abuse.

The provision of physical care has cultural implications. For example, the skin of African Americans sometimes requires special care to remove ash, and some lotions are very effective in maintaining skin integrity. However, do all nurses take the time to learn about these needs and products? African Americans also have special hair care needs. Yet, all too often, health care providers consider hair care a routine part of daily care and do not question patients about their preferences or needs. We must involve patients in their care and demonstrate our respect for their unique needs by asking them how they wish to be treated or what specific routines they prefer. Unless we make a concerted effort to identify and address the needs of different populations, we will fail to provide the best care we are capable of providing.

Even the best efforts can be hampered by assumptions and stereotyping. Health care workers from community health centers can encourage cultural sensitivity training to avoid the stereotypical thinking typified in the following incident involving a Hispanic patient. The woman had been diagnosed with terminal cancer and wanted to renew her marriage vows. Employees assumed that the woman, who had 11 children, was Catholic and called a priest to perform the ceremony— but the patient was Baptist.

Not all African American women want to wear their hair in cornrows or platting. Not all women shave their legs. Not everyone finds solace in hearing about God or religion at a time of death. To be truly patient-centered, we must be open to subtle clues, recognize the possibility of differences, and ask when we are not sure we know our patient's values and beliefs.

How then do nurses integrate these concepts into their practice? JoEllen Koerner, MSN, RN, FAAN, a national expert on cultural diversity and a member of the Expert Panel on Culturally Competent Health Care of the American Academy of Nursing, makes four recommendations for dealing with transcultural issues in American practice settings (Koerner, 1992). First, she recommends promoting understanding on a local level. Health professionals concerned about transcultural practice should start by determining which minority population in their area is the largest. This can be done by looking at admitting statistics or community-wide demographics. Second, the effort should be made to get to know that population and to offer staff education on issues specific to that culture, including physical needs.

Third, many cultures have specific beliefs about health and healing. Once these are known to the health care providers, efforts should be made to incorporate these traditional healing techniques into the patient's care. With the Sioux Indians, Koerner's staff tries to incorporate healing techniques from the Sioux belief system into modern medicine. For example, they have a traditional medicine man visit the hospital. As long as these treatments are not harmful to the patient, they encourage and respect the patient's use of traditional healing techniques in conjunction with prescribed medication. Other beliefs may be less dramatic, such as the use of candles, holy water, relics, or prayer services, but they are nonetheless important to the patient and the family.

And finally, to achieve this level of practice, transcultural issues should be addressed in staff development. Koerner's staff has founded a Transcultural Nursing Club to encourage awareness of these issues. They discuss ways to deliver care most appropriately to people from different cultures. They have guests from different cultures present their beliefs and traditions and discuss their cultures' views of health care. For example, Mennonites have very different views about modesty, which should be known and respected in health care delivery. Most requests made by patients, such as the gender of the health care provider or the type of draping or clothing provided, can be met if we grasp the importance and the complexity of delivering culturally sensitive care.

In an effort to demonstrate cultural sensitivity, it is incumbent upon the nurse to:

1. Learn how to pronounce the names of patients and staff correctly.
2. Allow for formality when being addressed until a relationship can be formed.
3. Be aware that flattery and praise are not appropriate in all cultures—it is not always seen as a reward.
4. Use caution in rejecting gifts or food. These may be offered as an expression of gratitude and deference.
5. Be aware that speaking softly is not always an indicator of meekness.

THE WORK FORCE

An understanding of cultural diversity is crucial not only in dealing with patients but in the management of health care staff. According to Wil Ternoir and Marcia Macaulay in their book *Workforce 2000: A Common Destiny*, as America evolved into a multicultural society, prejudice and intolerance contributed to a pattern of discrimination against many racial and ethnic groups. Unfortunately, legislation cannot change how people feel. The intolerance which made equal employment opportunity (EEO) laws necessary still functions within society as a whole. The workforce is a reflection of society, and if racism and ethnic stereotypes are present in society, they exist in and impact on the workplace.

Managers and supervisors need to be alert for and sensitive to attitudes and behaviors that perpetuate racial and ethnic stereotypes and negatively affect the ability to communicate and build trust. A culturally skilled manager understands that racial and ethnic differences can impact an individual's communication style, approach to learning and authority, motivation, and response to rewards or criticism. Conversely, understanding and valuing differences can build trust and enhance communications and production, training, and motivation strategies.

Every nurse who wishes to deal successfully with cultural diversity must be willing to value and learn about differences. The successful nurse respects the fact that individuals are sensitive about how they are described and classified. Commonly applied labels are not necessarily accurate or appropriate, especially if the person indicates another preference.

Persons of color come from many different cultures. Black Americans may wish to be referred to as "black" or as "African American." Cubans of African descent and other persons who might be considered "black" may strongly resent that label. Their response may be, "I am not black, I am Cuban, Nigerian," and so forth.

Persons labeled as "Asian" represent many separate Asian and Pacific Island nations and cultures. Most consider themselves to be Korean, Chinese, Japanese, and so forth—not "Asians."

Those called "Hispanic" come from a variety of Spanish-speaking cultures. A common language does not mean common culture or that every person from a Spanish-speaking culture thinks of himself or herself as "Hispanic."

North America is home to hundreds of distinct cultures referred to as "Native Americans." Whereas some persons may be comfortable with that term, others may prefer to identify with their tribal heritage (eg, Chippewa, Blackfoot, or Cheyenne).

Assumptions based on geographical origin can be misleading, especially when combined with misinformation. For instance, persons from Iran are not Arabs and may strongly resent being referred to as such. Persons from Iran are "Persian" and belong to a distinct culture.

Culture also affects how nonverbal communications, such as use of space, touching, and gestures, are perceived. A skilled manager considers the following issues in dealing with staff:

Proximity/Spacing: People from some cultures may tend to stand very close to a person with whom they are communicating. This can cause discomfort for someone with a different perspective on appropriate spacing.

Touching: Any physical contact or touching that is part of an individual's communication style can create problems or discomfort for people from many cultures. This *does not* mean that managers and supervisors should abandon a "pat on the back" as a means of showing approval. Rather, your employees should feel empowered to tell you if such casual touching makes them uncomfortable.

Gestures: People from some cultures may be more animated than others, using gestures and body language to communicate their message. In addition, gestures that have a positive meaning in one culture may be insulting and rude in another.

Eye Contact: Traditionally, Americans have valued direct eye contact as a sign of confidence and respect, whereas not making eye contact has negative connotations. However, in many cultures, making eye contact with an authority figure is considered an insult.

Use of Silence: People from some cultures are uncomfortable with silence (particularly as an element of one-on-one communications), preferring active verbal interaction. Other cultures may value periods of contemplative silence. When the two types attempt to communicate, both may misunderstand the other's communication style and motivation.

Body Language: The body is one of the more subtle ways people communicate meaning and sincerity. If a manager or supervisor is uncomfortable dealing with persons from a certain group, the tension is likely to be reflected in body language. It is not unusual for a manager or supervisor to *say* all the right things while unconsciously sending a different message through facial expressions.

Language/Accent: A common mistake is to judge or stereotype an individual based on an accent or an inability to speak "articulate" English. It is a grave mistake to make negative assumptions about persons who have not mastered the English language or who speak with an accent. Allowing an employment atmosphere in which employees joke about or imitate an employee's accent can send the message that differences are not respected or valued.

The skilled nurse recognizes that discrimination and harassment can occur between persons within the same minority group. Unfortunately, within some minority groups there exist subtle and even overt attitudes about issues such as skin color, national origin, or tribal affiliation. It is important to remember that persons who fall within the same minority classification (eg, Native American, African American, Asian American, or Hispanic American) are not necessarily culturally linked.

Managers and supervisors should take prompt action to deal with *any* incidents involving racial or ethnic harassment or other inappropriate behaviors that might create an uncomfortable working environment. Managers and supervisors should lead by example. You can create the *perception* that you are racially biased by participating in, agreeing with, or ignoring inappropriate attitudes toward race or ethnicity. Inaction may be interpreted as overall indifference or, even worse, as support of such attitudes, signaling the go-ahead for other inappropriate behaviors. If the behaviors continue, failure to address them promptly can lead to an uncomfortable or offensive working environment, in which minority employees may be more likely to challenge your decisions as racially biased.

Managers and supervisors must be aware of and respect an employee's past experiences and must develop management skills that will begin building trust. The ultimate goal is to establish mutual communication and create a relationship in which the employee begins to *trust* that your motivation is positive and sincere—even though you may make a mistake or unintentionally say or do something the employee feels is insensitive.

Mistrust and suspicion can form a divisive wall that inhibits communication and frustrates effective management. Trust begins when people learn to communicate honestly, using mutual respect as a basis for resolving problems or conflicts caused by differences. Managers and supervisors can take a lead role by using awareness, flexibility, and good management skills to treat employees as individuals who are worthy of trust and respect.

SUMMARY

The viability of any health care practice depends on the ability of its employees to work together as a team and to appreciate the uniqueness of people—patients, visitors, and coworkers. We must be cautious, however, that our emphasis on ethnic pride and the positive aspects of diversity does not bring with it a new politically correct intolerance that results in division rather than unity.

Although understanding diverse cultures is difficult, nurses must work at valuing patients and coworkers that they perceive as different from themselves. Because of the changing demographics, we all have to accept this challenge and learn to deal with cultural, racial, ethnic, and religious differences in a sensitive, understanding, and positive manner. The sooner we do, the sooner we will achieve quality patient-centered and patient-valued care, and the better off we will be as a positive and productive society.

DISCUSSION QUESTIONS

1. Describe the need for nurses to understand cultural diversity as it relates to patient care and to staff support.

2. Develop a picture of the future work force as in changes in cultural mix.
3. Develop a plan to explore cultural diversity as a critical factor in professional nursing.

REFERENCES

Boumbulian, P. J., Day, M. W., Delbanco, T. L., Edgman-Levitan, S., Smith, D. R., & Anderson, R. J. (1991). Patient-centered patient-valued care. *Journal of Health Care for the Poor and Underserved*, 2(3), 338–346.

Koerner, J. E. (1992). Culturally competent nursing. *Q-Quality Assessment Quarterly*, 2(3), 2.

Ternoir, W. J., & Macaulay, M. (1991). Managing diversity. *Workforce 2000: A Common Destiny—Management Reference Guide*. Minneapolis, MN: Professional EEO Consultants.

SUGGESTED READING

Bahr, H. M., Chadwick, B. A., & Strauss, J. H. (1979). *American ethnicity*. Lexington, MA: DC Heath.

Casse, P. (1981). *Training for the cross-cultural mind*. Washington, DC: Society of Intercultural Education, Training and Research.

Daniel, N. (1975). *The cultural barrier*. Edinburgh: Edinburgh University Press, 1975.

Harris, P. R., & Moran, R. T. (1979). *Managing cultural differences*. Houston: Gulf Publishing.

Lewan, L. S. (1990). Diversity in the workplace. *HR Magazine on Human Resource Management* 35(6), 42–45.

Overman, S. (1991). Managing the diverse work force. *HR Magazine on Human Resource Management* 36(4), 32–39.

Thiederman, S. (1991). *Bridging cultural barriers for corporate success*. Lexington, MA: Lexington Books.

INDEX

Note: Page numbers in *italics* indicate illustrations; those followed by d indicate display material; those followed by t indicate tables.